Preventing Abuse and Neglect in the Lives of Children with Disabilities

E. Paula Crowley

Preventing Abuse and Neglect in the Lives of Children with Disabilities

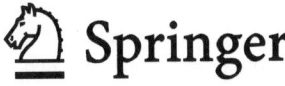 Springer

E. Paula Crowley
Department of Special Education
Illinois State University
Normal, IL, USA

ISBN 978-3-319-30440-3   ISBN 978-3-319-30442-7   (eBook)
DOI 10.1007/978-3-319-30442-7

Library of Congress Control Number: 2016935703

Printed on acid-free paper

This Springer imprint is published by Springer Nature
The registered company is Springer International Publishing AG Switzerland

To children with disabilities, their parents, families, neighbors, friends, and the professional personnel who care about them.

Foreword

The world can be a dangerous place for children with and without disabilities. When we are aware and understood those dangers, we act to prevent potential injury. For example, we recognize the danger of car accidents, so we require children to be placed in appropriate car seats. We recognize the danger of drowning, so we establish nationwide programs to teach children how to swim as well as mark potentially unsafe places for swimmers. We recognize the danger of fires, so we establish fire prevention codes concerning clothing, furniture, and structures. More recently, we recognized the danger of bullying, so we now expect, or legislatively require, our schools to establish anti-bullying programs. Unfortunately, we do not recognize, understand, discuss, or act to prevent childhood dangers that are simply so horrific that they essentially become taboo topics of conversation. These are the dangers of child neglect, physical, sexual, and emotional abuse. E. Paula Crowley has written a courageous text, and her work addresses a significant gap in our knowledge base.

Each year, approximately 3.5 million referrals, involving 6.4 million children with and without disabilities suspected of experiencing abuse and neglect are made to Child Protective Services in the United States. News broadcasts, newspaper articles, and YouTube videos yield a daily deluge of stories of children who are starved, beaten, violated, and emotionally harmed by individuals from within or known by their families. The stories are frequently so outrageous and so distasteful that we attempt to erase them from our minds. Unfortunately, children who experience these circumstances do not have this option; instead, they often pay a very heavy lifelong "price" for something that might have been prevented. That price may include poor physical health, inappropriate behavior (e.g., withdrawn, aggressive, over compliant, etc.), risky social behavior (e.g., drug abuse, sexually activity, running away, etc.), learning problems, academic failure or even death. Data from the Center for Disease Control (CDC) entitled "The Adverse Childhood Experience (ACE) Study" indicate that the impact of abuse and neglect is not limited to childhood. Adults who experienced childhood abuse and neglect demonstrate lifelong accelerated risks for psychological problems, drug addiction, life threatening illness, and suicide. The dangers and impact of childhood neglect, physical, sexual, and psychological abuses are both real and prevalent. The question becomes, what can we do to prevent, or at least reduce the occurrence, duration, and impact of child neglect and abuse?

Paraphrasing the Serenity Prayer by Reinhold Niebuhr (1892–1971), we must accept the things we cannot change, change the things we can, and have wisdom to know the difference. Child abuse and neglect most frequently occurs in families experiencing a litany of problems including:

- Economic distress
- Spousal abuse
- Mental health problems
- Drug addiction
- Criminal behavior
- Insecure and chaotic housing and participants (i.e., individuals coming into and leaving the home)
- Prior history of child abuse
- Inadequate parent/child bonding, parenting skills, social network, and coping strategies

These problems are prevalent throughout all segments of society. A family's ethnicity, wealth, education, or social standing do not preclude, or inherently predict, whether a child will, or will not, experience abuse or neglect. Perpetrators are often trusted individuals either within or known by families. In the context of the "Serenity Prayer," we cannot change the families into which children are born. Nor, can we identify, understand, and resolve all family problems. What can we do? We can learn the signs, or the indicators that a child may be experiencing abuse and/or neglect. We can be on the "lookout" for the occurrence of those signs in the children we see in the store, church, neighborhood, school, or playground. We can call 1-800-FOR-A-CHILD 24/7 to have a confidential conversation with a counselor to figure out whether our suspicions merit a call to the local Child Protective Services. We can also identify those children who are at greatest risk for experiencing abuse and/or neglect. Given that information, we can then work to give children who are vulnerable the knowledge and skills they need to recognize, avoid, and report abusive and neglectful situations.

Children with disabilities experience abuse and neglect at a rate that is three to four times greater than that experienced by their nondisabled peers. Existing evidence indicates that 27 % of children with disabilities will experience abuse and 90 % will experience bullying before age 19. As a result, it is for this group, i.e., students with disabilities, that we are most challenged to accept abuse and neglect prevention responsibilities.

The purpose of this text is to give caregivers and professionals the depth of knowledge required to understand, design, implement, and evaluate programs designed to prevent, recognize, and report abuse and neglect in the lives of children with disabilities. The challenge is to integrate prevention efforts within the context of the children's day-to-day lives at home, in school, and the community. Inherent within the prevention design for children with disabilities is early intervention programming. Efforts to enhance parent/child bonding, enrich parent/child interactions, deepen human understanding, and strengthen family support systems will contribute to the prevention of abuse and neglect in the lives of children with and without disabilities.

Within school settings it is critical that children with disabilities learn: (1) that they have the right to say "NO" and to express that right, how that right changes over time, and what to do if that right is not respected; (2) how families and friends love and interact with their children; (3) the language needed to express their feelings and to share the who, what, when, how, and where of their day-to-day experiences; (4) how to make and keep age appropriate friends; (5) that while keeping "surprises" is good, keeping "secrets" is not; (6) to tell an adult if they are experiencing neglect, abuse, and/or bullying; and (7) how their emerging sexuality affects their bodies and their emotions.

Children with disabilities and their families have unique legal rights. These rights mandate their access to the necessary resources and services designed to meet their individual needs. Their Individualized Family Service Plans, Individual Education Plans, and 504 Plans are individualized legal documents that are designed to guide their education. Unfortunately, most education and related service professionals lack the training or resources needed to use the children's educational documents effectively so to prevent, recognize, report, and respond appropriately to their maltreatment experiences, including abuse, neglect, and bullying. This text represents a significant effort to address this problem.

Kent State University   Harold A. Johnson
Kent, OH, USA

Preface

The news cycle reveals story after story about the abuse and neglect of children with and without disabilities in the United States. Memories fade quickly. We listen to the transfixing stories of Adam Lanza, Trayvon Martin, Amanda Berry, Gina DeJesus, Michelle Knight, Terrell Campbell, Kajaunce Morton, Michael Bloodson, and so many more. Every day, countless children are abused and neglected go unnamed and unrecognized. At best, they are acknowledged in national and state statistics. At worst, there is no record at all. We rarely acknowledge the human suffering and life-long toll left behind by abuse and neglect during childhood.

Current estimates of the extent to which children with disabilities are abused and neglected are mired in issues that compromise their accuracy. Researchers have known for almost two decades that children with disabilities are three to four times more likely to be abused and neglected than their nondisabled peers. Also, many children who experience abuse and neglect are later diagnosed with disabilities. Many are abused and neglected in the contexts of their families as well as in the context of personnel and environments entrusted with their care and welfare.

In June 2012, Governor Patrick Quinn of Illinois signed into law reforms that are designed to protect thousands of children and adolescents with disabilities who live in nursing home facilities. This was in part a response to the *Chicago Tribune* reporters' well-documented 10-year pattern of abuse and neglect at Alden Village Nursing Home in Chicago. Among these reforms are stiffer fines for abuse and neglect, fewer obstacles to shuttering facilities following evidence of abuse and neglect, stricter procedures for the administration of psychotropic medicines, and stronger requirements for detailed reports following child deaths. Some state officials and advocates for persons with disabilities described the legislation as the most significant effort in a generation.

In May 2010 Park Forest police in Illinois faced the spectacle of a 6-year-old boy who dialed 911. He sought help having been left alone for hours with his 8-year-old cousin, a girl with cerebral palsy and who was unable to speak. She was chained to a bed and covered in human waste. The children were found living in squalor and without running water. Following this incident, the children were removed from the home and their adult caregivers were each charged with criminal neglect of a disabled person and endangering the life or health of a child.

At first glance, most people would find a story like this surprising and even shocking. They do not want to think about such stories any further. They quickly dismiss them and forget the details. Somehow, many people in the United States have come to believe that children and adolescents with disabilities were abused and neglected in some bygone era. Indeed, children were once abandoned or even the victims of filicide if they were born with a disability. Have we come a long way since the days of *Titicut Follies* and *Christmas in Purgatory?* The stories reported in the newspaper coverage remind us of the ongoing abuse and neglect of children with and without disabilities. But at what point does the shock wear off and we forget? In this book we will delve in layer-by-layer into the complex world of abuse and neglect in the lives of children with disabilities.

It all began for me as a teacher of children with emotional and behavioral disorders in a residential treatment center during the 1980s. The stories of abuse and neglect in the clinical files of some of the children I worked with defied the most vivid imagination. I will not forget reading about the repeated parental discipline that 9-year-old David received. His father used a rope to tie his feet together. He then tied him, upside down to the branch of a tree and beat him with a stick time-and-time again. Among my priorities was to teach David long division and to comprehend the next piece of text he read. David's academic and social behaviors were atypical. He was an intelligent and a highly aggressive child. David was among many other children who exhibited atypical social and academic behaviors. Laurie, John, Ricky, Diva, Joey, Brett, Jason, Melody, and so many more often befuddled the clinical and the educational staff. Somehow we all passed through our reading of clinical files and went on with our work. The children's lives went on too, and I wonder how they fare today.

It all came back to me in 2004. The abuse and neglect of young children came to my attention while teaching a course on the assessment of young children with disabilities. I invited Laura Beavers, a guest speaker from a clinical setting to talk with my students about the child behaviors they might encounter and the importance of their own professional observations.

Much to my surprise, Laura spent most of her time focusing on the soft signs of abuse and neglect among young children. Subsequently, I began to study the link between abuse and neglect and disability in childhood. Daily newspaper articles popped to my attention. I began to gather these articles and found myself analyzing their content. This effort grew into a content analysis research study that I continue to this day.

Children with disabilities are a particularly vulnerable population. They are at a much higher risk of abuse and neglect than their nondisabled peers. The more we know about their characteristics, the forms, the outcomes, the perpetrators, and the contexts of their abuse and neglect, the better prepared we are to understand them and engage in our roles as professionals. Furthermore, the more we know about child abuse and neglect, the better prepared we are for our roles as specialists in child abuse and neglect prevention.

This book is divided into three main sections. The first four chapters describe the extent of the problem, the characteristics of the children, the forms of abuse and neglect, and its observable outcomes. The next three chapters focus on knowing the perpetrators. The last three focus on predicting and preventing abuse and neglect in the lives of children with disabilities.

More specifically, Chap. 1 begins with an overall discussion of the evidence on the abuse and neglect of children and adolescents with disabilities and a description of the study that provided a foundation for this book. The findings of the analysis of the newspaper coverage is threaded through each subsequent chapter. Chapters 2, 3, 4, 5, 6, 7, 8, and 9 contain data from national and international reports and from literature in this area. The findings in each chapter are illustrated stories from the *Chicago Tribune* newspaper covering a 10-year span beginning in 2004. Each chapter contains a set of reflection and critical thinking exercises. These exercises are designed to promote dialogue. They may be useful in seminars designed for students in related fields of study such as law, medicine, education, social work, nursing, and related professional fields. We conclude each chapter with a set of recommendations for research and practice.

Having completed the initial mandatory report, how would you as a special educator, school administrator, social worker, school nurse, parent, guardian, medical professional, or an abuse and neglect prevention specialist, on a daily basis, respond to a child or an adolescent with a disability who has been abused or neglected? How would you, in your role, address the complicated variables that permeate the evidence found in the literature on the abuse and neglect of children and adolescents with disabilities? Do we think that our jobs are done once we complete mandatory reports? Is it possible that children and adolescents with disabilities who have been exposed to violence interact differently with the world around them? Is it possible that there are good, bad, and indifferent ways to interact with these children?

At best, we can prevent the abuse and neglect of all children and adolescents with and without disabilities. At worst, we can perpetuate systems, attitudes, behaviors, and the series of known risk factors that set up children and adolescents with and without with disabilities for the abuse and neglect they encounter. Realistically what can we do? I hope the scenarios and reflection questions in this book will generate discussion, as well as, inspire new ideas and a new commitment to protect the lives of children with disabilities from abuse and neglect.

I undertook the task of writing this book with the hope that it will go beyond the numbers and give readers a chance to reflect on the lives of real children and adolescents with disabilities who have been abused and neglected. It is important to recognize that this book is databased. Data from the United States Department of Health and Human Services maltreatment reports as well as the research in this area are integral parts of this text. The stories selected from the newspaper coverage over a 10-year span focus on children with disabilities who have been abused and neglected. These stories include case descriptions of children and adolescents with disabilities who have been abused and neglected. They are not hypothetical.

My hope is that uncovering these stories and the known details of their contexts will facilitate the preparation of more aware and responsive researchers and clinicians in an assortment of disciplines. I trust that those who read it will work more effectively to prevent when possible, and ameliorate when necessary, the senseless and often deadly abuse and neglect in the lives of children and adolescents with disabilities. Furthermore, my hope is that the questions, observations, and concerns that arise from awareness of this information will inform the work of researchers and policymakers in law, medicine, education, and related fields.

In conclusion, we must remain optimistic that we can live in a world that protects children and adolescents, especially those with disabilities, who are at greater risk of abuse and neglect. The only way to develop such a world is for individuals and communities, one-by-one, to uncover this problem, reveal the truth of what we know, and face its implications for caregiving, for necessary databased understanding, and for the development of policies and procedures that will prevent it. We must celebrate our efforts to work together to develop a world that protects children and adolescents with disabilities from the lifelong and often deadly harm caused by abuse and neglect.

Normal, IL, USA   E. Paula Crowley

Acknowledgements

Thanks to all at Springer who made this book come to life. Thank you to Miranda Dijksman, Esther Otten, and Myriam Poort who initially accepted this manuscript. Your comments and suggestions greatly enhanced the contribution of this work. Thank you to Hendrikje Tuerlings, Sindhuja Gajendran, and their staff who worked on the last steps of this project. I appreciate their professionalism and courtesy all along the way. I would like to extend my endless gratitude to the diligent reporters at the *Chicago Tribune* without whom so much would never be known. I would like to thank my colleagues at Illinois State University who in many important ways contributed to this project. First, thank you to Trish Klass, Lin Zeng, and graduate assistants – Christina Cabrera, Kelsey Cushman, Melanie Weber, and Brianne Petry – who all contributed uniquely to this work. I thank my colleague Harold Johnson, for his interest and support of this project from the outset. I appreciate his keen awareness and ongoing commitment to the work of stopping abuse and neglect in the lives of children with disabilities. I thank Mark Zablocki for his contributions to the first drafts of Chaps. 3, 5, and 7. I thank an anonymous reviewer who stated that an article I submitted to a journal years ago, needed to be a book instead. I thank students and colleagues who attended my presentations on this subject at professional conferences for many years now. I thank the librarians at Illinois State University's Milner Library who make so much work possible. I thank my sister Ethel Crowley for her good example, care, encouragement, and guidance during critical junctures of this project. I thank my colleagues and friends Maribeth Lartz, Lucille Eckrich, Marcia Rossi, Helen Bowen, and many friends and acquaintances for their continued interest and encouragement along the way. Finally, I thank my husband Daniel Deneen and son Patrick Deneen for their abiding patience, understanding, and love during my long absences.

Contents

Expanded Table of Contents

**Preventing Abuse and Neglect in the Lives of Children
with Disabilities**

Illinois State University   E. Paula Crowley
Normal, IL, USA

Part I
Abuse and Neglect in the Lives of Children with Disabilities

Chapter 1
The Abuse and Neglect of Children with Disabilities: The Extent of the Problem

The world is a dangerous place, not because of those who do
evil, but because of those who look on and do nothing.
(Albert Einstein, Theoretical Physicist, 1879–1955.)

Abstract We begin this chapter with a brief examination of the current statistics on the abuse and neglect of children with and without disabilities. We place this issue in a historical context. Then we examine the inherent challenges to an accurate count of these children. We show how differences among definitions challenge the development of an accurate understanding of abuse and neglect in the lives of children with disabilities. We examine what we know about this topic based on data from national and international databases as well as from the professional literature. We provide a description of the study and the methodology used in the research that provides the foundation for this book. Following a discussion of organizations dedicated to preventing abuse and neglect among children, we close this chapter with a set of recommendations for research and practice.

The U.S. Department of Health and Human Services (U.S. DHHS, 2013) data from 2012 indicate a national estimate of 3,438,000 referrals (46.1 children per 1,000) of children under 17 years old to child protection services (CPS). Following these child referrals, an estimated 2,111,000 (28.3 children per 1,000) were screened-in. Screened-in referrals received dispositions following their investigations. CPS dispositions determine the specific details about the child victims of the abuse and neglect. CPS dispositions also determine whether there is a need for an alternative response such as the initiation of family supports and services. Therefore, in 2012 an estimated 1,327,000 children were referred but were not investigated further. An estimated 17.8 children per 1,000 referrals were screened-out and were not investigated further.

Data from the U.S. DHHS indicate that the number of children who received dispositions has been climbing since 2008. An estimated 26.8 children per 1,000 received dispositions from CPS in 2008, and in 2012 28.3 children per 1,000 received dispositions from CPS. This increase is also observable in the data on the abuse and neglect of children with disabilities (ANCD). Between 2011 and 2012 alone the U.S. DHHS data indicated an increase from 11.2 to 13.3 % of children with disabilities who were abused and neglected. Many researchers observe that these

© Springer International Publishing Switzerland 2016

E.P. Crowley, *Preventing Abuse and Neglect in the Lives of Children with Disabilities*, DOI 10.1007/978-3-319-30442-7_1

statistics represent an underestimate of the extent of this problem for reasons that we will discuss later in this chapter.

What do we know about the ANCD? Who are these children? Who are their perpetrators? In what circumstances does ANCD occur? Is this a modern social development? Or, have children with disabilities been abused and neglected for as long as we can remember? To what extent are they abused and neglected today? What may we hope for tomorrow and into the future? Individuals and groups of researchers across multiple disciplines, including historians, anthropologists, sociologists, medical and educational researchers, among others have long devoted their knowledge and skills to the study of the ANCD.

Our History

During the 1970s the study of the bioarchaeology of care emerged. This new field of study links our distant past with our growing and developing understanding of ourselves and the world in which we live. Forensic anthropologists rely on bones to tell the tales of human existence. The Index of Care recently developed by Tilley and Cameron (2014) is designed to identify and interpret the provision of health care in prehistory. This instrument represents the attempts of modern bioarchaeologists to examine caregiving and disability in prehistoric times. Forensic anthropologist:

> ... Clyde Snow liked to say that bones made good witnesses, never lying, never forgetting, and that a skeleton, no matter how old, could sketch the tale of a human life, revealing how it had been lived, how long it had lasted, what traumas it had endured and especially how it had ended. (McFadden, 2014)

Using the tools of anthropology to study the horrors of mass graves among other human atrocities, Snow and his colleagues devoted their careers to the quest for knowledge and understanding of human rights' violations internationally.

Tilley (2012) found evidence to support the observation that cultures in the distant past provided humane treatment for individuals with disabilities. In his article in the *New York Times* "Ancient Bones That Tell a Story Of Compassion" (December 18, 2012) James Gorman made it very clear that though abuse and neglect of people with disabilities, including the youngest children, is as old as the earliest humans, so is the culture of caring for persons with disabilities.

In his article, Gorman discussed the work of researchers Tilley and Oxenham of the Australian National University in Canberra who found that among skeletons laying straight, the skeleton of a man in Burial 9 who lived 4,000 years ago South of Hanoi who was laid to rest in a fetal position, suggesting physical disabilities. Tilley and Oxenham concluded that this man had weak bones, and they found other evidence that suggested he had little, if any use of his arms and that he could not have fed himself or kept himself clean. Based on the available evidence, these researchers concluded that people took time to care for the man in Burial 9, and they tended to his every need.

Despite evidence to show caring for individuals with disabilities in cultures more than 45,000 years ago (Gorman, 2012), century after century and decade after decade, across the medical and social sciences' literature, data and commentary on the abuse and neglect of children, adolescents and adults with disabilities may be found. Ancient civilizations have been known to let the members of their communities with disabilities ramble into the wilderness where they would eventually die (Sobsey, 1994). They may have been intentionally, the victims of starvation, attack, exhaustion, or of under- or over-exposure or a combination of any of these.

Our More Recent History

European physicians and educators took the lead in the search for humane treatment of children with disabilities. In the summer of 1800, disheveled, naked and filthy, Victor at 12 years old was found in the French countryside by a group of hunters (Hallahan, Kauffman, & Pullen, 2015; Kanner, 1964). Victor got the attention of Philippe Pinel, a prominent French physician, and Jean-Marc Itard, a physician and an authority on diseases of the ear and on the education of students who are deaf (Hallahan et al., 2015). Pinel advised Itard, who began teaching communication skills to Victor. After 5 years he developed language and became more socialized. Pinel and Itard were among the scholars of the French Enlightenment and they laid the foundation for the individualized education of children with disabilities (Verstraete, 2005). While the reason Victor was living alone in the woods remains unknown, it would not be surprising to discover that he was indeed abandoned.

Kempe, Silverman, Steele, Droegemueller, and Silver first published "The Battered-Child Syndrome" in 1962. Due to its importance, this article was reprinted in 1984. The battered-child syndrome described the condition of young children with indicators of serious physical abuse. Kempe and his medical team regarded this abuse as a cause of childhood disability and death. Furthermore, they observed that in most hospitals child abuse was seldom recognized, infrequently diagnosed and not brought to the attention of appropriate authorities.

Over the years researchers, writers, reporters, photographers, and filmmakers continued their efforts to unveil the conditions of abuse and neglect of persons with disabilities. These efforts may be observed in two haunting exposés: the photographic essay, *Christmas in Purgatory* (Blatt & Kaplan, 1966) and in the film *Titicut Follies* (1967) directed by Frederick Wiseman.

Christmas in Purgatory: A photographic essay on mental retardation by Burton Blatt and Frederick Kaplan (1966) is based on direct observations in five unnamed state institutions for children and adults with disabilities in four eastern states. Blatt and Kaplan's photographic essay contains commentary and photographs that depict abuse, neglect, and generally inhumane treatment of thousands of children and adults with disabilities. The photographs in *Christmas in Purgatory* were instrumental in bringing public attention to facts that could not be denied. *Christmas in Purgatory* paved the way for the passage of the groundbreaking Public Law 94–142 (now IDEA, 2004) that, for the first time in the history of the United States, gave every child with a disability a right to a free, appropriate, and public education.

American filmmaker and documentarian, Frederick Wiseman observed life at the Bridewater State Hospital for the criminally insane in Massachusetts in the 1960s. The controversial film *Titicut Follies* was filmed in 1967 but was banned from public viewing until 1992. Though Wiseman had been granted permission to make this film, Massachusetts Superior Court judge Harry Kalus ordered all copies of the film to be destroyed while claiming that the film invaded the inmates' privacy. We may conclude that in reality this ban was merely a way to avoid the uncomfortable truth about the inhumane treatment of persons with disabilities that this film exposed.

These two major contributions to the literature in the social sciences illuminated the inhumane treatment of children, adolescents, and adults with disabilities in the United States and all over the world that continues to this day. Still, many individuals remain unaware that children and adults with disabilities are abused and neglected in the United States and across the world on a daily basis.

Exercise 1.1: Reflection

Following a review of the film, Titicut Follies (1967) and the book, Christmas in Purgatory, by Blatt and Kaplan (1966) consider what surprised you most? What do you believe were the most important contributions of this film and book? Do you agree that these two publications constitute a significant contribution to the professional literature? Do you believe that they provide an important historical perspective for future professionals? Do you agree that if we disregard our history, we are bound to repeat it?

Challenges to the Accuracy of Our Data

Challenges to the accuracy of child abuse and neglect (CAN) and ANCD data are rooted in issues related to definition, identification, and reporting procedures (Fallon, Trocmé, Fluke, MacLaurin, Tonmyr, & Yuan, 2010). The term child maltreatment encompasses CAN. Federal legislation in the United States provides guidance to states by defining minimum acts or behaviors that constitute child maltreatment – abuse and neglect. In the Child Abuse Prevention and Treatment Act (CAPTA) (2010) child maltreatment – CAN is defined as:

> ... *at a minimum, any recent act or failure to act on the part of a parent or caretaker which results in death, serious physical or emotional harm, sexual abuse or exploitation, or an act or failure to act which presents an imminent risk of serious harm'. (p. 6)*

The federal definition of CAN refers specifically to parents and caregivers and a "child" who is defined as a person that is 18 years old and younger. Throughout these chapters we will use "child" or "children" to refer to children and adolescents less than 18 years of age. Legislation at the federal level sets minimum standards for each state to develop its own unique definition of abuse and neglect that fits within the civil and criminal statutes of that state. As a result, among the challenges to our understanding of the extent and dimensions of CAN are the varying definitions of abuse and neglect throughout the United States and across the world.

Exercise 1.2: Critical Thinking
Compare and contrast the definition of CAN in Illinois, Texas, Virginia and Vermont. Can you find common features among these definitions? Which definition seems the most appealing to you? Would you support a common definition of CAN embraced by every state throughout the United States? Analyze how the International Society for the Prevention of Child Abuse and Neglect define child abuse?
You will find links to these definitions at the end of this chapter.

The term 'child with a disability' means a child from 3 to 21.11 years old who has a disability as defined in section 602 of the Individuals with Disabilities Education Act (2024 U.S.C. 1401) (2004). The term infant or toddler from birth to 3 years old, with a disability as defined in section 632 of such Act (202 U.S.C. 1432). The 13 categories of childhood disability as defined in the Individuals with Disabilities Educational Improvement Act (IDEA, 2004) include children with autism, deaf-blindness, deafness, emotional disturbance, hearing impairment, intellectual disability (formally mental retardation), multiple disability, orthopedic impairment, other health impairment, specific learning disability, speech or language impairment, traumatic brain injury, and vision impairment including blindness. As in the case of the definitions of abuse and neglect and while guided by the Federal definition, each state develops its own definition of the categories of childhood disability. Furthermore, there is a lack of consensus on the definitions of some childhood disabilities, such as learning disability, across the professional disciplines of medicine, law, education, and their related disciplines.

Exercise 1.3: Critical Thinking
Are you surprised that the definition of disability remains a professional frontier? Perhaps commonly shared definitions of disabilities represent an unrealistic expectation. Yet, a shared vocabulary is essential to the development of any discipline. *What can we do to move our professional communities forward without a shared vocabulary?*

Defining disability in the context of ANCD offers additional unique challenges to researchers, policymakers, and professional personnel. We will discuss these challenges in the following section.

Documenting precisely the manifestations of disability in childhood is complex and so is the terminology associated with it. To begin, the same disability may be manifested differently from one child to another. Depression in childhood may appear as withdrawn and reclusive behavior or it may appear as acting-out and aggression behavior (Walker & Gresham, 2014). Additionally, the same child may be regarded as disabled among some professionals and not among others. For example, a child may be diagnosed with a learning disability in school and may not have a medical diagnosis. In their classic textbook, *Exceptional children: An introduction to special education (13th ed.),* Hallahan, Kauffman, and Pullen (2015) include children and adolescents with attention deficit with/without hyperactivity disorder, as well as children and adolescents with special gifts and talents. The *Maltreatment Report* (U.S. DHHS, 2013) and the IDEA Regulations of (2004) exclude both of these groups of children.

The Report generated by the U.S. Department of Health and Human Services (U.S. DHHS, 2013) Children's Bureau is based on the data generated by the National Council of Abused and Neglected Children (NCANDS). NCANDS recognizes only seven disability categories, namely, behavior problem, emotionally disturbed, learning disability, intellectual disabilities (formally, mental retardation), other medical condition, physically disabled, and visually or hearing impaired.

When compiling these data generated by NCANDS, researchers at the U.S. DHHS combined the categories of learning disability with the IDEIA categories of specific learning disability, speech or language impairment and traumatic brain injury. Furthermore, the categories of visually or hearing impaired combine the two IDEIA categories of deaf-blindness and deafness. In conclusion, the professional challenges inherent in defining, observing, documenting, and reporting CAN among children with disabilities pose unique threats to the reliability and validity of child maltreatment data.

The Dual Challenges of Identifying Disability and Reporting ANCD

Challenges to an accurate count of children with disabilities who are abused and neglected include the failure to identify child disability in the first place. Many children who have disabilities remain unidentified (Billmire & Myers, 1985; Hallahan et al., 2015; Hershkowitz, Lamb, & Horowitze, 2007). Mild disabilities, including learning disabilities and some emotional and behavioral disorders may go unnoted throughout a child's life and even into adulthood.

Additional challenges to an accurate count of the ANCD include staff shortages, financial constraints and reporting procedures. Interagency collaboration is required in order to provide data for the development of reports. For example, states submit data to NCANDS on a voluntary basis. There are no requirements or penalties imposed for unreported data. Data may be missing or incomplete due lack of personnel or time constraints.

Furthermore, children with disabilities who are abused and neglected may go unnoticed. Disability may be so blended with CAN that it disappears. Caseworkers may be unable to tell whether disability preceded or followed the abuse and neglect. While the focus remains on the trauma of abuse and neglect, the presence of disability may become lost in the emergency at hand.

The identification of disability in childhood is frequently confined to educational settings and may be unnoted in the medical or clinical context. On the other hand, some children will be identified with disabilities by the medical professionals and they may not be identified with disabilities by education professionals. Children may be diagnosed with visual impairments or hearing losses by medical professionals and these may be unnoted in educational settings.

The protection of family privacy as well as the isolation that disability frequently brings about in families contributes to the nonreport of abuse and neglect in the lives of some children with disabilities. These children often remain hidden from the routines of family life, friendships, and life in the community. Often they do not circulate in the routines of life in childhood and adolescents. Instead many live in isolation, whereby their abuse and neglect is often unknown and therefore unacknowledged.

The characteristics of children with disabilities constrain reporting to appropriate authorities. For example, children with communication disorders, autism, blindness, deafness, or with emotional or behavioral disorders are frequently unknown in their neighborhoods largely due to the difficulties these children have making friends and engaging in social exchanges. They may be the targets of abuse and neglect, and no one will ever know. For example, on September 13, 2011 Gutowski, Sadovi, and Jaworski described such isolation, abuse and neglect in a story in the *Chicago Tribune*:

> Price's children were rarely seen, and when they did come to the backyard, it was often at odd hours, the neighbors said.
>
> On Thursday, one of those children was found unresponsive in the yard wearing only a T-shirt and was later pronounced dead of natural causes related to bronchopneumonia.
>
> Authorities said the mentally disabled boy and his four siblings, ranging from 12 to 18, never went to school and were forced to live in filth among more than 200 animals -- many of them dead. The home, officials said, was covered with feces and infested with spiders.

Exercise 1.4: Reflection

Why do you think the neighbors did not report the abuse and neglect of Ms. Price's children? What clear indicators might they have noticed and included in a report to appropriate authorities? Would it have been important to mention that one of the children had a disability? *The challenges inherent in the definition of abuse and neglect as well as in the definition of disability might contribute to a neighbor's hesitation to make a report. Do you agree? Disagree? Explain your rationale. The discussion below offers further explanations.*

Reporting the abuse and neglect of any child remains a daunting task for many adults. The threats afforded by the mandate to report the ANCD may be less of a threat because of the confounding variables presented by the disabilities of the child targeted. For example, the hesitation to report the abuse and neglect of a child with a disability may be grounded in the expectation that the child and the parent or caregiver are not held to the same expectations as peer children or caregivers. This is captured in the following statement from the story above by Gutowski et al. "Lydia Price's neighbors said Monday that they thought something was amiss inside her small brick bungalow on South Lombard Street in Berwyn" and they did not report their concerns. The truth became known following the death of a child with an intellectual disability.

What Do We Know About CAN and ANCD in the United States?

During 2012, the estimated referral rate of CAN was higher than it has been in years. The *Child Maltreatment Report* (U.S. DHHS, 2013) indicates that, on average, documented referrals were made for an estimated 46.1 children per 1,000 in 2012 and this number has steadily increased from 42.1 in 2008, 41.6 in 2009, 42.2 in 2010, and 43.9 in 2011. We must be concerned about this trend. More and more children per 1,000 are maltreated in the United States. Researchers estimate that 32 % or more of these children have disabilities (Bones, 2013; Leeb, Bitsko, Merrick, & Armour, 2012). According to ChildHelp (2014):

> Children are suffering from a hidden epidemic of child abuse and neglect. Every year more than 3 million reports of child abuse are made in the United States involving more than 6 million children (a report can include multiple children). The United States has one of the worst records among industrialized nations – losing on average between four and seven children every day to child abuse and neglect.

CPS investigated more child maltreatment referrals in 2012 than in the years prior. The U.S. DHHS (2013) observed that "The national rate of reports that received a disposition was 28.3 per 1,000 children in the national population, a 5.6% increase since 2008 when the rate was 26.8 per 1,000 children in the population" (p. 6). In 2012, an estimated 62.0 % of all referrals were screened-in for further investigation of child maltreatment. We may well wonder whether an infrastructure needs to be put in place to support the 38.0 % that were screened-out for further investigation.

What will stop the needless, life changing, and costly abuse and neglect of children with and without disabilities? How can we document the trends in CAN among children with and without disabilities as accurately as possible in order to intervene when necessary and prevent when possible?

Taking a Closer Look at National Trends

Every 10 years the Census is taken on the number of people living in the United States (United States Census, 2010). These data report overall state populations, as well as, population density per square mile/kilometer. The U.S. DHHS (2013) report contains state-by-state statistics on the rate of screened-in reports per 1,000 children. The trend among these data indicates that the rate of screened-in CAN referrals is higher than the National average in states with the highest and lowest population densities.

In 2012, the six most densely populated states were New Jersey, Rhode Island, Massachusetts, Connecticut, Maryland, and Delaware. An estimated 52.8 children per 1,000 were screened-in cases of abuse and neglect in these states, whereas the national average is estimated at 46.1 children per 1,000 (U.S. DHHS, 2013)

Table 1.1 Screened-in CAN in highest population density in the United States

Highest population density states	People per square mile	People per square kilometer	Rate of abuse and neglect per 1000 children
New Jersey	1,205	465	29.9
Rhode Island	1,016	392	56.7
Massachusetts	852	329	53.8
Connecticut	741	286	53.9
Maryland	606	234	41.5
Delaware	471	161	81.5
Average	*815*	*Average*	*52.8*
		National average	*46.1*

Data from the U.S. DHHS, 2013

Table 1.2 Screened-in CAN in lowest population density in the United States

Lowest populated density states	People per square mile	People per square kilometer	Rate of abuse and neglect per 1000 children
New Mexico	17	7	63.2
South Dakota	11	4	78.5
North Dakota	10	4	24.4
Montana	7	3	59.3
Wyoming	6	3	47.8
Alaska	1	<1	90.8
Average	*8.6*	*Average*	*60.6*
		National average	*46.1*

Data from the U.S. DHHS, 2013

(see Table 1.1). We discuss the context in which the ANCD occurs in Chap. 8 of this book.

The six states with the lowest population density, according to the 2010 Census, are New Mexico, South Dakota, North Dakota, Montana, Wyoming, and Alaska. In these states and in contrast with the National average of 46.1 children, an estimated average of 60.6 children per 1,000 were screened-in cases of abuse and neglect (see Table 1.2). Tables 1.1 and 1.2 contain specific details relative to the estimated number of children who were screened-in cases of abuse and neglect per most and least densely populated state. Why is the estimated rate of child maltreatment referrals per 1,000 children higher (60.6 children per 1,000) in less densely populated states than it is in the most densely populated states (52.8 children per 1,000)? It is important to note that these data are not disaggregated; therefore, it is not possible to know how many child maltreatment referrals concerned children *with* and *without* disabilities? In subsequent chapters we will focus directly on finding out as much as we can about the ANCD.

Before we leave the National statistics, we turn our attention to trends in the estimated number of CAN screened-in referrals per 1,000 in the most highly

Table 1.3 Screened-in CAN in the six most highly populated states in the United States

Most highly populated states	People per square mile	People per square kilometer	Rate of abuse and neglect per 1000 children
California	243	94	38.5
Texas	99	38	29.1
New York	417	161	Not reported
Florida	365	141	56.9
Illinois	232	90	22.4
Pennsylvania	285	110	Not reported
Average	*273.5*	*Average*	*36.7*
		National average	*46.1*

Data from the U.S. DHHS, 2013

populated states. Based on the U.S. Census data from 2010 these States include California, Texas, New York, Florida, Illinois, and Pennsylvania. The estimated average rate of child maltreatment screened-in referrals in these states was 36.7 children per 1,000 – lower than the National average (46.1 children per 1,000). Why is the estimated rate of screened-in referrals of CAN per 1,000 children lower in the most highly populated states? The U.S.- DHHS report an estimated 52.8 screened-in CAN referrals per 1,000 in the most densely populated states and the estimated 36.7 CAN referrals in geographically large and highly populated states. For example, New Jersey is the most densely populated state and the estimated rate of CAN referrals per 1,000 is lower (29.9) than the National average (46.1) (see Tables 1.1, 1.2, and 1.3).

In the most highly populated states, such as California, Texas and New York with lower population densities (273.5), the estimated rate of referral per 1,000 children is lower (36.7) in both the most densely (815) populated states, such as New Jersey and Rhode Island (52.8) and least densely (8.6) populated states, such as New Mexico and South Dakota (60.6). This is further clarified by a careful analysis of screened in CAN referrals in such states as Vermont – that ranks 30th in density and estimates 117.9 CAN referrals per 1,000 in 2012 while the National average is 46.1 referrals per 1,000 children. Estimates in Alaska, which ranks 50th in population density, indicate 90.8 CAN referrals per 1,000 children. What explains the trend toward more screened-in CAN referrals per 1,000 children in states with lower population densities?

Taking a Closer Look at National Trends in ANCD

The estimated number of children with disabilities who were victims of CAN increased from 355,435 in 2010 to 522,483 in 2011. This represents an increase in the maltreatment of 167,048 children with disabilities from 2010 to 2011. In 2012, 503,943 children with disabilities were abused and neglected in the United

States. For context, the 503,943 children with disabilities who were abused and neglected in 2012 would fill 8,400 busses carrying 60 children per bus. The human toll associated with these human losses will never be fully known.

Child Fatality and CAN

An estimated 1,593 children died as a result of CAN in 2012 (U.S. DHHS, 2013). In the same year, the National rate of child fatality was 2.2 per 100,000 children. These children were mostly under 3 years of age (70.3 %), more frequently boys – 2.5 per 100,000 and girls – 1.9 per 100,000 died following CAN. These children were White (38.3 %), African-American (3.9 %) and Hispanic (15.3 %). Their deaths were perpetrated primarily by either one or two parents (see Chap. 6).

In a state-by-state analysis of the fatality rates among 100,000 children, not disaggregated for childhood disability, no reported data were reported from Idaho, Maine, and Massachusetts, and a fluctuation from 00 in Vermont to 4.6 in Arkansas. The overall National and state-by-state statistics on child fatality are subject to such limitations as the nature of the reporting procedures used. We will never know how many children die of unacknowledged, unrecognized, and undocumented CAN and ANCD. Additionally, child fatality estimates do not include a breakdown of children with and without disabilities. Based on the evidence provided by Jones et al. (2012) and from generations of researchers, we may conclude that for every one child who dies as a result of CAN, among them are three to four children with disabilities.

What Else Do We Know? Current Literature on the ANCD

Based on the findings of a meta-analysis of observational studies, Jones et al. (2012) estimate that up to a quarter of children with disabilities experience physical and sexual violence and that children with disabilities are three to four times more likely to be victims of violence than are their nondisabled peers.

Over the years, study after study, at national and international levels, again and again establish that children and adolescents with disabilities are abused and neglected more frequently than their peers without disabilities (Bones, 2013; Gore & Janssen, 2007; Hibbard & Desch, 2007; Stalker & McArthur, 2012; Sobsey, 1994, 2002; Sullivan, 2009; Sullivan & Knutson, 1998, 2000; Verdugo, Bermejo, & Fuertes, 1995). Ammerman et al. (1989) found the overall incidence of child maltreatment to be 39 % in 150 children with multiple disabilities who were admitted to a psychiatric hospital. Of those children 60 % had been physically abused, 45 % had been neglected, and 36 % had been sexually abused. Sullivan and Knutson (2000) found that children with disabilities are 3.79 times more likely to be physically abused, 3.76 times more likely to be neglected, and 3.14 times more likely to be sexually abused than their nondisabled peers.

Clearly, the protection of children with disabilities from CAN remains an enormous challenge in the United States. The information in each chapter provides clear evidence that a much greater effort is needed in order to prevent both CAN and ANCD. Consider the following critical thinking exercise:

Exercise 1.5: Critical Thinking
Based on the data generated by Sullivan and Knutson (2000) we can expect differences in abuse and neglect patters among children with and without disabilities:

Disability status	Physical abuse	Neglect	Sexual abuse
No disability	10 children	10 children	10 children
With a disability	37.9 children	37.6 children	31.4 children

Translate these data into real-life situations. What are these numbers telling you?

It is difficult to face the challenges and the questions posed to us while studying CAN and in particular the ANCD. The proper care and protection of all children is possible. The first step in making this happen is the development of a clear understanding of the scope and dimensions of our failures to do so (see Chap. 9). Here we continue this effort by describing the study that provided stories from a 10-year analysis of newspaper coverage of children with disabilities who were abused and neglected.

Exercise 1.6: Critical Thinking
Child growth and development theorists make it very clear that from their prenatal days and onward through their childhood years, children need a secure and nurturing relationship with at least one parent and ideally two. They need to be protected from serious, debilitating trauma and chronic stress. *Write at least six major contributing factors that, for you, explain why so many children across the world are born into circumstances that no child can live and grow in safely and securely? Why are so many children malnourished physically, emotionally, intellectually, and spiritually? Why do you think that so many children fail to grow to adulthood and realize at least some if not all of their potential as human beings?*

Newspaper Coverage of Child Abuse and Neglect and Disability

What is the role of newspapers in the digital age? Is a study of newspaper coverage relevant in the age of Twitter and other social media? Ju, Jeong, and Chyi (2014) reassure us that newspapers have an essential role in modern society. John F. Sturm (n.d.), President of the Newspaper Association of America stated that:

More than 104 million adults read a print newspaper every day, more than 115 million on Sundays. That's more people than watch the Super Bowl (94 million), American Idol (23 million) or that typically watch the late local news (65 million).

61 percent of 18–24 year olds and 25–34 year olds read a newspaper in an average week and 65 percent of them read a newspaper or visited a newspaper website in the past week.

The news media provide information about current events and issues occurring in the local community, as well as at state, national, and international levels. According to the Newspaper Association of America 73 % of adults read a newspaper or visit a newspaper web site in an average week. Researchers observe that newspapers have considerable influence in the development of public awareness (Bogart, 1981; Epstein, 1981; Ju et al., 2013; McNergney, Hallahan, Keller, & Crowley, 1992; Schulte, 1983).

Newspapers and other public media have a role in raising awareness of such issues as, the role of disability as a risk factor for abuse and neglect, as well as the role of abuse and neglect as a risk factor for disability (Ammerman, 1991; Bones, 2013; Carty & Ratcliffe, 1995; Kelly, 1992; Leeb et al., 2012; Reece & Sege, 2000; Sobsey & Varnhagen, 1989; Sullivan & Knutson, 1998; Taylor, 1987). To what extent is the public aware that children and adolescents with disabilities are more likely to be neglected, physically abused, and sexually abused than are children without disabilities?

To what extent does the abuse and neglect of children and adolescents with disabilities get newspaper coverage? This text is designed to address our lack of knowledge about ANCD. The following chapters contain analyses of the literature in this area, as well as the findings of a study that focused on a content analysis of newspaper coverage of the abuse and neglect of children and adolescents with disabilities. The data were generated from stores in the *Chicago Tribune* from January, 2004 to December, 2013. Also included in each chapter, are reflection and critical thinking exercises that are designed to prepare a reader to consider this content on a deeper and more personal level. These reflections may also constitute the foundation for the development of dialogue on critical issues relevant to the abuse and neglect of children with disabilities.

Exercise 1.7: Critical Thinking

The *Chicago Tribune* is a large circulation newspaper located in a large metropolitan area. When combined the 368,145 (printed copies) and the 46,785 (digital copies) represent a total average circulation of 414,930 newspapers per day. *Do you expect that the stories about the abuse and neglect of children with disabilities in the Chicago Tribune differ from those in medium and small circulation newspapers? Do you expect that the overall themes found in these stories might be similar to those found in large, medium, and small circulation newspapers? State three reasons to support your observations.*

Procedures for Generating Newspaper Data

This content analysis focused on the newspaper coverage of the types of abuse and neglect to which children with disabilities are exposed; the outcomes of their abuse and neglect; the age, gender, and disability characteristics of these children; the age, gender, disability, and relationship characteristics of the perpetrators of their abuse and neglect; and the circumstances in which this abuse and neglect occurred.

We selected the *Chicago Tribune*, a large Midwestern metropolitan area newspaper with a circulation of more than 350,000 copies daily. We used the *News Bank* electronic database to identify newspaper articles on the abuse and neglect of children and adolescents with disabilities from January, 2004 to December, 2013. Using the index of *Exceptional Learners* (Hallahan & Kauffman, 2003) we developed a list of terms frequently used to describe disability categories. We used the keywords "abuse" and "neglect" to narrow the focus of our search. We combined the following key words for the search (child maltreatment or child abuse) and (disabilit* or autism or blind or deaf or retard* or handicap* or Down syndrome or ADHD or special education or disorder or gifted or talented). We included all sections of the newspapers in our search for articles on the abuse of children and adolescents with disabilities and excluded only advertisements, announcements, obituaries, movie reviews, opinion pages, and sales. Two raters reviewed each article and established 100 % agreement on the appropriateness of the articles for inclusion in this study.

Coding Procedures and Data Analysis

Following the selection of newspaper articles, two independent raters analyzed each article independently using a coding form for each article in the following areas:

Type of Abuse/Neglect Based on our pilot study of a sample of the 2004 newspaper articles, varying types of abuse and neglect take place, including, physical abuse, sexual abuse, drug abuse, emotional abuse, neglect, sexual photography, and discrimination. We also included a category for types of abuse not included in these categories.

Outcome of Abuse/Neglect The categories that described the outcome of the abuse, neglect and maltreatment included disability, victim removed from the family, death, under investigation, and "other" for outcomes not included in these categories.

Who and What Disability In our pilot study, it was clear that some articles discussed the child/victim as having a disability and in other articles the adult perpetrator had the disability. Furthermore, we documented the type of disability discussed in the article.

Type of Article The three types of articles we found included specific case descriptions, personal stories of individuals who reflected on their own abuse, and informational articles, for example, descriptions of programs designed for victims of abuse.

Number and Description of Age and Gender We coded the number of children included in the article, as well as, the age and gender of victims and the perpetrators. When age and/or gender were not specified, we left the space for that entry blank.

Perpetrator Relationship Our pilot study indicated varied relationships between perpetrators and victims. We coded father/mother, legal guardian, school personnel, special education teacher, stranger, relative, foster parent, priest/minister, family friend, and "other" for relationships not included in this list.

Reason Given for the Abuse/Neglect The coding system for the reason given for the abuse included lack of knowledge or inability to care for the child with a disability, perpetrator was under the influence, perpetrator had a diagnosed disability before the incident, perpetrator claimed "mentally unstable," no reason given, and specify "other" for reasons not included in the above categories.

Coders checked more than one option when appropriate. The researchers checked the coding of all the articles and established 100 % agreement on the coding of each article.

Initial Findings

In all, 149 stories met the criteria for inclusion in this study and of these, 36 represented extended coverage of previously published stories. The remaining 113 stories represented unique coverage across three story types namely, unique stories about children with disabilities relative to their abuse and neglect, stories that provided information to readers relative to the abuse and neglect and child disability and the final group of unique stories involved the sharing of personal reflections and experiences relative to abuse and neglect and disability. Seventy eight (69.0 %) of these stories described unique cases of ANCD; 47 (41.6 %) of these stories provided information about abuse and neglect relative to disability; and 10 (8.8 %) described personal reflections of abuse and neglect relative to disability. Eighteen stories (15.9 %) of the stories described cases of abuse and neglect and also provided information to readers. Two stories provided both personal reflection and information to readers. One story described a personal case as well as provided information about the ANCD (see Table 1.4).

Table 1.4 Type of newspaper story (n = 113)[a]

Case situational	78
Informational	47
Personal stories	10
Case and informational	18
Personal and informational	2
Case and personal and informational	1

[a]n exceeds the number of stories involving different story types
Data from the study of the newspaper coverage of ANCD in the *Chicago Tribune*

Organizations Dedicated to Preventing CAN

The International Society for the Prevention of Child Abuse and Neglect (ISPCAN) is a multidisciplinary organization that was founded in 1977 to bring together professionals who are concerned about CAN globally. The mission of ISPCAN is to support individuals and organizations who work to protect children from abuse and neglect worldwide. The Society's objectives include raising awareness about CAN, disseminating information, promoting the human rights of children, improving the identification, treatment and prevention of CAN, promoting the professional exchange of best practices of ISPCAN members internationally and designing and delivering comprehensive training programs to professionals and volunteers who are engaged in treating and preventing child abuse.

The first goal of ISPCAN focuses on increasing awareness of the extent, the causes, and possible solutions for all forms of child abuse. At this time, ISPCAN does not differentiate priorities for children with and without disabilities in its mission or objectives at this time.

The most common strategies used by ISPCAN to increase awareness of CAN internationally are advocacy, professional training, print and electronic media campaigns, and the prosecution of child abuse offenders. Newspapers have a unique role in the mass media and therefore, have a unique role in the prevention of the abuse and neglect of children and adolescents with disabilities.

Exercise 1.8: Reflection

Review the ISPCAN website and consider its contribution to our efforts to prevent CAN. *If you were to join this professional organization today, what considerations would convince you to do so? What stumbling blocks, if any, would you have to overcome in order to join this organization?*

Prevent Child Abuse America was founded in Chicago, Illinois in 1972. It was founded to:

> ... ensure the healthy development of children nationwide. The organization promotes that vision through a network of chapters in 50 states and nearly 600 Healthy Families America home visiting sites in 39 states, the District of Columbia, American Samoa, Guam, the Northern Commonwealth of the Marianas, Puerto Rico, US Virgin Islands, and Canada. A major organizational focus is to advocate for the existence of a national policy

framework and strategy for children and families while promoting evidence-based practices that prevent abuse and neglect from ever occurring.

Exercise 1.9: Reflection

Review the Prevent Child Abuse America website and find out how you may become involved in preventing the abuse and neglect of children with disabilities. *Consider the unique contribution you might make to the prevention of abuse and neglect of children with disabilities.*

What Can We Do? Implications for Research and Practice

Awareness of the disproportionate amount of abuse and neglect in the lives of children with disabilities is essential for parents, guardians, professionals, and related personnel who occupy designated and essential roles in the lives of children with disabilities. This awareness is the first step toward the appropriate care, protection, education, and overall treatment of children with disabilities. The following section contains 12 recommendations for promoting health and safety in the lives of children with disabilities. These recommendations focus on three aspects of each of the following: the legal rights and human dignity of children despite their incidental characteristics; what parents, guardians, extended family, and community members can do to prevent abuse and neglect in the lives of children with disabilities; and what researchers and professionals can do to prevent abuse and neglect in the lives of children with disabilities.

Affirm Children's Human Dignity and Rights

A focused awareness that affirms the human dignity and the rights of children, regardless of their incidental characteristics, is essential in order to prevent their abuse and neglect. The life of each child, with or without disabilities, has an undeniable right to be treated with human dignity and respect. Therefore:

Recommendation 1.1: Affirm the human dignity of every child, regardless of such incidental markers as race, ethnicity, and disability.

***

Are provisions made for children with disabilities that facilitate their full membership in their local communities? Do they have access to the community? Is there sufficient knowledge, understanding and flexibility among community members to encourage their community participation, to the fullest? Is there sufficient infrastructure, such as ramps and transportation, as well as encouragement to participate in programs that promote their self-expression, inclusion and integration whenever possible? We recommend, in particular, an analysis of community strengths and weaknesses relative to the needs of children with disabilities and their families. Need based public awareness programs that promote understanding, compassion, and caring would go a long way to protect children from maltreatment in its every form. Community leaders and child advocates must work together in order to:

Recommendation 1.2: Develop public awareness programs at the community level in order to enhance understanding, awareness, and integration of children with disabilities.

***

Children with disabilities who learn how to self-advocate are in a better position to fulfil their potential as human beings as well as to protect themselves from abuse and neglect. Those who know themselves and the unique challenges of their disabilities will, more likely, develop the self-confidence that comes with self-knowledge and self-acceptance. They will more likely ask for what they need, articulate why they feel safe or unsafe, and request assistance appropriately when in need.

When children with disabilities cannot self-advocate their health and safety is at increased risk. Their increased vulnerability adds to their need for additional appropriate supports and services. When children learn about their disabilities and the unique challenges inherent in them they:

Recommendation 1.3: Develop self-advocacy skills so that they can communicate their wants, needs and preferences more clearly.

***

What is more tragic than CAN? What more clearly represents the lowest ebb of human existence than to observe a child who has been abused and neglected? It seems even more intolerable to consider abuse and neglect in the lives of children with disabilities – such as those who cannot communicate their fears, cannot walk or run to safety, or cannot tell what happened even if requested to do so. Despite the unimaginable tragedy of abuse and neglect in the lives of children with and without disabilities, it occurs every minute of every day in every corner of the world. It is time to:

Recommendation 1.4: Redouble our commitment to stop abuse and neglect in the lives of children with and without disabilities all over the world by empowering families, extended families, and communities members

***

When children have unique physical, emotional, and learning needs, due to their disabilities, they require specialized care in their homes and communities.

Knowledgeable parents, guardians, extended family, and community members in the lives of children with disabilities will better protect them from abuse and neglect. When they understand their children's unique needs and develop a set of carefully constructed guidelines for their daily routines, they are protecting their children from abuse and neglect. This knowledge and skills will guide day-to-day decision-making during interactions with children with disabilities. The provision of appropriate personnel, training, and ongoing resources and support is essential in order to meet the needs of children with disabilities. Children's safety and protection is more assured when caregivers:

Recommendation 1.5: Understand and accept their children and their disabilities.

***

Why are parents, members of extended families and communities so reluctant to speak about CAN and ANCD? Too often this is a moot subject that commands silence and at most hushed conversations. The longer we remain unable to face the truth of the vulnerability of children to abuse and neglect, particularly those with disabilities, we perpetuate it. Awareness and understanding are both essential in the prevention of abuse and neglect in the lives of children with disabilities. We advocate for support of programs such as Prevent Child Abuse America as well as Prevent Child Abuse Chapters all over United States and the International Child Abuse Network (ICAN) and International Society for the Prevention of Child Abuse and Neglect (ISPCAN) . We advocate for increased:

Recommendation 1.6: Awareness that children with disabilities are at a higher risk of for abuse and neglect.

***

Parents, family and community members have essential roles in protecting the health and safety of children. The safety and protection of children with disabilities requires their caregivers to have additional knowledge and heightened awareness. For example, some children with autism have unique difficulty in noisy or crowded spaces. Children with intellectual disabilities may not understand when they are at-risk or when they put others at-risk. The cost of caring for some children with disabilities defies the imaginations of some parents – medical costs in particular may render some families unable to care for their child or children with disabilities. Children with disabilities are best served when their parents, guardians, extended family, and community members have an ongoing and persistent:

Recommendation 1.7: Commitment and willingness to advocate for the needs of children with disabilities.

***

Parents, guardians, family, and community members promote the health, safety and wellbeing of their children with disabilities when they encourage their participation in their own homes, their local communities and in all the routines of family life. Access to the routines of daily life normalizes the lives of children with and without disabilities. During their participation in daily routines, children learn essential vocabulary and skills. Children with disabilities are ill-served when they are denied age appropriate experiences that link them to the lives of their peers and to the lives of adults they might encounter during daily routines. For example, children with disabilities will be well-served by being included in grocery shopping trips, library visits, and play sessions. Their lives are enhanced and strengthened by engaging in age appropriate family and community routines. They are well-served when parents and caregivers make it possible for children with disabilities to:

Recommendation 1.8: Participate and integrate, to the extent possible, in their own homes and local communities, as well as in the big world around them.

***

Roles of Researchers and Professionals in the Prevention of CAN

A carefully constructed set of research questions will provide data for ongoing innovation and development in the area of abuse and neglect and child disability. Such innovation will guide program development and service delivery. When the quality of life increases for children with disabilities, everyone wins! With appropriate home, school, and community education and treatment, children with disabilities can more properly grow to be happy, healthy and contributing members of society. Continued innovation and development of our understanding of disability in childhood is essential in order to maximize the potential of each child with a disability. We suggest that researchers and professionals:

Recommendation 1.9: Establish an interdisciplinary research agenda that focuses on the quest to understand, predict, and intervene therapeutically in the lives of children with disabilities who have been exposed to abuse and neglect.

***

Professional challenges that are based on difficulty with conceptual understanding of abuse, neglect, disability and accompanying terminology perpetuate abuse and neglect in the lives of children with disabilities. The data from the U.S. DHHS

(2013) indicate that only about 20 % of CAN reports are substantiated. We might well wonder why. Is it not clear when a child is abused? When does appropriate care end and neglect begin? What constitutes disability? We lack professional consensus on these questions. Too often our lack of consensus leads to child fatality (see Chap. 4). Continued engagement in professional debate is essential in order to refine our terminology and:

Recommendation 1.10: Use data based methods to identify the unique needs of each child with a disability. This knowledge will guide decision-making about how to meet children's needs in the home, school and community.

***

Ignorance perpetrates abuse and neglect in the lives of children with disabilities. To what extent does the general public know that children with disabilities are abused and neglected at higher rates than their nondisabled peers? How much do people know about the needs of children with autism, spina bifida, deafness, blindness, cerebral palsy, and attention deficit disorder with or without hyperactivity? Do members of the general public know that young children have anxiety disorders, depression, as well as other severe emotional and psychiatric disorders at mild, moderate and severe levels? When we understand the effects of disability in childhood we will more readily contribute to the prevention of abuse and neglect in the lives of these children. Efforts to keep children with disabilities safe from abuse and neglect necessitates that we continue to:

Recommendation 1.11: Build professional interdisciplinary consensus around such terminology as abuse, neglect and disability through collegiality and focus on solving real problems in a collaborative and interdisciplinary manner.

***

The corporal punishment of children must stop. Violence by adults in the name of child discipline is a blithe on our society and this must be acknowledged. Unchecked violence begets more violence and this cycle continues to escalate and move forward from one generation to the next. The discontinuation of corporal punishment of children requires a cultural shift that is interdisciplinary in nature, thus requiring reforms in our educational, medical and legal systems.

Educational, medical and legal systems have protections of the human dignity and rights of children in place. Still, existing protections fail children in countries all over the world. The voices of children with disabilities are muffled even further by people and systems that, too often, misunderstand or intentionally disregard their needs and the needs of their caregivers. It is a myth that the rights of children with and without disabilities are protected sufficiently by established professional procedures. The voices of children with disabilities are denied a hearing in courtrooms, hospitals and schools. Children with disabilities are physically beaten or restrained into submission too often. Corporal punishment of children with and without disabilities is legally protected in countries all over the world. We suggest that:

Recommendation 1.12:   Reforms in educational, medical and legal systems are essential as long as children with and without disabilities are denied a hearing and as long as there is continued support of corporal punishment in homes, schools and communities all over the world.

***

The Focus of This Book

The following chapters contain the findings of an analysis of the data from the U.S. DHHS, the professional literature and the findings from an analysis of the newspaper coverage in a large circulation newspaper. We get behind the numbers and provide case examples of children with disabilities who were abused and neglected. We provide case examples of their perpetrators and the context of their abuse and neglect. We conclude each chapter with a set of recommendations for research and practice.

The next eight chapters address specific dimensions of what we know about abuse and neglect in the lives of children with disabilities. Chapters 2, 3, and 4 focus specifically on the children and adolescents with disabilities, the forms of their abuse and neglect, the outcomes of this exposure and their prevailing age, gender and disability characteristics. Chapters 5, 6 and 7 focus on the age, gender, and disability characteristics of the perpetrators of the ANCD. Chapters 8 and 9 focus on predicting abuse and neglect in the lives of children with disabilities. More specifically, Chap. 8 focuses on understanding the context in which ANCD happens, Chap. 9 focuses on professionals as perpetrators of ANCD. Chapter 10 concludes this text with a singular focus on prevention. This chapter provides a data based, three dimensional and comprehensive system that focuses the disciplines of education, medicine, and law on the prevention of ANCD. Exercises for reflection and analysis are distributed throughout all the chapters of this text. Finally, each chapter concludes with a set of 12 recommendations for research and practice and a set of references for continued study in this area.

Chapter Summary

We began this chapter with a reflection on the current status of CAN and ANCD in a historical context. We examined major challenges to the accuracy of these data. We discussed the contributions of definition issues, as well as identification and reporting procedures. We discussed what we know based on the national data and we reviewed the professional literature on abuse and neglect in the lives of children with disabilities. We provided a description of the newspaper study and the initial findings of this study. We discussed major organizations that are dedicated to the prevention of abuse and neglect in the lives of children with and without disabilities. We closed this chapter with a set of recommendations for researchers and practitioners.

References

Ammerman, R. T. (1991). The role of the child in physical abuse: A reappraisal. *Violence and Victims, 6*(2), 87–101. Retrieved from http://www.ingentaconnect.com/content/springer/vav/1991/00000006/00000002/art00001

Ammerman, R. T., Van Hasselt, V. B., Hersen, M., McGonigle, J. J., & Lubetsky, M. J. (1989). Abuse and neglect in psychiatrically hospitalized handicapped children. *Abuse & Neglect, 13*(3), 335–343. doi:10.1016/0145-2134(89)90073-2

Billmire, M. E., & Myers, P. A. (1985). Serious head injury in infants: Accident or abuse? *Pediatrics, 75*, 340–342. Retrieved from http://pediatrics.aappublications.org/content/75/2/340.short

Blatt, B., & Kaplan, F. (1966). *Christmas in Purgatory: A photographic essay on mental retardation*. Boston, MA: Allyn & Bacon.

Bogart, L. (1981). *Press and public: Who reads what, when, where and why in American newspapers*. Hillsdale, NJ: Lawrence Erlbaum.

Bones, P. D. C. (2013). Perceptions of vulnerability: A target characteristics approach to disability, gender, and victimization. *Deviant Behavior, 34*(9), 727–750. doi:10.1080/01639625.2013.766511

Carty, H., & Ratcliffe, J. (1995). The shaken infant syndrome. *British Medical Journal, 310*(6976), 344–345. Retrieved from http://www.ncbi.nlm.nih.gov/pmc/articles/PMC2548758/

Child Abuse Prevention and Treatment Act (CAPTA). (2010). (42 U.S.C. §5101 (42 U.S.C. A. §5106 g). Retrieved from http://www.acf.hhs.gov/sites/default/files/cb/capta2010.pdf

ChildHelp. (2014). *National child abuse statistics*. Retrieved from http://www.childhelp.org/pages/statistics

Epstein, E. J. (1981). The selection of reality. In E. Abel (Ed.), *What's news: The media in American society* (pp. 119–132). San Francisco, CA: Institute for Contemporary Studies.

Fallon, B., Trocmé, N., Fluke, J., MacLaurin, B., Tonmyr, L., & Yuan, Y. Y. (2010). Methodological challenges in measuring child maltreatment. *Child Abuse & Neglect, 34*(1), 70–79. doi:10.1016/j.chiabu.2009.08.008

Gore, M. T., & Janssen, K. G. (2007). What educators need to know about abused children with disabilities. *Preventing School Failure, 52*(1), 49–55. doi:10.3200/PSFL.52.1.49-55

Gorman, J. (2012, December 18). Ancient bones that tell a story of compassion. *The New York Times*, p. A1. http://www.nytimes.com/2012/12/18/science/ancient-bones-that-tell-a-story-of-compassion.html?pagewanted=all&_r=1&

Gutowski, C., Sadovi, C., & Jaworski, J. (2011, September 13). Mother charged after boy's death. *Chicago Tribune*. Retrieved from http://articles.chicagotribune.com/2011-09-13/news/ct-met-berwyn-hoarding-charges-0913-2-20110913_1_animal-hoarding-animal-hoarding-exotic-animals

Hallahan, D. P., & Kauffman, J. M. (2003). *Exceptional learners: An introduction to special education* (8th ed.). Boston, MA: Allyn & Bacon.

Hallahan, D. P., Kauffman, J. M., & Pullen, P. C. (2015). *Exceptional learners: An introduction to special education* (13th ed.). Upper Saddle River, NJ: Pearson.

Hershkowitz, I., Lamb, M. E., & Horowitze, D. (2007). Victimization of children with disabilities. *American Journal of Orthopsychiatry, 77*(4), 629–635. doi:10.1037/0002.9432.77.4.629

Hibbard, R. A., & Desch, L. W. (2007). Maltreatment of children with disabilities. *Pediatrics, 119*(5), 1018–1025. doi:10.1542/peds.2011-0323

Individuals with Disabilities Education Improvement Act. (2004). 20 USC 1400. Retrieved from http://nichcy.org/wp-content/uploads/docs/PL108-446.pdf

Jones, L., Bellis, M. A., Wood, S., Hughes, K., McCoy, E., Eckley, L., ... Officer, A. (2012). Prevalence and risk of violence against children with disabilities: A systematic reviewand meta-analysis of observational studies. *Lancet, 380*(9845), 899–907. doi:10.1016/S0140-6736 (12)60692-8

Ju, A., Jeong, S. H., & Chyi, H. I. (2014). Will social media save newspapers? Examining the effectiveness of Facebook and Twitter as news platforms. *Journalism Practice, 8*(1), 1–17. doi:10.1080/17512786.2013.794022

Kanner, L. (1964). *A history of the care and study of the mentally retarded.* Springfield, IL: Charles C. Thomas.

Kelly, L. (1992). The connections between disability and child abuse: A review of the research evidence. *Child Abuse Review, 1*(3), 157–167. doi:10.1002/car.2380010305

Kempe, C. H., Silverman, F. N., Steele, B. F., Droegemueller, W., & Silver, H. K. (1962). The battered-child syndrome. *Journal of the American Medical Association, 181*, 17–24.

Kempe, C. H., Silverman, F. N., Steele, B. F., Droegemueller, W., & Silver, H. K. (1984). The battered-child syndrome. *JAMA, 251*(24), 3288–3294. doi:10.1001/jama.1984. 03340480070033

Leeb, R. T., Bitsko, R. H., Merrick, M. T., & Armour, B. S. (2012). Does childhood disability increase risk for child abuse and neglect? *Journal of Mental Health Research in Intellectual Disabilities, 5*(1), 4–31. doi:10.1080/19315864.2011.608154

McFadden, R. D. (2014). Clyde Snow, a sleuth who read bones from King Tut's to Kennedy's, is dead at 86. *New York Times*, May 16. Retrieved from http://www.nytimes.com/2014/05/17/us/clyde-snow-forensic-detective-who-found-clues-in-bones-dies-at-86.html

McNergney, R. F., Hallahan, D. P., Keller, C. E., & Crowley, E. P. (1992). Improving communication between educational researchers and journalists. In R. F. McNergney (Ed.), *Education research, policy, and the press: Research as news* (pp. 75–87). Boston, MA: Allyn & Bacon.

Reece, R. M., & Sege, R. (2000). Childhood head injuries: Accidental or inflicted? *Achieves of Pediatric and Adolescent Medicine, 154*(1), 11–15. doi:10-1001/pubs

Schulte, H. F. (1983). Mass media as vehicles of education, persuasion, and opinion making in the Western world. In L. J. Martin & A. G. Chaudhary (Eds.), *Comparative mass media systems* (pp. 113–146). White Plains, NY: Longman.

Sobsey, D. (1994). *Violence and abuse in the lives of people with disabilities: The end of silent acceptance?* Baltimore, MD: Brooks.

Sobsey, D. (2002). Exceptionality, education, and maltreatment. *Exceptionality, 10*(1), 29–46. doi:10.1207/S15327035EX1001_3

Sobsey, D., & Varnhagen, C. (1989). Sexual abuse of people with disabilities. In M. Csapo & L. Gougen (Eds.), *Special education across Canada: Challenges for the 90s* (pp. 199–218). Vancouver, The Netherlands: Center for Human Development and Research.

Stalker, K., & McArthur, K. (2012). Child abuse, child protection and disabled children: A review of recent research. *Child Abuse Review, 21*(1), 24–40. doi:10.1002/car.1154

Strum, J. F. (n.d.). *The reality about newspapers.* Retrieved from http://www.naa.org/Newspaper-Ads/Sturm_Open-Letter-Ad.pdf

Sullivan, P. M. (2009). Violence exposure among children with disabilities. *Clinical Child and Family Psychology Review, 12*(2), 196–216. doi:10.1037/0002-9432.77.4.629

Sullivan, P. M., & Knutson, J. F. (1998). The association between child maltreatment in a hospital-based epidemiological study. *Child Abuse & Neglect, 22*(4), 271–278. doi:10.1016/S0145-2134(97)00175-0

Sullivan, P. M., & Knutson, J. F. (2000). Maltreatment and disabilities: A population-based epidemiologic study. *Child Abuse & Neglect, 24*(10), 257–1273. doi:10.1016/S0145-2134(00)00190-3

Taylor, S. J. (1987). Observing abuse: Professional ethics and personal morality in field research. *Qualitative Sociology, 10*(3), 288–302. doi:10.1007/BF00988991

Tilley, L. (2012). The bioarchaeology of care. *The SAA Archaeological Record, 120*(3). http://onlinedigeditions.com/article/The_Bioarchaeology_Of_Care/1078681/113770/article.html

Tilley, L., & Cameron, T. (2014). Introducing the index of care: A web-based application supporting archaeological research into health-related care. *International Journal of Paleopathology, 6,* 5–9. doi:10.1016/j.ijpp.2014.01.003

United States Census. (2010). *2010 census data.* Retrieved from http://www.census.gov/2010census/data/

U.S. Department of Health and Human Services, Administration for Children and Families, Administration on Children, Youth and Families, Children's Bureau. (2013). *Child maltreatment 2012.* Retrieved from http://www.acf.hhs.gov/programs/cb/research-data-technology/statistics-research/child-maltreatment

Verdugo, M. A., Bermejo, B. G., & Fuertes, J. (1995). The maltreatment of intellectually handicapped children and adolescents. *Child Abuse & Neglect, 19*(2), 205–215. doi:10.1016/0145-2134(94)00117-D

Verstraete, P. (2005). The taming of disability: Phrenology and bio-power on the road to destruction of otherness in France (1800–60). *History of Education, 34*(2), 119–134. doi:10.1080/0046760042000338746

Walker, H., & Gresham, F. (2014). *Handbook of evidence-based practices for emotional and behavioral disorders.* New York, NY: Guilford.

Wiseman, F. (1967). *Titicut follies.* Retrieved from http://litmed.med.nyu.edu/Annotation?action=view&annid=13015

Helpful Resources for Further Study

International Child Abuse Network (ICAN). Retrieved from http://www.yesican.org/

International Society for the Prevention of Child Abuse and Neglect (ISPCAN). Retrieved from http://www.ispcan.org/

Prevent Child Abuse America (PCAA). Retrieved from http://www.preventchildabuse.org/

U.S. Department of Health and Human Services Administration for Children and Families Administration on Children, Youth and Families Children's Bureau. *Child abuse and neglect fatalities 2009: Statistics and interventions.* Retrieved from http://www.childwelfare.gov/pubs/factsheets/fatality.pdf

U.S. Department of Health and Human Services, Administration for Children and Families, Administration on Children, Youth and Families, Children's Bureau. (2011). *Child maltreatment 2010.* Retrieved from http://www.acf.hhs.gov/programs/cb/stats_research/index.htm#can

U. S. Government Accountability Office. (2011). *Child maltreatment: Strengthening national data on child fatalities could aid in prevention (GAO-11-599).* Retrieved from http://www.gao.gov/new.items/d11599.pdf

Disability Definitions

Illinois definition of child abuse and neglect. http://www.ilga.gov/legislation/ilcs/ilcs3.asp?ActID=1460&ChapterID=32

Individuals with Disabilities Education Improvement Act. (2004). 20 USC 1400. Retrieved from http://nichcy.org/wp-content/uploads/docs/PL108-446.pdf

Texas definition of child abuse and neglect. https://www.oag.state.tx.us/ag_publications/txts/childabuse1.shtml

Vermont definition of child abuse and neglect. http://dcf.vermont.gov/taxonomy/term/283/0

Virginia's definition of child abuse and neglect. http://www.dss.virginia.gov/files/division/dfs/cps/intro_page/manuals/07-2011/section_2_definitions_of_abuse_and_neglect.pdf

Chapter 2
Age, Sex, Disability, and Other Characteristics of Children with Disabilities Who Are Abused and Neglected

I have a dream that my four little children will one day live in a nation where they will not be judged . . . (Martin Luther King, Jr., American Activist, 1929–1968)

Abstract People who know the demographic trends among children with disabilities who are abused and neglected are poised to develop more effective intervention and prevention programming. In this chapter we examine the U.S. DHHS data on the age, sex, and disability characteristics of children with disabilities who are abused and neglected. We analyze the related peer reviewed literature in this area. We present the data from our analysis of the newspaper coverage of abuse and neglect of children with disabilities (ANCD). We get behind the numbers and provide stories from the newspaper coverage which illustrate the prevailing demographics of children with disabilities who are abused and neglected. We conclude this chapter with a set of recommendations for researchers and practitioners.

Demographics matter. The age, sex, and other characteristics such as race and ethnicity of children with disabilities determine a great deal about their life experiences. Are some children with specific disability characteristics particularly vulnerable to abuse and neglect? Are they particularly susceptible to specific kinds of abuse or neglect? What are the characteristics of children with disabilities who are most vulnerable to abuse and neglect? Are boys with disabilities more susceptible to specific kinds of abuse and neglect than girls with disabilities? What demographic characteristics increase the vulnerability of children with disabilities to abuse and neglect? Do we observe trends in ethnicity and socioeconomic status among children with disabilities who are abused and neglected?

Exercise 2.1: Critical Thinking

Select a question from above that is most important to you? *Given what you know at this point, hypothesize what you expect to be true.*

Targeted and creative programming in child abuse prevention and intervention for children with disabilities requires data based decision-making. The more we know about children with disabilities who are abused and neglected, the greater the

© Springer International Publishing Switzerland 2016

E.P. Crowley, *Preventing Abuse and Neglect in the Lives of Children with Disabilities*, DOI 10.1007/978-3-319-30442-7_2

probability of developing focused and effective abuse and neglect prevention and intervention programs. The more we know about the children with disabilities who are at-risk for abuse and neglect, the better chance we have of focusing, more sensibly, the insufficient staff and resources we assign to abuse and neglect intervention and prevention programming. In the end, with reliable data and a clearer understanding of the abuse and neglect potential of some children with disabilities, the higher the chance we have of preventing their maltreatment from occurring in the first place. Furthermore, we must do all we can to stop its repetition, over and over again, among some children with disabilities.

In this chapter we will focus on what we know about children with disabilities who are abused and neglected. What are their prevailing characteristics? We will analyze the data on the age, sex, and disability characteristics of children with disabilities and determine whether and how these characteristics increase the abuse and neglect potential of children with disabilities. How old are these children? Are there predictable patterns based on their age characteristics? We will make observations about what professionals can learn in order to recognize child abuse and neglect (CAN) potential based on identified age, sex, and disability characteristics. We will begin with a brief discussion of mandated reporters and the most recent data from the U.S. DHHS (2013). We will then analyze the literature on the demographics of children with disabilities who are abused and neglected. We will present the findings from the study of the *Chicago Tribune* newspaper coverage over a 10-year span and end this chapter by getting behind the numbers to observe the lives of the children with disabilities who have been abused and neglected.

Mandated Reporters of the Abuse and Neglect of Children with Disabilities

Mandated reporters are those who have frequent contact with children with disabilities.

They commonly include social workers, teachers, principals, and other school personnel. Medical staff, such as physicians, nurses, and other health-care workers, counselors, therapists, and other mental health professionals, are commonly designated mandated reporters. Child care providers, medical examiners or coroners and law enforcement officers are typical mandated reporters.

In the United States some states designate mandated reporters and these include individuals involved in commercial film and photograph processing, computer technicians, and volunteers at organized activities for children including camps, day camps, youth centers, and recreation centers. Domestic violence workers, animal control or humane officers, court-appointed special advocates, and members of the clergy are also among mandated reporters in some states. Finally, in some states faculty, administrators, athletics staff, and other employees and volunteers at institutions of higher learning, including public and private colleges and universities and vocational and technical schools are on the list of mandated reporters.

If a mandated reporter suspects that a child with a disability is abused and neglected they have a legal obligation to report their observations. "Approximately 48 states, the District of Columbia, American Samoa, Guam, the Northern Mariana Islands, Puerto Rico, and the Virgin Islands designate professions whose members are mandated by law to report child maltreatment" (Child Welfare Information Gateway, 2014).

Data on the Maltreatment of Children with Disabilities in the United States

The 23rd *Child Maltreatment* report (U.S. DHHS, 2013) provides the most recent data on the disability category designation of children with disabilities who were abused and neglected in the United States and the District of Columbia. These data clearly underestimate the extent to which these children are abused and neglected for reasons we discussed in Chap. 1. In addition to these reasons, this U.S. DHHS report provides statistics from only 39 states (78.0 %), the District of Columbia and Puerto Rico. Even then, there is a 2.1 % increase in the number of children with disabilities who were abused and neglected in the United States from 2011 to 2012. In 2011, 11.2 % of children with disabilities were abused and neglected and in 2012 this increased to 13.3 %.

Exercise 2.2: Reflection
Personnel in Alabama, Colorado, Idaho, Iowa, Louisiana, Michigan, New York, North Carolina, North Dakota, Pennsylvania, and Virginia did not provide data on the number of children with disabilities who have been abused and neglected in their states in 2012. *If personnel in these states had reported their numbers, do you expect that a different outcome would be observed in the prevailing trends in these data? Provide a rationale for your response.*

Age and Sex Characteristics of Children with Disabilities Who Are Abused and Neglected

At this time the U.S. DHHS (2013) provide data on overall age and sex characteristics of children who are abused and neglected in the United States. They do not provide specific data on the age and gender characteristics of children with disabilities who are abused and neglected. This is a loss for professionals who want to know how to target prevention and intervention programming in the area of the ANCD. We cannot assume that the data on overall abuse and neglect trends in the areas of age and sex characteristics are the same for all children, including those with disabilities.

Table 2.1 The age of children who were abused and neglected in the United States in 2012

Age in years	# of children	% of children
<1	86,747	12.8
1	47,277	7.0
2	47,469	7.0
3	46,465	6.8
4-10	264,681	38.9
11-15	143,748	21.2
16-21	42,423	6.2
Total	678,810	100

Data from the U.S. DHHS (2013)

Table 2.2 The sex of child victims in the United States in 2012

Sex	# of children	% of children
Boys	330,620	48.7
Girls	345,823	50.9
Unknown	2,367	0.3
Total	678,810	100.0

Data from the U.S. DHHS (2013)

What Do We Know?

The U.S. DHHS (2013) indicate that very young children are most vulnerable to CAN (see Table 2.1). Among these children 12.8 % were under 1 year old and 33.6 % were 3 years and younger. Children from birth to 11 months old accounted for 44.4 % of child fatality resulting from CAN. Based on the prevailing evidence which we reported in Chap. 1, we can expect that children with disabilities are disproportionately represented among these children.

Girls are abused and neglected more frequently than boys (see Table 2.2). The U.S. DHHS does not report both the age and sex of children with disabilities who are abused and neglected. We do not know whether girls with disabilities are more or less vulnerable to abuse and neglect when they are young or whether these statistics change as girls grow older. We do know, in general, that girls are more vulnerable to abuse and neglect. We may wonder whether boys and girls with disabilities are more vulnerable to different types of abuse and neglect. Who is most likely to be neglected? Who is most vulnerable to sexual abuse? Who is more vulnerable to physical abuse? These and many more questions linger.

Do Disability Characteristics Matter Among Children with Disabilities?

The U.S. DHHS (2013) reported on the ANCD in only seven disability characteristics namely, behavior problem, emotionally disturbed, learning disability, mental

Table 2.3 U.S. DHHS (2013) categories

Behavior problem
Emotional disturbance
Learning disability
Intellectual disability
Other medical condition
Physically disabled
Visually or hearing impaired

Table 2.4 Disability categories IDEA (2004)

Autism	Multiple disabilities
Deaf-blindness	Orthopedic impairment
Deafness	Other health impairment
Developmental delay	Specific learning disability
Emotional disturbance	Speech and language impairment
Hearing impairment	Traumatic brain injury
Intellectual disability	Visual impairment, including blindness

retardation, other medical condition, physically disabled, and visually or hearing impaired (see Table 2.3). Questions arise immediately. In what group do we find children with autism? Where are the data on children who have attention deficit disorder (ADD) and attention deficit hyperactivity disorder (ADHD)? These data count children with visual disabilities, blindness, hearing impairments, and deafness all in one group.

The U.S. DHHS reports the maltreatment of children with "behavior problems" and "emotionally disturbed" separately. IDEA defines students with "emotional and behavior problems" as a single category. Though they are not counted separately in the 2013 *Child Maltreatment* report, in the United States Individuals with Disabilities Education Act (2004) children with autism, deaf-blindness, and deafness, multiple disabilities, speech or language impairment, traumatic brain injury and blindness have legally mandated educational rights.

At this time the abuse and neglect of some children with these disabilities is not reported in a manner that represents their separate categorical designation in IDEA (see Table 2.4). Though the disabilities of these children are not distinguished separately, it is probable that the broad categories used by U.S. DHHS include them. For example, based on these data, we do not know how many children with autism are abused and neglected, though we may expect that they are counted among those designated as "behavior problem" or "emotional disturbance". Examine Tables 2.3 and 2.4 for a comparison of the disability categories of IDEA (2004) and U.S. DHHS (2013). May we anticipate consistency among definitions of disability and reporting procedures across federal agencies? Who among us cares sufficiently that we identify accurately children with disabilities who are at-risk for abuse and neglect?

Table 2.5 Victims of abuse and neglect with a reported disability in 2012

Disability category	Total victims 2011	Total victims 2012	% of Total victims 2011	% of Total victims 2012
Other medical condition	3.8	4.3	33.9	32.3
Behavior problem	2.6	3.2	23.2	24.0
Emotional disturbance	2.1	2.5	18.8	18.8
Learning disability	1.0	1.1	8.9	8.3
Visually or hearing impaired	0.7	1.0	6.3	7.5
Physically disabled	0.6	0.7	5.4	5.3
Intellectual disability	0.4	0.5	3.6	3.8
Total disabilities	11.2	13.3	100.1	100

Data from the U.S. DHHS (2013)

To make this matter even more complicated, in the United States, the assigned reporting personnel voluntarily report child disability category assignment. This information is not required of reporters to the National Child Abuse and Neglect Data System (NCANDS) and at this time, these reporters provide the data for the annual *Child Maltreatment* reports of U.S. DHHS. The issues go on. Children with disabilities are often diagnosed with disabilities in more than one category. One child may have both a learning disability *and* a behavioral disorder. Based on the data from 2012 (U.S. DHHS, 2013), most children with disabilities who are abused and neglected were assigned to the other medical condition category. Of the 13.3 % children with disabilities who were abused and neglected in 2012, a total of 4.3 % were assigned to the other medical condition category – an increase from 3.8 % in 2011. In 2012, this category accounted for 32.3 % of the total children with disabilities who were abused and neglected (see Table 2.5).

Exercise 2.3: Critical Thinking
Are you surprised to find that children with other medical conditions are those who are most frequently reported as abused and neglected? Who might be the children in this category? What medical conditions would you expect to observe? Which type of abuse and neglect would you expect these children to be exposed to most frequently?

The search for patterns requires us to examine these data closely. The U.S. DHHS (2013) data indicate that children with behavioral problems and those designated with emotional disturbance are the second and third largest groups of children with disabilities reported to have been abused and neglected. Of the 13.3 % of children with disabilities who were reported to have been abused and neglected, a combined total of 42.8 % were identified with either behavior problems or as emotionally disturbed. Together children diagnosed with behavior problems

(23.7 %), emotionally disturbed (18.7 %) and with other health impartments (32.6 %) account for 75.0 % of all children with disabilities who are abused and neglected.

To some professionals there is very little difference between the children who have behavior problems and those who are emotionally disturbed. A plethora of disorders are represented in these categories and reliable differentiation between them is often not possible (Walker & Gresham, 2013). For example, both children with behavior problems and those who are emotionally disturbed might internalize or externalize conflict and pain. Children in either category might exhibit behaviors that are characterized either by aggression or depression. They might act-in or act-out. They might have anxiety, attention deficit disorders, posttraumatic stress disorder, or they might have fears or phobias. They might have autism and additionally they might have communication disorders. Because so many different disabling conditions of childhood are all reduced to these seven categories, it is tempting to discredit this report (see Table 2.4). Despite the limitations of these data, from them we learn about the prevailing disability characteristics among children with disabilities who are abused and neglected. We may conclude that among children with disabilities, those who have been diagnosed with medical conditions, behavior problems, and those who are designated as emotionally disturbed are at increased risk for CAN.

Exercise 2.4: Reflection

The *Maltreatment Report* (2013) includes a separate data set that describes the disability categories relative to children who were abused and neglected in the United States during 2012. Beyond these data, we know few specifics. *What additional data would you like to see in the annual report on child maltreatment?*

The Literature on Abuse and Neglect and Age, Sex, Child Disability, and Other Characteristics

Among adults and children with disabilities, demographics matter. Bones (2013) found that males and females with disabilities are subjected to victimization by perpetrators of abuse and neglect differently. Males with disabilities are protected from abuse and neglect by dominant cultural stereotypes. Bones found that the perceived physical strength and autonomy of adult males with disabilities acts as a protective factor. Furthermore, these data indicate that females with disabilities appear to be especially vulnerable to victimization. We may further conclude that the dominant cultural stereotypes of women set them up for sexual victimization. In the following sections we will examine the role of age, sex, and disability characteristics as potential indicators for the ANCD.

Age and Child Abuse Potential

To what extent does the age of a child with a disability dispose them as potential targets of CAN? Do you predict that young children with disabilities are at serious risk of being abused and neglected? Is it possible that age acts as a protective factor, in that, when children with disabilities grow older they can more readily escape potential perpetrators of their abuse and neglect? When they act as self-advocates, do they solicit the care and protection of responsible adults?

Age matters among children with disabilities. Researchers over the years consistently observe that youngest children with disabilities, especially those under the age of 1 year are at the highest abuse and neglect potential (Douglas & Mohn, 2014; Esernio-Jenssen, Tai, & Kodsi, 2011; McLeod, Uemura, & Rohrman, 2012; Sobsey, Randall, & Parrila, 1997). Sobsey and his colleagues found that boys with disabilities up to the age of 12 years old are physically abused more often than girls with disabilities. Based on their findings, these data change as girls grow older. Girls between the ages of 12 and 17 were physically abused more frequently than were males with disabilities. Adolescents with disabilities are more vulnerable to online victimization than their nondisabled peers (Wells & Mitchell, 2013).

Girls between 1 and 5 years old and adolescent girls between 12 and 17 years old were more frequently sexually abused than were their male counterparts. Boys ages 6–11 were sexually abused more frequently than were their female counterparts. Boys with disabilities from 1 to 17 years were neglected more frequently than were girls with disabilities. Sobsey and his colleagues found that boys with disabilities between the ages 6 and 11 were more frequently emotionally abused than were girls with disabilities of the same age. However, they found no differences in the emotional abuse of younger and older boys and girls with disabilities. Boys with disabilities between the ages of 1 and 11 were more frequently subjected to abuse of all kinds than were girls with disabilities. Finally, perhaps not surprisingly, girls with disabilities between 12 and 17 years of age were more frequently subjected to physical abuse and sexual abuse than were their male counterparts with disabilities.

The Webster dictionary defines filicide first as "the act of murdering one's child" and second as "a parent who does this". In a study by Coorg and Tournay (2013), 22 children with disabilities who died as a result of filicide were prevailingly males between the ages of 10 and 14 years (45.4 %) and females between the ages of 3 and 17 years (18.1 %). The next largest was a group of males from birth – 9 years (36.3 %). Four children with disabilities who died as a result of filicide (18.1 %) were between 15 and 18 years of age. These findings are consistent with the observations of Soylu and his colleagues (2013) relative to the level and severity of abuse to which males and females with disabilities are subjected, and they are consistent with the observations of Bones (2013) relative to the stereotypic physical strength of males with disabilities that acts as a protective factor.

Sex and Child Abuse Potential

Gender matters. Data indicate that there are differences in the ways that girls and boys with disabilities are abused and neglected (Balogh et al., 2001; Banks, 2014; Coorg & Tournay, 2013; Firth et al., 2001; Mueller-Johnson, Eisner, & Obsuth, 2014; Nalavany, Ryan, & Hinterlong, 2009; Sobsey et al., 1997). Years ago now, Sobsey and his colleagues observed that boys with disabilities are at increased risk for physical abuse and neglect while girls are at increased risk for sexual abuse and emotional abuse. More recent studies indicate that males with disabilities are subjected to harsher and more dangerous forms of abuse and neglect and they are at increased risk of death following abuse and neglect. Coorg and Tournay (2013) found that the deaths of boys with disabilities (81.8 %) outnumbered the deaths of girls with disabilities (18.1 %). Most frequently gunshot wounds (40.9 %) were the cause of the deaths of these children. Males with disabilities died (88.8 %) as a result of gunshot wounds more frequently than did females (11.1 %) with disabilities.

Both boys and girls with disabilities are subjected to sexual abuse and prevailingly females with disabilities are the most frequent targets (Hershkowitz, Lamb, & Horowitz, 2007; Sobsey et al., 1997; Soylu, Alpaslan, Ayaz, Esenyel, & Oruc, 2013). Soylu et al. (2013) found that among 102 children from 6 to 16 years old (33 males and 69 females) with disabilities who had been sexually abused, 67.6 % were females and 32.4 % were males. Comparatively males and females with intellectual disabilities were exposed to more frequent and more severe forms of sexual abuse than were their nondisabled peers. For example, males and females with intellectual disabilities experienced vaginal, anal, and oral penetration (69.6 %) more frequently than their peers without disabilities (35.7 %). Pregnancy emerged more frequently among sexually abused females with intellectual disabilities (6.9 %) than among their nondisabled peers (0.6 %).

Child Disability Characteristics and Abuse and Neglect Potential

Leeb, Bitsko, Merrick, and Armour (2012) analyzed research on the increased risk potential of children with disabilities for abuse and neglect. Leeb and colleagues observed that much research remains to be done in order to establish this link unequivocally. However, though punctuated with inherent methodological challenges, in study after study, across disciplines and over time, data indicate that childhood disability characteristics predisposes them for increased risk of abuse and neglect and conversely abuse and neglect predispose children for increased risk of disability. In this section, we discuss what the literature tells us about childhood disability characteristics that dispose children to be at heightened risk for abuse and neglect. We will address such questions as, does child disability category assignment increase the abuse and neglect potential of children with disabilities?

Researchers observe over and over again and through the years – children across all disability categories are abused and neglected more than their nondisabled peers. Based on available data we may conclude that children with disabilities are abused and neglected five to seven times more than their nondisabled peers (Akbas et al., 2009; Alriksson-Schmidt, Armour, & Thibadeau, 2010; Banks, 2014; Douglas & Mohn, 2014; Knutson, Johnson, & Sullivan 2004; Kvam, 2004; Kvam, 2000; Soylu, Alpaslan, Ayaz, Esenyel, & Oruc, 2013; Spencer et al., 2005; Stalker & McArthur, 2012; Sullivan, 2009; Sullivan & Knutson, 2000a; 2000b; Ulloa Flores & Navarro Machuca, 2011).

The abuse and neglect of children with intellectual disabilities, manifested in physical, sexual, emotional abuse as well as neglect have long been the focus of many researchers (Blatt & Kaplan, 1966; Sobsey et al., 1997; Soylu et al., 2013; Vig & Kaminer, 2002). Soylu et al. compared the sexual abuse of children with intellectual disabilities and their nondisabled peers and found differences in the type and severity of the sexual abuse experienced by these children. For example, more intrusive forms of sexual abuse, including vaginal and anal penetration occurred among children with intellectual disabilities (64.7 %) than occurred among their peers without disabilities (35.1 %). Among children with intellectual disabilities, abuse disclosures occurred less often (25.4 %) than for their peers without disabilities (57.8 %). Furthermore, accidental witness occurred more frequently among children with intellectual disabilities (34.3 %) than among their peers without disabilities (22.1 %), and child abduction of sexually abused children with intellectual disabilities (16.7 %) occurred more often than among their peers without disabilities (11.7 %).

Prevailingly among their peers with disabilities and across the disciplines of social work, psychology, sociology, medicine, among others, children with emotional and behavioral disorders as well as those with communication disorders are most frequently and consistently the group of children who are associated with abuse and neglect. Govindshenoy and Spencer (2006) found that children with conduct disorders and learning disabilities were most strongly associated with all forms of abuse and neglect. Furthermore, these researchers found that children with speech and language disorders were associated with abuse and neglect more frequently, and they were less frequently exposed to sexual abuse.

From April 2004 to June 2010 McDonald, Milne, Knight, and Webster (2013) studied the disability characteristics of children, ranging in age from 14 months to 55.3 months. These children had been abused and neglected and placed in a preschool for young children in protective custody. These children were 55 % male and 45 % female – 91 % of these children had significant behavioral problems. A global developmental delay was observed in 38 % of these young children and girls were more likely (p = .03) to receive this diagnosis. Emotional and behavioral disorders were observed in 85 % of the children and internalizing behaviors were more common than externalizing behaviors. Among these young children, four were diagnosed with autism.

Children with emotional and behavioral disorders and those with communication disorders exhibit varied disabilities such as depression, anxiety, antisocial disorders, psychosis, autism, as well as deafness, speech and language disorders, and more. According to Flores and Machuca (2011) children with ADHD and children with conduct disorders are most frequently abused and neglected. Children with externalizing disorders include those who exhibit aggression toward people, animals, and property and these children are most frequently physically abused. Internalizing disorders in childhood are reflected in such behaviors as depression, disabling fears, phobias, anxieties, as well as socially withdrawn behaviors – even to the point of social isolation.

Khalifeh, Howard, Osborn, Moran and Johnson (2013) examined the violence perpetrated against 16-year-olds and older with disabilities. They found that those who had a long-term mental illness and physical disabilities experienced violence and victimization more frequently than those with nonmental disabilities and those without disabilities. Khalifeh et al. also found that those with mental illness experienced violence three times more than their nondisabled peers, and two times more than their peers with disabilities who were not associated with mental illness. These findings are consistent with the literature that individuals with emotional and behavioral disorders are most vulnerable to violent abuse and neglect.

Kvam (2000; 2004) and Sebald (2008) found that children with behavioral disorders and communication disorders are most frequently abused and neglected, children with learning disabilities, sensory impairments and concentration problems are also at-risk for physical abuse and children who are deaf are at increased risk for sexual abuse.

The study of disability characteristics relative to the abuse and neglect of children with physical disabilities offers unique challenges to researchers and clinicians (Govindshenoy & Spencer, 2006). Children with physical disabilities are at increased risk of physical injury and additional disabilities due to poor coordination and balance. In a study designed to differentiate the bruising frequency and patterns among children with and without disabilities, Goldberg et al. (2009) found that children with physical disabilities have increased bruising frequency as well as different bruising patterns than their nondisabled peers. Children with physical disabilities 10 years and older exhibit increased bruising in the back (lumbar region) and abdomen/pelvis areas, more typically protected areas among their peers without disabilities. Goldberg and her colleagues found that for children with physical disabilities, orthotics were not associated with bruising and instead they served as protective devices. These researchers caution caregivers to be alert to bruising on the neck, ears, chin, anterior chest, or buttocks areas as well as to unusual and unexplainable bruising frequency and patterns which may indicate abuse and neglect of children with physical disabilities.

Benedict, White, Wulff, and Hall (1990) studied the maltreatment reports of 53 children with multiple disabilities, including profound intellectual disabilities, cerebral palsy or other physical disabilities, seizure disorders, severe vision and hearing disabilities and found that 67.6 % were the targets of physical abuse;

including cuts, bruises, welts (29.4 %); skull and bone fractures (23.5 %); burns and scalds (14.7 %) and sexual abuse (8.8 %). Benedict et al. found neglect among 100 % of these children and this was manifested by lack of supervision (21.1 %); medical neglect (21.1 %); inadequate housing (15.8 %); hygiene neglect (15.8 %); and other neglect (26.3 %).

In summary, data from the professional literature indicate that child demographics matter. Child gender, age and disability category assignment differentially dispose children with disabilities to increased risk for different types and levels of severity of abuse and neglect. They are exposed to all types of abuse and neglect more frequently than are their nondisabled peers. Boys with disabilities are more frequently exposed to all types of abuse and neglect than are females with disabilities. Adolescent females with disabilities are at increased risk of physical abuse, and sexual abuse. Overall, males with disabilities between 10 and 15 years tend to be abused and neglected more frequently than their younger and older counterparts. Among children with disabilities across all disability categories, those with emotional and behavioral disorders as well as those with intellectual disabilities seem to be the most frequently and most severely abused and neglected children.

Newspaper Coverage of the Disability Characteristics of Children with Disabilities Who Are Abused and Neglected

The Age and Sex Characteristics

Age matters. Children with disabilities across the age span from birth to 18 are uniquely vulnerable to abuse and neglect. Data indicate, prevailingly, that children under the age of 1 year and those with disabilities are uniquely vulnerable and their abuse and neglect. This group of children accounted for over 7.3 % of the newspaper coverage. Stories of ANCD at every age appeared in the newspaper coverage and they did not lessen significantly as the children grew older (see Table 2.6). Children between 4 and 15 years old were the focus of 63.3 % of the stories about the ANCD. Gender matters too. A content analysis of the newspaper coverage indicates that most stories focused on males with disabilities. This finding holds whether the newspaper story described the abuse and neglect of a single child with a disability, or whether the story covered two, three, four or more children (see Table 2.7). Males from birth to 18 years were represented in 57.7 % stories and females were represented in 42.3 % of the stories. When stories focused on only one child, 55.0 % were males and 45.0 % were females. The newspaper coverage also included stories of large groups of children including, 5, 11, 29 and more children and included no male and female designation. When gender was known, males with disabilities were consistently more frequently represented among children with disabilities who were abused and neglected than were females with disabilities.

Table 2.6 Age characteristics of children with disabilities abused and neglected (n = 108 stories[a])

Age in years	# of children	%
<1 year	8	7.3
1–3	13	12.0
4–10	25	23.0
11–15	44	40.3
16–18	18	17.4
Total	109	100.0 %

[a]Potentially more than one child per story
Data from a study of the newspaper coverage in the *Chicago Tribune*

Table 2.7 Gender characteristics by story and number of children involved (n = 108 stories[a])

# of children	Number of stories	% Male	% Female
A single child	77	55.0	45.0
Two children	19	54.5	45.5
Three children	9	54.5	45.5
Four children	3	66.8	33.3

[a]Potentially more than one child per story
Data from a study of the newspaper coverage in the *Chicago Tribune*

Disability Characteristics

To what extent does newspaper coverage reflect the findings in the national databases and in the professional literature on the prevailing characteristics of children with disabilities who are abused and neglected? Newspaper stories prevailingly report the abuse and neglect of children with emotional and behavior disorders, children with multiple disabilities, and those with other health impairments (See Table 2.8). Together these three groups of children accounted for 62.8 % of all the stories about the abuse and neglect of children with disabilities which were published in the *Chicago Tribune* over the 10-year period, 2004–2013. The disabilities of the children were unspecified in 9.6 % of the stories. In these stories reporters referred to children with disabilities as those who have special needs, disabilities or receive who receive special education services.

Consistent with the data in the *Child Maltreatment* (U.S. DHHS, 2013) report, the data on the newspaper coverage indicates that stories about the abuse and neglect of children with emotional and behavioral disorders top the list. This is also consistent with the data in the professional literature that we have already discussed in this chapter.

Other stories about children with disabilities who were abused and neglected spanned the IDEA categories of autism, deaf-blindness, deafness or hearing impairment, emotional disturbance, intellectual disability, multiple disabilities, orthopedic impairment, other health impairment, and specific learning disability. Though not a separate category in IDEA, two stories focused on the emotional abuse of

Table 2.8 Known disability of child victim (n = 94)

Disability	# of children	%
Emotional disturbance/Behavior disorder	31	33.0
Multiple disabilities	15	16.0
Other health impaired	13	13.8
Unspecified (special education student, disability, etc.)	9	9.6
Intellectual disability	8	8.5
Autism	7	7.4
Orthopedic impairment	5	5.3
Deaf-blindness	3	3.2
Gifted	2	2.1

Data from a study of the newspaper coverage in the *Chicago Tribune*

children who were gifted. Most surprisingly however, no newspaper coverage of children with disabilities who were abused and neglected focused specifically on children with speech and language impairment.

Beyond the Numbers: Stories of Real Children Exhibit the Evidence – Age, Gender, and Disability Characteristics

David Jackson (2008, July 17) described a 15-year-old who "repeatedly raped his 12-year-old roommate at Illinois' largest psychiatric hospital." Stacey, mother of the 15-year-old brought him to "Riveredge seeking treatment for his sexual aggression. He had been molested by a man and begun acting out wildly … In police reports and [in] a Tribune interview, Stacey said she repeatedly warned Riveredge not to house her son with another child." Despite this mother's request, sexual abuse ensued and "the abuse ended when a Riveredge worker interrupted an attack … and the 12-year-old was treated for injuries and trauma at Loyola University Medical Center." Jackson added that "Stacey's son, who according to a police report is bipolar, was adjudicated for sexual assault in juvenile court … now is housed in a Downstate facility that treats adolescent sex offenders."

Exercise 2.5: Reflection
Read the complete story referenced at the end of this chapter by Jackson (2008), "A mother mourns 2 lost futures." *What is your analysis of what happened? What does this story tell you about the age, gender, and disability characteristics of children with disabilities who are abused and neglected? Are you surprised by any aspect of this story? Was the abuse predictable? Was it preventable? What might have caused the staff to ignore Stacey's request? What good, bad, and indifferent consequences might result from this story in the Chicago Tribune on July 17, 2008?*

On March 24, 2004, *Chicago Tribune* reporter, Rachel Osterman, described the sexual abuse of a 9-year-old girl who had diagnosed learning disabilities and attention deficit hyperactivity disorder who attended Bartlett Elementary School in Bartlett, Illinois. In court this child testified that Mr. Kevin Kilgallen, her 36-year-old male teacher sexually abused her by repeatedly luring her out of the Safe School after-school program and into his classroom in exchange for candy both before and after school.

When testifying in court she barely raised her voice above a whisper and stated that in the classroom after school her teacher would put a towel on her eyes, whispered sexual innuendos and told her to participate in sexual acts. On the same day a second 10-year-old girl testified in court and stated that she was sexually abused by the same teacher.

The evidence provided by children with disabilities is often disregarded. Disability becomes a centerpiece for determining the outcomes of stories like these. For example, in his opening remarks in the courtroom that day, Mr. Kilgallen's attorney stated that the accusations against his client were misleading and he "tried to poke holes in the witnesses' (two girls) testimony, suggesting said that the girl's learning disabilities –attention deficit-hyperactivity disorder – inclined her 'to act out' and that the mother and Levan (child's interviewer at the Children's Advocacy Center) had only second-hand knowledge of the alleged incidents" (Osterman, 2004).

At the outset Mr. Kilgallen denied the charges but resigned from his teaching responsibilities at the school. He was charged with one count of aggravated criminal sexual abuse and predatory criminal sexual assault and one count of aggravated criminal sexual assault. In this case, initially the teacher faced 50 years in prison according to Illinois Criminal Code. Following a jury trial, though still claiming innocence, he was convicted and he is currently serving a 30-year prison sentence for predatory criminal sexual assault and aggravated criminal sexual abuse (Reeder, 2007).

Exercise 2.6: Reflection

Mr. Kilgallen, the teacher who sexually abused a 9-year-old girl with learning disabilities and attention deficit hyperactivity disorder discredited the girls' testimony. Read the complete story by Scott Reeder. *How do you feel? Did you know things like this happen? Why? Are you surprised by any part of this story? Does it propel you to action in any way?*

Implications for Research and Practice

In this chapter we focused on the age, sex, and disability characteristics of children with disabilities who are abused and neglected. How old are these children? Are they boys or girls? What do we know about the extent to which boys with disabilities are abused and neglected? Are girls and boys with disabilities abused and neglected differently? Do specific disability characteristics predispose boys and girls with disabilities to be more vulnerable to abuse and neglect?

Awareness of prevailing trends in these data is essential for caregivers, professionals and related personnel who work with children with disabilities. Here we provide a set of recommendations to guide the work of researchers and practitioners. These recommendations focus on the need for continued research on the characteristics of children with disabilities who are abused and neglected, the needs of families and children with disabilities, and the need for school-based programs that promote the health and safety of children with and without disabilities.

Research on the Characteristics of Children with Disabilities who are Abused and Neglected

Continued clarification on the characteristics of children with disabilities who are abused and neglected is essential. Data from the U.S. DHHS consistently indicate that children with emotional and behavioral disorders constitute the highest percentage of children who are exposed to trauma during childhood. Children with emotional and behavioral disorders constitute a diverse group of children. Some of them have autism. Others have ADHD. Some of these children have learning disabilities. Focused research projects would clarify the characteristics of children with emotional and behavioral disorders who are most vulnerable to abuse and neglect.

Increased clarity about the age, gender, and disability characteristics of children who are most susceptible to different forms of abuse and neglect will provide for more focused research and more enlightened clinical practice. We will not stop the abuse and neglect of children with disabilities until we:

Recommendation 2.1: Generate data in order to clarify more precisely the characteristics of the children with disabilities who are vulnerable to abuse and neglect.

***

At this time the U.S. DHHS does not disaggregate children with disabilities who are abused and neglected according to age, sex, or disability characteristics other than those included in seven categories. The data provided by U.S. DHHS do not provide specifics on the ages of the children with disabilities who are abused and neglected. Neither do we know whether these children are boys or girls. The data from the U.S. DHHS fail to reflect the number of children with such commonly diagnosed disabilities as autism and attention deficit disorders. We may only assume that these children are included among those with emotional and behavioral disorders or perhaps among those diagnosed with other health impairments. Therefore we must:

Recommendation 2.2: Develop targeted and interdisciplinary research projects in order to identify the prevailing trends in child disability characteristics that increase their vulnerability to abuse and neglect.

***

How can we increase public awareness of the variables that contribute to disability prevention in the first place? How can preparenting adults be educated to engage in behaviors that reduce the potential for disability among young children? To what extent are people in the general public aware of the steps they can take to lessen the risk of disability in childhood? For example, programs that warn women about the dangers of using alcohol and cigarettes during pregnancy encourage them to avoid the neglectful behaviors that cause disability in childhood. Exposure to toxins in the environment, poor prenatal medical attention, and poor prenatal nutrition dispose pregnant women to have babies with disabilities. How can we get the word out on these facts as well as effect behavior change? Information about disability prevention in babies and very young children must be provided to parents, young adults who are planning to become parents, educators, members of the medical and law enforcement communities, extended family members, neighbors, service providers across disciplines, members of the clergy, among others. We must work to find the most effective ways to:

Recommendation 2.3: Disseminate research findings about disability prevention among babies and very young children while using multiple media, multiple audiences, and across multiple disciplines.

***

Future professionals in the area of medicine, law, education, social services, and related areas will be well served by an awareness of the nexus of abuse, neglect and disability in childhood. They need to be able to answer questions like, what are the characteristic of childhood autism? What ways do children with autism need specialized care and education? What disability characteristics differentiate the 13 categories of disability in childhood included in IDEA? General knowledge and realistic expectations of children with disabilities will protect both children and their adult caregivers. Professionals who understand the effects of a variety of disabilities in childhood will be able to articulate the unique needs of the children in their care. We propose that professional preparation programs:

Recommendation 2.4: Integrate the data that illustrate the nexus of abuse and neglect and childhood disability and consider the implications of these data in professional decision-making.

***

Focus on the Needs of Parents and Caregivers

Children with disabilities who are under the age of four are the most vulnerable of all children to abuse and neglect in its most severe forms. CAN fatality rates due to abuse and neglect are highest in this particular age group. We provide details from the research on child fatality resulting from abuse and neglect in Chap. 4 of this text. Young children with disabilities are particularly vulnerable to abuse and neglect for several reasons. Early detection of disability frequently implies a more severe disability. For example, when children are diagnosed with disabilities as babies or as very young children, this usually implies that their disabilities are more severe. It is also possible that their caregivers do not understand their needs as these children are new arrivals to their lives. The challenges of providing care to babies and very young children with disabilities cut across caregivers' social, economic, and educational levels. The high numbers of very young children who are abused and neglected necessitates that we:

Recommendation 2.5: Develop focused and targeted programs to address the needs of parents and caregivers of young children with disabilities.

***

Children with emotional and behavioral disorders demand unique understanding of those around them and they are among the most frequently abused and neglected children. These children look like everyone else in that there are no external markers attributable to their special emotional and behavioral needs. Conversely, the unique needs of many children with sensory disabilities and those with physical disabilities are readily apparent. Children with emotional and behavioral disorders are confusing to the neighbors. They incite such comments as "Why can't Johnny behave?" "Does she *always* act like that in the grocery store?" "He has an attitude!" Children with emotional and behavioral disorders exhibit their disabilities in their behaviors. Children communicate their thoughts and feelings through their behaviors. Some children who are afraid act aggressively. Some children who are angry withdraw. This may be their best effort to let others know that something is wrong. We might wisely understand these behaviors as children's expressions of overwhelming and unmanageable feelings. It is easy to disconnect them from a child's response to trauma. Cooling down strategies such as – "take a deep breath and count from ten to one – and then, when you feel ready, let me know what is happening." Children with emotional and behavioral disorders have disabilities just as those who are blind, deaf, or cerebral palsy or spina bifida. Awareness of their needs will be more readily available in the general public when we:

Recommendation 2.6: Develop targeted programs that focus on understanding and addressing the needs of children with emotional and behavioral disorders.

***

When children with disabilities are around peers and adults who do not understand their disabilities, they are handicapped further. Peers and adults who do not understand disability in childhood may either over- or under-estimate the needs of children and their parents. They under-estimate the needs of children with disabilities when they speak for them, disregard their input, or when they fail to include them in the routine of every-day-life. For example, it is unrealistic to expect a child with an anxiety disorder to attend a dental appointment without consideration of the child's diagnosis. It is also unrealistic to consider that a child with autism will not engage in stereotypic behaviors which might include the manipulation of sensory objects. It is just as unrealistic to ignore the input of a child with cerebral palsy who relies on a communication board or other augmentative communication device. It is therefore essential that we:

Recommendation 2.7: Develop educational programs and encourage the participation of parents, family members, and professionals across disciplines about realistic expectations of children with disabilities.

***

CAN and ANCD Awareness and Training Programs in Schools

Key considerations for CAN prevention programming in schools include a clearly focused target population, regard for the diverse needs of the child population, inclusion of children with disabilities, children who exhibit problem sexual or aggressive behaviors, and children from low socioeconomic backgrounds (Brassard, & Fiorvanti, 2015; Scholes, Jones, Stieler-Hunt, Rolfe, & Pozzebon, 2012). Additionally, school personnel will wisely consider issues associated with the age and gender of students. Boys should be targeted as they may be less likely to report abuse due to stigmatization and they are more likely to be abused in group situations (i.e. summer camp). The age of the child should be considered because younger children are more vulnerable to CAN and ANCD, and they are more likely to use passive or escape forms of protection. Older children typically retain more information than younger children. Differences in cognitive development, relations to authority figures, and moral development should also be considered as well as developmental issues for groups such as preschoolers. Thus when developing abuse and neglect prevention programs, school personnel are advised to:

Recommendation 2.8: Design comprehensive programs that address the unique age, gender and developmental needs of targeted children.

***

Effective abuse and neglect prevention programs for children in schools have specific characteristics (Brassard & Fiorvanti, 2015; Scholes, et al. (2012). These include:

- active participation of targeted students
- explicit skills training
- group training
- standardized key messages taught by trained instructors
- integration into the school curriculum
- repeated presentations in programs and follow-up training
- an affirmation of the multisystemic nature of the programs including parental involvement and teacher education and
- the inclusion of features known to enhance learning and retention of prevention education (e.g., improve self-esteem and problem solving)

These skills are required by children with disabilities too and they may be taught to them in an age appropriate manner and while using accommodations and modifications to meet their individualized educational needs. Data indicate the necessity for:

Recommendation 2.9: School programming that is designed to prevent abuse and neglect among children with disabilities. This programming includes the development and enhancement of the self-care, self-advocacy and community support of these students while meeting their individual educational needs.

***

Bowman-Perrott et al. (2013) observed that children with emotional/behavioral disorders and attention-deficit/hyperactivity disorders were most likely to get suspended or expelled from schools. These children, among others with disabilities, may be so accustomed to denial of school privileges that they do not know what is right and what is wrong, what is normal and what is not normal. They may accept maltreatment as part of daily life. They do not readily recognize physical, emotional, sexual abuse and/or neglect.

When designing abuse and neglect preventing programs for children with and without disabilities in school environments it is essential to include intended key domains and messages. Brassard and Fiorvanti (2015) and Scholes, et al. (2012) indicate the need to teach children skills and strategies in order to develop their own self-protection. These researchers recommend that children:

- Develop a support network of trusted adults
- Ask trusted adults to be part of their support network
- Build rapport within their networks
- Develop a healthy self-concept
- Understand safe body rules
- Build confidence to stop and report unsafe behavior
- Learn ways to reject inappropriate and unwanted touching
- Know what to do if they experience abuse

- Build appreciation of individuality and differences.
- Respect of self and others

They also suggest that students learn how to use their support networks in order to practice appropriate self-disclosure; and increase their awareness that abuse and neglect are not acceptable and that it is not their fault. Based on the available data we recommend that school personnel:

Recommendation 2.10: Teach children the important role of participation in trusted networks where they experience acceptance and learn the knowledge and skills they need to protect themselves from the victimization that is associated with CAN and ANCD.

***

Is it possible that children who participate in abuse and neglect prevention programming in school environments might experience negative side effects? Is it possible that reteaching is an essential part of this programming? Might children forget how to talk about their abuse and neglect or about the abuse and neglect of their peers? Educators who are aware of students' unique learning needs at the acquisition, fluency, maintenance and generalization levels (Alberto & Troutman, 2013) will be in a better position to navigate the daily routine with these children. Teachers engaged in abuse prevention programming may expect that some children may not want to know about this devastating human reality. They may resist the knowledge that is available to them while learning about abuse and neglect in their lives. Teachers and parents wisely reassure children that this information is critical to their safety. Parents and caregivers have a unique role in the reaffirmation of school programming at home. We observe the necessity to:

Recommendation 2.11: Reteach and support children while they learn to protect their own safety and welfare. Enhance the maintenance and generalization of their newly acquired skills.

***

Programs designed to teach children about abuse and neglect must be data-based and evaluated rigorously on an ongoing basis. This will ensure that best practices are being implemented and that children and families are attaining the intended benefits. We observe that it is necessary to engage in:

Recommendation 2.12: Ongoing evaluation of school abuse and neglect prevention programming, in order to ensure that children and their families are receiving essential knowledge and skills that enhances their lives with the intended outcomes.

***

Exercise 2.7: Analysis
Conduct a thorough literature search in your library on the subject of the ANCD. Make a list of keywords including gender and age and constrain your search using peer-reviewed academic articles only. *How many articles were you able to find? Choose one and write a synopsis of the research article. In groups, discuss the main finding of the articles that you discovered.*

Chapter Summary

In this chapter we examined the age, sex, and disability characteristics of children with disabilities who are abused and neglected. Data from large national databases, as well as from studies in this area indicate that young children with disabilities are particularly vulnerable to child fatality following their abuse and neglect. Childhood fatality occurs most frequently among children under 1-year-old. As boys with disabilities age they are protected by their perceived strength. Girls with disabilities are sexually abused more frequently than boys. Children with disabilities who exhibit challenging emotional and psychological behaviors as well as those who exhibit other medical conditions are abused and neglected more frequently than their peers with other disability characteristics. We illustrated these data with stories from the newspaper coverage on the ANCD. We concluded this chapter with a set of recommendations for researchers and practitioners.

References

Akbas, S., Turla, A., Karabekirog˘lu, K., Pazvantog˘lu, O., Keskin, T., & Bo˘ke, O. (2009). Characteristics of sexual abuse in a sample of Turkish children with and without mental retardation, referred for legal appraisal of the psychological repercussions. *Sexuality & Disability, 27*, 205–213. doi:10.1007/s11195-009-9139-7

Alberto, P. A., & Troutman, A. C. (2013). *Applied behavior analysis for teachers* (9th ed.). Columbus, OH: Pearson.

Alriksson-Schmidt, A., Armour, B. S., & Thibadeau, J. K. (2010). Are adolescent girls with a physical disability at increased risk for sexual violence? *Journal of School Health, 80*(7), 361–367. doi:10.1111/j.1746-1561.2010.00514.x

Banks, N. (2014). Sexually harmful behaviour in adolescents in a context of gender and intellectual disability: Implications for child psychologists. *Educational & Child Psychology, 31*(3), 9–21. Retrieved from http://eds.a.ebscohost.com/eds/pdfviewer/pdfviewer?vid=3& sid=a13b4a23-6290-4f3e-a8c1-250410b08020%40sessionmgr4005&hid=4213

Balogh, R., Bretherton, K., Whibley, S., Berney, T., Graham, S., . . . Firth, H. (2001). Sexual abuse in children and adolescents with intellectual disability. *Journal of Intellectual Disability Research, 45*(3), 194–201. doi:10.1046/j.1365-2788.2001.00293.x

Benedict, M. I., White, R. B., Wulff, L. M., & Hall, B. J. (1990). Reported maltreatment in children with multiple disabilities. *Child Abuse & Neglect, 14*, 207–217. doi:10.1016/0145-2134(90)90031-N

Blatt, B., & Kaplan, F. (1966). *Christmas in Purgatory: A photographic essay on mental retardation*. Boston, MA: Allyn & Bacon.

Bones, P. D. C. (2013). Perceptions of vulnerability: A target characteristics approach to disability, gender, and victimization. *Deviant Behavior, 34*(9), 727–750. doi:10.1080/01639625.2013.766511

Bowman-Perrott, L., Benz, M. R., Hsu, H.-Y., Kwok, O.-M., Eisterhold, L. A., & Zhang, D. (2013). Patterns and predictors of disciplinary exclusion over time: An analysis of the SEELS national data set. *Journal of Emotional and Behavioral Disorders, 21*(2), 83–96. doi:10.1177/1063426611407501

Brassard, M. R., & Fiorvanti, C. M. (2015). School-based child abuse prevention programs. *Psychology in the Schools, 52*(1), 40–60. doi:10.1002/pits.21811

Child Welfare Information Gateway. (2014). Mandatory reporters of child abuse and neglect. Retrieved from https://www.childwelfare.gov/systemwide/laws_policies/statutes/manda.cfm

Coorg, R., & Tournay, A. (2013). Filicide-suicide involving children with disabilities. *Journal of Child Neurology, 28*(6), 742–748. doi:10.1177/0883073812451777

Douglas, E. M., & Mohn, B. L. (2014). Fatal and non-fatal child maltreatment in the US: An analysis of child, caregiver, and service utilization with the National Child Abuse and Neglect Data Set. *Child Abuse & Neglect, 38*(1), 42–51. doi:10.1016/j.chiabu.2013.10.022

Esernio-Jenssen, D., Tai, J., & Kodsi, S. (2011). Abusive head trauma in children: A comparison of male and female perpetrators. *Pediatrics, 127*(4), 649–657. doi:10.1542/peds.2010-1770

Firth, H., Balogh, R., Berney, T., Bretherton, K., Graham, S., & Whibley, S. (2001). Psychopathology of sexual abuse in young children with intellectual disability. *Journal of Intellectual Disability Research, 45*, 244–252. doi:10.1046/j.1365-2788.2001.00314.x

Goldberg, A. P., Tobin, J., Daigneau, J., Griffith, R. T., Reinert, S. E., & Jenny, C. (2009). Bruising frequency and patterns in children with physical disabilities. *Pediatrics, 124*(2), 604–609. doi:10.1542/peds.2008-2900

Govindshenoy, M., & Spencer, N. (2006). Abuse of the disabled child: A systematic review ofpopulation-based studies. *Child: Care, Health and Development, 33*(5), 552–558. doi:10.1111/j.1365-2214.2006.00693.x

Hershkowitz, I., Lamb, M. E., & Horowitz, D. (2007). Victimization of children with disabilities. *American Journal of Orthopsychiatry, 77*, 629–635. doi:10.1037/0002-9432.77.4.629

Individuals with Disabilities Education Improvement Act. (2004). 20 USC 1400. Retrieved from http://nichcy.org/wp-content/uploads/docs/PL108-446.pdf

Jackson, D. (2008, July 17). A mother mourns 2 lost futures. *Chicago Tribune*. Retrieved from http://articles.chicagotribune.com/2008-07-17/news/0807161200_1_juvenile-group-therapy-single-mother

Khalifeh, H., Howard, L., Osborn, D., Moran, P., & Johnson, S. (2013). Violence against people with disability in England and Wales: Findings from a national cross-sectional survey. *Plos One, 8*(2), 1–9. doi:10.1371/journal.pone.0055952

Knutson, J. F., Johnson, C. R., & Sullivan, P. M. (2004). Disciplinary choices of mothers of deaf children and mothers of normally hearing children. *Child Abuse & Neglect, 28*(9), 925–937. doi:10.1016/j.chiabu.2004.04.005

Kvam, M. H. (2000). Is sexual abuse of children with disabilities disclosed? A retrospective analysis of child disability and the likelihood of sexual abuse among those attending Norwegian hospitals. *Child Abuse & Neglect, 24*(8), 1073–1084. doi:10.1016/S0145-2134(00)00159-9

Kvam, M. H. (2004). Sexual abuse of deaf children: A retrospective analysis of the prevalence and characteristics of childhood sexual abuse among deaf adults in Norway. *Child Abuse & Neglect, 28*(3), 241–251. doi:10.1016/j.chiabu.2003.09.017

Leeb, R. T., Bitsko, R. H., Merrick, M. T., & Armour, B. S. (2012). Does childhood disability increase risk for child abuse and neglect? *Journal of Mental Health Research in Intellectual Disabilities, 5*(1), 4–31. doi:10.1080/19315864.2011.608154

McDonald, J. L., Milne, S., Knight, J., & Webster, V. (2013). Developmental and behavioural characteristics of children enrolled in a child protection pre-school. *Journal of Paediatrics & Child Health, 49*(2), 142–146. doi:10.1111/jpc.12029

McLeod, J., Uemura, R., & Rohrman, S. (2012). Adolescent mental health, behavior problems, and academic achievement. *Journal of Health and Social Behavior, 53*(4), 482–497. doi:10.1177/0022146512462888

Mueller-Johnson, K., Eisner, M. P., & Obsuth, I. (2014). Sexual victimization of youth with a physical disability: An examination of prevalence rates, and risk and protective factors. *Journal of Interpersonal Violence, 29*(17), 3180–3206. doi:10.1177/0886260514534529

Nalavany, B. A., Ryan, S. D., & Hinterlong, J. (2009). Externalizing behavior among adopted boys with preadoptive histories of child sexual abuse. *Journal of Child Sexual Abuse, 18*(5), 553–573. doi:10.1080/10538710903183337

Osterman, R. (2004, March 24). Girl, 10, testifies to sex abuse by teacher. *Chicago Tribune*. Retrieved from http://articles.chicagotribune.com/2004-03-24/news/0403240157_1_after-school-program-sexual-safe-school

Reeder, S. (2007). Experts disagree on frequency of sexual abuse of students. *Hidden Violations, Small Newspaper Group*. Retrieved from http://hiddenviolations.com/stories/?prcss=display&id=358899

Sebald, A. M. (2008). Child abuse and deafness. *American Annals of the Deaf, 153*(4), 376–383.

Scholes, L., Jones, C., Stieler-Hunt, C., Rolfe, B., & Pozzebon, K. (2012). The teachers' role in child sexual abuse prevention programs: Implications for teacher education. *Australian Journal of Teacher Education, 37*(11), 104–131.

Sobsey, D., Randall, W., & Parrila, R. K. (1997). Gender differences in abused children with and without disabilities. *Child Abuse & Neglect, 21*(8), 707–720. doi:10.1016/S0145-2134(97)00033-1

Soylu, N., Alpaslan, A. H., Ayaz, M., Esenyel, S., & Oruc, M. (2013). Psychiatric disorders and characteristics of abuse in sexually abused children and adolescents with and without intellectual disabilities. *Research in Developmental Disabilities, 34*(12), 4334–4342. doi:10.1016/j.ridd.2013.09.010

Spencer, N., Devereux, E., Wallace, A., Sundrum, R., Shenoy, M., Bacchus, C., et al. (2005). Disabling conditions and registration for child abuse and neglect: A population-based study. *Pediatrics, 116*(3), 609–613. doi:10.1542/peds.2004-1882

Stalker, K., & McArthur, K. (2012). Child abuse, child protection and disabled children: A review of recent research. *Child Abuse Review, 21*(1), 24–40. doi:10.1002/car.1154

Sullivan, P. M. (2009). Violence exposure among children with disabilities. *Clinical Child and Family Psychology Review, 12*(2), 196–216. doi:10.1037/0002-9432.77.4.629

Sullivan, P. M., & Knutson, J. F. (2000a). The prevalence of disabilities and maltreatment among runaway children. *Child Abuse & Neglect, 24*(10), 1275–1288. doi:10.1016/S0145-2134(00)00181-2

Sullivan, P. M., & Knutson, J. F. (2000b). Maltreatment and disabilities: A population-based epidemiologic study. *Child Abuse & Neglect, 24*(10), 1257–1273. doi:10.1016/S0145-2134(00)00190-3

Ulloa Flores, R. E., & Navarro Machuca, I. G. (2011). Estudio descriptivo de la prevalencia y tipos de maltrato en adolescentes con psicopatología. *Salud Mental, 34*(3), 219–225. Retrieved from http://www.scielo.org.mx/scielo.php?script=sci_arttext&pid=S0185-33252011000200005

U.S. Department of Health and Human Services, Administration for Children and Families, Administration on Children, Youth and Families, Children's Bureau. (2013). *Child maltreatment 2012*. Retrieved from http://www.acf.hhs.gov/programs/cb/research-data-technology/statistics-research/child-maltreatment

Vig, S., & Kaminer, R. (2002). Maltreatment and developmental disabilities in children. *Journal of Developmental and Physical Disabilities, 14*(4), 371–386. doi:10.1023/A:1020334903216

Walker, H. M., & Gresham, F. M. (Eds.). (2013). *Handbook of evidence-based practices for emotional and behavioral disorders*. New York, NY: Guilford Press.

Wells, M., & Mitchell, K. J. (2013). Patterns of internet use and risk of online victimization for youth with and without disabilities. *The Journal of Special Education, 20*(10), 1–10. doi:10.1177/0022466913479141

Chapter 3
The Forms of Abuse and Neglect of Children with Disabilities

> *Human kindness has never weakened the stamina or softened*
> *the fiber of a free people. A nation does not have to be cruel*
> *to be tough.* (Franklin D. Roosevelt, 32nd President of the
> United States, 1882–1945)

Abstract This chapter examines the forms of maltreatment, including physical abuse, sexual abuse, emotional, and psychological abuse, and neglect that prevail in the lives of children with disabilities. We analyze data from large data bases, including the U.S. DHHS and the available databased research in this area. We present our findings following an analysis of the newspaper coverage of the abuse and neglect of children with disabilities (ANCD) and illustrate these findings with stories about the children and adults represented by these numbers. We complete this chapter with a discussion of the implications of these findings for research and practice. We provide reflection and critical thinking exercises throughout the chapter.

Children with and without disabilities are maltreated – abused and neglected every day in the United States and all over the world. They endure maltreatment in the forms of physical and sexual abuse, emotional and psychological abuse, and neglect perpetrated by caregivers at home, in hospitals, schools, and other institutions. What constitutes child maltreatment? When do we decide that a child is maltreated? Who actually decides? What constitutes the abuse of a child? What is neglect of a child? Is violence against children the same as child maltreatment? We may indeed wonder why these become complex questions. Child-by-child differences among children with disabilities contribute to their complexities. For example, a child with autism may be emotionally traumatized by the same noise that other children would hardly notice. Likewise, the health and welfare of a child with cerebral palsy may be put at-risk by improper physical positioning.

We begin this chapter with an analysis of the terminology we use to communicate about child maltreatment. We examine what we know from the large national and international databases and analyze the literature on the prevailing forms of maltreatment to which children with disabilities are exposed. We examine the findings of the newspaper study and provide case examples that illustrate our

© Springer International Publishing Switzerland 2016   55
E.P. Crowley, *Preventing Abuse and Neglect in the Lives of Children with Disabilities*, DOI 10.1007/978-3-319-30442-7_3

findings. We conclude the chapter with a discussion of the implication of this information for research and practice.

Defining Child Maltreatment

The World Health Organization (WHO, 2014) defines child maltreatment as child abuse and neglect (CAN) that includes:

> ... all forms of physical and emotional ill-treatment, sexual abuse, neglect, and exploitation that results in actual or potential harm to the child's health, development or dignity. Within this broad definition, five subtypes can be distinguished – physical abuse; sexual abuse; neglect and negligent treatment; emotional abuse; and exploitation.

Child maltreatment – the abuse and neglect of children with and without disabilities is reported by the U.S. DHHS (2013) in the following categories, namely, medical neglect, neglect, physical abuse, psychological maltreatment, and sexual abuse. Statistics on children who are exposed to the different forms of maltreatment are not disaggregated to reflect how children with disabilities might be differently abused and neglected from their peers in the general child population.

Exercise 3.1: Critical Thinking
What forms of abuse and neglect do you expect that children with disabilities are exposed to most frequently? *Write three to five statements to support your observations.*

Physical Abuse of Children with Disabilities

Physical abuse of children with disabilities is characterized by harm that results from applying inappropriate physical force in effort to restrain or manage a child. Shaken baby syndrome results from the physical abuse of babies and causes serious trauma, severe disability, or even death. Babies who have been forcefully shaken as infants may be extremely irritable, have difficulty staying awake, and have trouble breathing.

Physical abuse of children with disabilities includes hitting, kicking, pulling hair, burning in water, or with fire; using physical force that results in physical or psychological harm; force feeding; forcing task performance that is beyond the child's strength; insufficient or too much clothing; failing to remove a child from danger; misusing prescribed or unprescribed medications; or inappropriately restraining or locking a child in a small space or room.

Observable indicators of physical abuse include discomfort with physical contact, being apprehensive when other children cry, extreme aggression or withdrawal, afraid of parents or afraid to go home, coming to school too early, staying late, complaining of soreness and chronically running away from home.

What is the difference between corporal punishment, cruel and unusual punishment, and physical abuse? The courts decide case-by-case. The use of physical punishments may be observed as a method to discipline children or as a consequence for childhood behavior that is deemed unacceptable. Cruel and unusual punishment crosses a line and shocks the moral sense of observers. Torture, cruelty, degrading, and confinement shock us all. The definitions blur differentiation between physical punishment and corporal punishment.

The use of both physical and corporal punishment has troubled professionals for a long time. Sadly, both remain in use today under the guise of child discipline procedures (Holden, Williamson, & Holland, 2014; Jones et al., 2012; Sandgrund, Gaines, & Green, 1974; Sobsey, 1994, 2002; Zirpoli, 1990). Holden et al. (2014) found that mothers of 2–5 year-old children use corporal punishment more frequently than fathers; they use it when young children do not heed their requests to "stop it"; and corporal punishment is administered 26.5 s on average following the child's perceived misbehavior.

Exercise 3.2: Critical Thinking

David is 10 years old. You heard him telling his peers in the classroom that he was caught shoplifting and as a result his father beat him with a belt. Later, you took David aside and told him what you heard. You requested that he allow the school nurse to examine him, and he agreed. The nurse found no bruises or marks. You called David's father and he confirmed that he hit David with a belt as a punishment for shoplifting. Next day his father picked him up from school as usual, and David seemed happy to see his father. *Do you have any further responsibilities as a professional? Explain your rationale.*

Scenarios like this provide real challenges for caregivers and professionals. Since David's and his father's version of events are the same and he does not seem fearful of his father, would you agree that this was an isolated incident of physical punishment? Would you agree that steps need to be taken in order to protect both David and his father from escalated physical violence?

Sexual Abuse of Children with Disabilities

Sexual abuse occurs when children with and without disabilities take part in sexual activities with one or more individuals. The engagement of children with and without disabilities in sexual activities in order to achieve sexual gratification constitutes sexual abuse.

Sexual abuse of children may involve touching, fondling or kissing; developing pornographic materials; or the failure of a parent, assigned caregiver or professional to protect a child when sexual abuse is suspected (Caldas & Bensy, 2014; Sommarin, Kilbane, Mercy, Maloney-Kitts, & Ligiero, 2014; Soylu, Alpaslan, Ayaz, Esenyel, & Oruc, 2013). Young children with and without disabilities who have been sexually abused may appear irritable and unengaged. They may also have difficulty eating, sleeping, and meeting expected developmental milestones. Older children may either withdraw or act out as a result of sexual abuse.

Behavioral and emotional indicators of sexual abuse may include age-inappropriate knowledge of sex, sexually explicit drawings, and unexplained fear of a person or a place. Other indicators include withdrawal behavior, self-image problems, depression, anxiety, mood swings, and shame.

Mueller-Johnson, Eisner, and Obsuth (2014) found that sexual abuse occurs more frequently among children with physical disabilities than among their peers both with other disabilities and among those without disabilities. Sexual abuse occurs more frequently among females with physical disabilities than among their male counterparts. Males with physical disabilities were physically abused with contact victimization three times more often than their nondisabled male peers. Mueller-Johnson and colleagues found that they were nearly twice as likely to experience noncontact sexual victimization than their nondisabled peers. Noncontact sexual abuse occurred among girls with physical disabilities 1.4 times more frequently than among their female peers without disabilities.

Children with autism spectrum disorders (ASD) are at greater risk to experience, as well as perpetrate sexual abuse than their nondisabled peers (Mandell, Walrath, Manteuffel, Sgro, & Pinto-Martin, 2005; Sevlever, Ross, & Gillis, 2013). Researchers also conclude that they are at higher risk of perpetuating sexual abuse as adults. Mandell and Walrath found that approximately 12 % (19 out of 156) of children with ASD experienced at least one episode of sexual abuse and an additional 4 % (7) of children experienced both sexual and physical abuse. Risk factors that increase the likelihood of their sexual abuse were poor communication and social skills. Researchers suggest that many service providers are in contact with children with ASD to assist in adaptive skills such as toileting and showering. Additional factors associated with increased risk of CAN include the readiness of some children with ASD to comply with sexually inappropriate requests. They are easy targets for sexual perpetrators of CAN because of inherent difficulty in identifying when abuse and neglect does and does not occur. Sevlever and her colleagues describe the dearth of research in this area and concluded by identifying the need for increased efforts to investigate sexual abuse among children with ASD.

Emotional or Psychological Abuse of Children with Disabilities

Emotional or psychological abuse of children with and without disabilities involves creating situations which bring about fear, anxiety, and even terror. Children who have been exposed to emotional abuse may wish to hide, withdraw, and reject common social exchanges. They may appear fearful, upset, and unhappy.

Bullying involves targeted emotional abuse and is expressed in negative and aggressive verbal exchanges toward an individual with a disability either in person or using electronic media. Among the many manifestations of emotional abuse is the use of verbal threats, swearing, shouting, and expressing deprecating statements, engaging in the delivery of verbal taunts, denying requests or preferences, or restricting access to family or friends.

Behavioral indicators of emotional abuse of children with and without disabilities may include habit disorders (sucking, rocking, or biting), conduct disorders, neurotic traits, self-destructive behavior/suicide attempts, cruelty; taking pleasure in hurting others and bullying their peers and adults. Bullying involves the use of quarrelsome and domineering behaviors that focus on others who are perceived as smaller and weaker. This is a form of emotional and psychological abuse to which children with disabilities are frequently exposed. Bullying may be observed as physical abuse and accompanied with emotional abuse. It is usually associated with peer perpetrators and victims. Bullying can be defined as repeated behavior intended to cause harm or intimidate someone who is considered less powerful (Zeedyk, Rodriguez, Tipton, Baker, & Blacher, 2014). The effects of bullying can include lowered academic performance, increased anxiety, low self-esteem, depression, suicide, absenteeism, or poor physical health (Weiner, Day, & Galvan, 2013; Wells & Mitchell, 2014). There is evidence to suggest that students with disabilities are bullied at higher rates than students without disabilities. In a comparative analysis of over 14,000 students with and without disabilities, Rose, Espelage, and Monda-Amaya (2009) found that students with disabilities had significantly higher rates of being the victims of bullies, fighting, and engaging in bullying behavior. In another study that investigated the bullying of deaf/hard of hearing youth, Weiner, Day, and Galvan (2013) reported that students who are deaf had significantly higher rates of being bullied than a comparative national sample of hearing students.

Exercise 3.3: Critical Thinking
Dave is a sophomore in high school and he is a starter on the basketball team. At a game you observed Dave's father criticizing and ridiculing him from the sidelines. He is so disruptive that during half-time, Dave and he got into a heated argument on the sidelines. Dave fouled out during the third quarter, and his father left the game in obvious disgust. Dave seemed relieved when his father left. He began to talk and joke with his teammates. *What are the indicators of emotional abuse in this scenario? What is your role as a professional person upon observation of this exchange?*

The forms of emotional abuse may manifest themselves differently or similarly among children. For example, a child who had been physically abused may bully another student at school while a child who has been emotionally abused may verbally threaten a peer in school. Alternately, students who are sexually abused may withdraw or they may exhibit inappropriate touching of peers or adults, or they may engage in exhibitionism.

Neglect of Children with Disabilities

Neglect of children with disabilities occurs when parents, caregivers, or professionals fail to respond to the unique individual needs of children or when they fail to take action that is in the children's best interest. Neglect may be intended or unintended and always compromises a child's health and safety. Deprivation of sufficient nourishment, clothing, shelter, medical care, and attention are examples of neglect. Neglect of children with disabilities may be observed in failure to provide protection from potential harm such as unsupervised play in swimming pools or playgrounds; unsupervised use of potentially dangerous equipment such as knives or scissors; deprivation of social and educational opportunities; leaving a child with a physical disability in bed all day; or any exposure to undue risk. Children with disabilities require increased protection due to the nature of their special needs. Children who are blind, deaf, have intellectual and emotional and behavioral disorders, communication disorders, learning disabilities, and those with physical disabilities all require very specialized care and attention from their adult caregivers.

Day-to-day observable indicators of child neglect include malnourished appearance, lethargy, poor hygiene, inappropriate dress for weather, lack of medical treatment for a serious illness, living in unhealthy or dangerous environments, and poor attendance. Behavioral and emotional indicators of neglect include begging for or stealing food, excessive absences, risky adolescent behavior, promiscuity, drugs, delinquency, "clingy" behavior, poor ability to relate to others, poor self-esteem, attachment difficulties, and difficulty setting personal boundaries.

Exercise 3.4: Reflection

Is it neglect? Read each of the following statements and circle "Yes" or "No"
following each one. Provide three reasons to defend your observation about
whether you believe the situation reflects neglect on part of the caregiver(s):
Neglect

Poverty – A child's parents cannot afford to get her needed prescription glasses.
Yes No

Home alone – 10-year-old Melissa is home alone every day after school until her mother comes home from work at 7:00 p.m. Yes No

Dirty child – Louis consistently comes to school dirty. Yes No

Substance abuse – Beth's mother abuses alcohol even though Beth seems well cared for. Yes No

Preventive health care – You discover that Peter has never been to the dentist.
Yes No

Educational neglect – Cynthia is truant from school. Yes No

Seat belts – Linda's mother never makes her wear a seat belt, and nor does she put her 2-year-old sister in a safety seat. Yes No

Viezel, Lowell, Davis, and Castillo (2014) examined the adaptive behavior of 160 children between 5 and 18 years old. Adaptive behaviors include daily living skills, social functioning, and communication skills. They observed the differences in the adaptive behavior of those who had been physically and sexually abused, and those who had been neglected. Forty two of these children were removed from their homes because of physical and sexual abuse, 118 were removed from their homes because of medical and educational neglect. The researchers compared the adaptive behavior scores of these children with those of a demographically matched comparison group of children.

Viezel and her colleagues used the Vineland Adaptive Behavior Scales (Sparrow, Cicchetti, & Balla, 2005) to compare the adaptive behaviors of children who were physically and sexually abused, and neglected with their peers in a typically developing comparison group. The Vineland evaluates skills in the domains of daily living skills, communication, and socialization. Viezel et al. found that, among the three groups, the comparison peer group had the highest adaptive behavior scores in all three domains. The children who were neglected had the lowest adaptive behavior scores. Those who were physically and sexually abused had higher scores than the neglect group and lower scores than the comparison group. Viezel et al. observed the largest functional difference among the children in the neglect group. Their daily living skills were the lowest among the groups. Following these were their low scores in the areas of communication and socialization.

Viezel and her colleagues found that children who were neglected exhibited more receptive, expressive, and written language skills deficits. These children exhibited limited daily living skills, such as, personal care, domestic tasks, and community living skills. Finally, children who were neglected exhibited delayed social skills, difficulty with play and leisure activities, and overall difficulty using coping skills.

A Closer Look at Definition Related Issues

The definitions of the forms of abuse and neglect differ across states. These definitions guide how CAN statistics are reported to the National Child Abuse Neglect Data System (NCANDS). Designated personnel in states are mandated to report CAN statistics in accord with the Child Abuse Prevention and Treatment Act (CAPTA, 2010, P. L. 111–320). CAPTA is the federal legislation that focuses on preventing and responding to CAN. CAPTA provides support to states for data collection activities and technical assistance. Child abuse is defined by CAPTA as:

> at a minimum any recent act or failure to act on the part of a parent or caretaker, which results in death, serious physical or emotional harm, sexual abuse or exploitation, or an act or failure to act which presents an imminent risk of serious harm.

CAPTA legislation defines this minimum standard, and states develop variations on this definition that result in inconsistencies in how data are reported across states. States are not required to submit data on the disability status of abused or neglected children. Variations in the way states define and collect these data makes it difficult to estimate accurately the extent to which children with disabilities are abused and neglected. For example, from 2008 to 2012, an average of 1.3 children per 1000 were maltreated in Pennsylvania. In the same time period, the District of Columbia reported an average of 24 victims of CAN per 1000 children (U.S. DHHS, 2013). We may well wonder about the implications of such disparity across state reports.

Exercise 3.5: Reflection
Carlos is usually an enthusiastic 6-year-old. Lately you observe that he is either withdrawn or very bossy with the other children. You intervene when you see Carlos grabbing a peer and yelling in his face. Carlos tells you not to call his mother or her new boyfriend who he thinks will get angry and hurt his mother. *Is there a concern here? What would you do if you observed Carlos engaging in this behavior?*

Forms of Child Maltreatment Indicated in the National Data

In 2012, the U.S. DHHS estimated a total of 678,810 unique victims of CAN and ANCD. During that year an estimated 9.2 children per 1000 children experienced physical abuse, sexual abuse, psychological abuse, and/or neglect (see Table 3.1). From 2008 to 2012 an estimated average of 698,000 children were maltreated annually – an estimated average 9.3 children per 1000 were maltreated each year. Less than 36.1 % of the child maltreatment reports are attributed to physical abuse, sexual abuse, and psychological maltreatment combined. We may well wonder why the reports of sexual abuse so dominates our cultural conversations. Additionally, why do we concern ourselves so infrequently about child neglect, that actually dominates the CAN and ANCD statistics?

Exercise 3.6: Reflection
In the United States the number of child maltreatment reports is higher than the number of unique victims of child maltreatment. For example, there were 865,478

Table 3.1 Maltreatment type [a] reported in 2012

Type of maltreatment	# of maltreatments	% by type
Neglect	531,241	78.3
Physical abuse	124,544	18.3
Sexual abuse	62,936	9.3
Psychological maltreatment	57,880	8.5
Medical neglect	15,705	2.3
Other	71,846	10.6
Unknown	1,326	0.2
Total maltreatments	865,478	127.5

[a]Reports may indicate more than one maltreatment type
Data from the U.S. DHHS, *Child Maltreatment Report*, 2013

total child maltreatments and 678,810 unique child victims. Do you find these statistics surprising? *What questions linger as you consider these numbers?*

We may wonder about what form of CAN was of concern among 73,172 (8.5 %) reports in the "other" and "unknown" maltreatment categories. What constitutes "other" as a form of abuse and neglect to which children with and without disabilities are exposed? Florida defines "other" as "threatened harm" and behavior that is not accidental and is likely to result in abuse. Florida does not include these threats with other forms of abuse such as psychological maltreatment. Alternately, Texas does not report "other" data claiming that reports are either "founded" or "unfounded." In Texas, CAN is reported using a coding system to categorize the levels of substantiated abuse. Finally, New York defines "other" as parental drug or alcohol abuse; a category that other states may define as neglect. Only Colorado, North Carolina, Oregon, Puerto Rico, and Texas use the "unknown" and "other" child maltreatment designation to report their statistics.

To what extent do these data fit with the maltreatment of children with disabilities? We may also wonder whether children with specific disability characteristics are maltreated differently. What forms of child maltreatment do you expect that children with disabilities are exposed to most frequently?

A Closer Look at the Neglect

The data on child maltreatment from the U.S. DHHS (2013) indicated that neglect tops the list of all maltreatment types. These data indicate that in 2012 maltreatment occurred among 9.2 % of the children in the United States from birth to 17 years old. These data are not disaggregated to reflect the unique maltreatment exposure of children with disabilities.

The combined CAN reports of medical neglect and generalized neglect are attributed to 80.6 % of all the child maltreatments in the general child population. Nationally, neglect represents the highest percentage of child maltreatment type reported by the U.S. DHHS in 2013. Separate statistics are reported for medical neglect and general neglect. An estimated total of 546,946 reports of child neglect were made in 2012. One child may have been the victim of more than one neglect type. Children were either neglected medically (2.3 %) or were the victims of general neglect (78.3 %). In the state-by-state analysis New York, California, Texas, Michigan, Florida, and North Carolina top the list among states with the highest incidents of child neglect. In all, 282,172 children were neglected in these six states (see Table 3.2).

Let us take an even closer look. We think of many, many children when we look at a number like 68,375 children in New York. What would this number of children look like if they were all to gather in one place? What would 76,026 children in California look like? How about gathering 62,551 children in Texas, 33,434 children in Michigan, 53,341 children in Florida, and 23,150 children in North Carolina? These numbers represent the highest counts of unique victims of CAN

Table 3.2 States reporting neglect most frequently in 2012

State	Unique victims	Total maltreatments	Medical neglect	General neglect	% of unique victims	% of total maltreatments
New York	68,375	109,072	4,093	74,055	114.3	71.6
California	76,026	91,574	*	65,900	86.7	72.0
Texas	62,551	72,007	1,649	52,062	85.9	74.6
Michigan	33,434	70,271	1,060	31,115	96.3	45.8
Florida	53,341	67,087	1,226	30,357	59.2	47.1
North Carolina	23,150	25,146	503	20,152	89.2	82.1
Total	316,877	435,157	8,531	273,641	Mean 88.6	Mean 65.3

Neglect represents 80.6 % of total child maltreatment reported nationally
*Data not available
Data from the U.S. DHHS, *Child Maltreatment Report*, 2013

among states in the United States in 2012. Together these numbers add to 316,877 children. To illustrate – it would take 5,282 school buses, transporting 60 children per bus, to transport them. How many school buses would it take to transport all the children who were neglected in 2012? Just imagine what the child neglect statistics alone would look like if we were to calculate them, not just for the United States, but for every country all over the world.

These statistics represent the count of unique victims of child neglect in six of the 50 states in the United States and the District of Columbia. We do not know how many times each child was victimized. As stated earlier, children with disabilities, including those with emotional and behavioral disorders, intellectual disabilities, autism, and physical disabilities are predictably more vulnerable to revictimization than their nondisabled peers.

Exercise 3.7: Reflection
Do you believe that a caregiver would give a boy with attention deficit disorder her own prescription medicine? *Write at least five scenarios under which this might actually occur.*

A Closer Look at Physical Abuse

The global effort to end corporal punishment began formally in 2001. Brazil ended this as a way to discipline children in 2014 (Global Initiative to End All Corporal Punishment of Children, 2014). Are you surprised to hear that corporal punishment remains an accepted way to discipline children in the United States? Farrell (2015) reports:

> …corporal punishment has declined sharply in recent years, but only 31 states (plus D.C. and Puerto Rico) have abolished it in public schools, either *de facto* or *de jure*.

Table 3.3 States reporting physical abuse most frequently in 2012

	Unique victims	Total maltreatments	Physical abuse	% of unique victims	% of total maltreatments
Ohio	29,250	34,555	12,351	42.2	35.7
Texas	62,551	72,007	11,876	19.0	16.5
Michigan	33,434	70,271	8,507	25.4	12.1
California	76,026	91,574	7,424	9.8	8.1
New York	68,375	109,072	7,312	10.7	6.7
Illinois	27,497	31,986	6,945	25.3	21.7
Total	297,133	409,465	54,415	Mean 22.06	Mean 16.78

Physical abuse represents 18.3 % of total child maltreatment reported nationally
Data from the U.S. DHHS, *Child Maltreatment Report*, 2013

Corporal punishment is still permitted in the other 19 states, and it remains a widespread practice in three of them, all in the South: Alabama, Arkansas and Mississippi.

When does corporal punishment become physical abuse? Some argue that deliberately hitting children will always constitute physical abuse while others argue that corporal punishment is a necessary part of child care while supported by Biblical references such as "spare the rod, spoil the child" (Proverbs 13:24).

Physical abuse is involved in 18.3 % of all the CAN in the United States (see Table 3.1). A total of 124,544 children were physically abused in 2012. If we were to transport these children in school buses we would need 2076 buses. Physical abuse occurred most frequently in Ohio, Texas, Michigan, California, New York, and Illinois (see Table 3.3).

A Closer Look at Sexual Abuse

The U.S. DHHS (2013) reported that 9.3 % of all child maltreatment involves sexual abuse (see Table 3.1). A total of 62,936 children less than 17 years of age were confirmed victims of sexual abuse in 2012. Texas, Ohio, Illinois, California, Indiana, and Tennessee reported the highest incidents of child sexual abuse in 2012 (see Table 3.4). If we were to transport all the children who were confirmed victims of sexual abuse in 2012 in school buses designed for 60 children, we would need 1,049 buses. We do not know how many of these children had disabilities prior to being sexually abused but based on the literature we may safely conclude that children with disabilities were disproportionately represented among these children. We may also conclude that children are physically and emotionally injured as a result of abuse and neglect. Some will acquire disabilities as a direct consequence of their exposure to abuse and neglect.

Table 3.4 States reporting sexual abuse most frequently in 2012

State	Unique victims	Total maltreatments	Sexual abuse reports	% of unique victims	% of total maltreatments
Texas	62,551	72,007	5,928	9.5	8.2
Ohio	29,250	34,555	5,490	18.8	15.9
Illinois	27,497	31,986	4,985	18.1	15.6
California	76,026	91,574	4,240	5.6	4.6
Indiana	20,223	23,094	3,061	15.1	13.3
Tennessee	10,069	11,212	2,986	29.7	26.6
Total	225,616	264,428	26,690	Mean 16.13	Mean 14.03

Sexual abuse represents 9.3 % of total maltreatment reported nationally
Data from the U.S. DHHS, *Child Maltreatment Report*, 2013

A Closer Look at Psychological Abuse

Psychological abuse accounts for 8.5 % of all the confirmed victims of CAN (see Table 3.1). Childhood psychological abuse is associated with childhood depression, learning difficulties, delinquency, emotion dysregulation, and interpersonal problems. This type of abuse is reported more frequently in Michigan than in any other state, it accounts for 43.6 % of all the unique victims of CAN (see Table 3.5). Additionally, the percentage of unique victims of psychological abuse in California, Georgia, Puerto Rico, Connecticut, and Utah is close to and more than double the national average.

A Closer Look at Child Fatality and CAN

Children die as a result of abuse and neglect. Data from the U.S. DHHS (2013) indicate that child deaths occur most frequently in contexts that are characterized by the neglect (69.9 %) and physical abuse (44.3 %) (see Table 3.6). Overall, combined neglect including medical neglect account for 78.8 % of child fatality associated with CAN in the United States in 2012.

Psychological abuse and sexual abuse combined account for 3.0 % of child fatalities in 2012.

We do not know how many children have diagnosed disabilities prior to their deaths following abuse and neglect. The data from the U.S. DHHS are not disaggregated to represent children with and without disabilities.

Table 3.5 States reporting psychological abuse most frequently in 2012

State	Unique victims	Total maltreatments	Victims of psychological abuse	% of unique victims	% of total altreatments
Michigan	33,434	70,271	14,581	43.6	20.7
California	76,026	91,574	13,931	18.3	15.2
Georgia	18,752	21,496	4,375	23.3	20.4
Puerto Rico	8,470	12,991	3,758	44.4	28.9
Connecticut	8,151	10,921	2,720	33.4	24.9
Utah	9,419	11,843	2,671	28.4	22.6
Total	154,252	219,096	42,036	Mean 31.9	Mean 22.1

Data from the U.S. DHHS, *Child Maltreatment Report*, 2013

Table 3.6 Child fatalities by type of abuse and neglect in 2012[a]

Type of abuse	# of child fatalities[b]	% of fatalities by maltreatment type
Neglect	919	69.9
Physical abuse	582	44.3
Other[c]	329	25.0
Medical neglect	117	8.9
Psychological abuse	29	2.2
Sexual Abuse	10	0.8

[a]Exposed to more than one maltreatment type
[b]Total Child Fatalities 1,315; Total Maltreatments 1,986
[c]Other is not explained in the U.S. DHHS (2013) report
Data from the U.S. DHHS, *Child Maltreatment Report*, 2013

Childhood Disabilities Precede and Follow CAN

Childhood physical, emotional, intellectual, and sensory disabilities may either precede or follow child maltreatment. Some typically developing children encounter and survive abuse and neglect and often go on to live lives that may appear to be unscathed. Other children go on to live with mild, moderate, or severe disabilities following their abuse and neglect. Many of these children have emotional and behavioral disorders, intellectual disabilities, sensory disabilities such as deafness, blindness, and other medical conditions. Though the U.S. DHHS report statistics on child fatality relative to those who have been exposed to CAN, statistics are not available on children who acquire disabilities following their exposure to CAN. Child fatality statistics that result from acquired disabilities are also not available.

Exercise 3.8: Reflection
Do you find it difficult to think about the maltreatment – neglect, physical, emotional, and sexual abuse of children with and without disabilities? *Do you think it is important to learn as much as you can about this subject? Why? Why not?*

The Newspaper Coverage of ANCD

According to our analysis of 113 unique newspaper stories – some of which were repeated stories – about the ANCD in a large, mid-western urban area, the ANCD is covered mainly in stories involving criminality. Law enforcement personnel, the incarceration of perpetrators, the citation of parents, school personnel, and hospital and long-term placements are examples of the focus of 69 % of the newspaper coverage of ANCD (see Table 3.7). Information stories that provided readers with knowledge and insight about ANCD was the focus of 41.6 % of the newspaper stories. These constituted articles about how to avoid fetal alcohol syndrome, create therapeutic environments for children with disabilities who have been abused and neglected, and special programs to rehabilitate those in need of protection and care. Personal stories of children who had been abused and neglected constituted 8.8 % of the newspaper coverage of ANCD. These stories described children and families who engaged in special education programs, or described adults who had been abused or neglected as children, who have now come to terms with the disabilities that followed.

Neglect of children with disabilities is reported in the newspaper coverage more frequently than any other form of child maltreatment (see Table 3.8). Neglect was the focus of 62.8 % of all the stories of child maltreatment involving children with disabilities. Physical abuse was the focus of 62.0 % of the stories involving the

Table 3.7 Newspaper coverage type of story

Newspaper articles (n = 113)[a]		
Type of story[b]	n	% of total
Criminal case	78	69.0
Informational story	47	41.6
Personal story	10	8.8

[a]Some stories were repeated in subsequent articles and were counted as one story
[b]Percentages over 100 % because some stories combined story types
Data from a study of the newspaper coverage in the *Chicago Tribune*

Table 3.8 Types of maltreatment of children with disabilities

Newspaper articles (n = 113)[a]		
Abuse type[b]	n	% of total
Neglect	71	62.8
Physical Abuse	70	62.0
Sexual Abuse	30	26.5
Psychological Abuse	15	13.2

[a]Some stories were repeated in subsequent articles and were counted as one story
[b]Some stories involved children who were exposed to more than one abuse type
Data from a study of the newspaper coverage in the *Chicago Tribune*

ANCD. Sexual abuse was the focus of 26.5 % of the stories involving ANCD. Stories about abuse and neglect in the lives of children with disabilities also focused on psychological abuse, drug abuse, and discrimination. These types of abuse and neglect also converged in the stories of ANCD, in that some children were neglected and sexually abused, neglected and physically abused, or psychologically abused and physically abused.

In the following section we get behind the numbers in order to examine the newspaper coverage of the ANCD. We will describe the lives of children with disabilities who were exposed to varied forms of abuse and neglect. We will provide case examples of the different types of newspaper coverage, as well as, provide case examples of the physical abuse, sexual abuse, psychological abuse, and neglect to which children with disabilities were exposed.

Getting Behind the Numbers and Meeting the Children and the Adults

Concern about the lives of children who are exposed to abuse and neglect was captured on August 15, 2012. Readers of the *Chicago Tribune* got a lesson in an information newspaper article by reporter Melissa Healy (2012). She stated:

> A child who is spanked, slapped, grabbed or shoved as a form of punishment runs a higher risk of becoming an adult who suffers from a wide range of mental and personality disorders, even when that harsh physical punishment was occasional and when the child experienced no more extreme form of violence or abuse at the hands of a parent or caregiver, says a new study.
>
> Among adults who reported harsh physical punishment short of physical or sexual abuse, psychiatric disorders including depression, anxiety disorders, mania and drug or alcohol dependency were between 2 and 5 percent more common. And more complex psychiatric illnesses marked by paranoia, antisocial behavior, emotional dependency and narcissism were between 4 and 7 percent more likely, according to the study published in the journal *Pediatrics*.

Healy went on to affirm that pediatricians discourage harsh physical punishment and that parents should learn how to use positive reinforcement and other parenting approaches. She concluded her article by stating:

> The current study found that reports of harsh physical punishment were more common in African-American homes than in Caucasian, Asian-American or Pacific Islander households. But researchers also found what they described as "a surprising finding": that as an adult's reported education and income levels increased, so did his or her likelihood of having experienced harsh physical punishment as a child.
>
> The practice of spanking seems to be widespread in the U.S.; a parent's right to discipline a child physically – short of hits that leave bruises or worse – rarely brings legal repercussions. But in recent years, videos of parents spanking or striking their children with repeated blows have sparked angry public debates.

Exercise 3.9: Critical Thinking
Would you agree that Healy provides an example of the potential of a newspaper to educate its audience? *What are your thoughts when you read this article? Does it give you hope for the future?*

In a story that combined information and criminal case the *Chicago Tribune* reported on October 21, 2013 that:

> Pamela Jacobazzi of suburban Bartlett has spent the last 14 years in prison for violently shaking 10-month-old Matthew Czapski to death. The 58-year-old former home day care operator is among hundreds of people nationwide convicted in recent decades on the basis of what doctors call "shaken baby syndrome." That diagnosis gained prominence in the 1980s and '90s, as publicity campaigns warned of the dangers of shaking infants.
>
> In September, though, DuPage County Judge Robert Kleeman rejected her bid for a new trial. He didn't rule on the validity of shaken baby syndrome. Instead, he said her trial attorneys had possessed all available medical evidence and had presented a reasonable defense. But a question lingers here and in similar cases across the U.S.: Is shaken baby syndrome based on shaky science?

This is the most recent development in a long story of a baby boy who died on August 11, 1994. Over the years, Ms. Jacobazzi insisted on her innocence. She denied that she harmed Matthew. In 2005, the lead prosecutor in the case stated that "the swelling in Matthew's brain was so severe that the skull began to shift." Matthew lay in a vegetative state for more than one year before he died. He had taken a fall and had a bump on his head a few days before the shaking incident. Pediatric records also showed that he had a blood disorder that could have predisposed him to injuries. Jacobazzi stated that Matthew had a developmental disability. He could not crawl when he was in her care. She was shocked that she was accused and denied ever shaking Matthew. She is due to be released from prison in 2015.

Lee Scheier (June 12, 2005) of the *Chicago Tribune* reported that thousands of Americans have been sent to prison over the past two decades due to shaken baby charges. Scherer stated that some of these people are guilty of child abuse resulting in shaken baby syndrome but others may be in prison for a crime they did not commit. Scheier stated that critics observe "scientific analysis fails to support shaken baby syndrome and that other causes, such as an accidental fall or a pre-existing medical condition, could be responsible." Shaken baby syndrome is difficult to prove since it most likely occurs without witnesses. The National Center for Shaken Baby Syndrome "using data from U.S. children's hospitals, estimates there are between 1200 and 1400 cases of the syndrome per year in this country, of which 25 % are fatal."

Exercise 3.10: Critical Thinking

Read the newspaper coverage of the case of Pamela Jacobazzi in the *Chicago Tribune* since 1994. You will find nine articles covering this story. *What is your analysis of this story? The medical community and the legal community grabble with cases like this while people in prisons believe that they are innocent. How will this situation be resolved? Make at least three recommendations for future practice in the proper care and treatment of children with disabilities as well as in just and fair legal and medical practice.*

The sexual abuse of girls with disabilities is illustrated in a story in the *Chicago Tribune* on August 31, 2007. The story began "A former Hoffman Estates High School student was sentenced Thursday to 11 years in prison after pleading guilty to molesting a 7-year-old boy and assaulting four mentally handicapped female students." The perpetrator of their sexual abuse was 15 years old when he sexually abused the boy and less than 1 year later he was charged with the abuse of the four girls. The newspaper coverage indicated that:

> Christopher D. Girard, 18, entered the plea to charges of aggravated criminal sexual assault and criminal sexual assault in a hearing before Cook County Circuit Judge Thomas Fecarotta Jr. in the Rolling Meadows courthouse. Fecarotta recommended that Girard, who was 15 at the time of the initial incident but charged as an adult, undergo sex offender counseling in prison. Girard will have to register as a sex offender for life.

The stories of the sexual abuse of males and females are abundant in the newspaper coverage. On November 8, 2009 Lisa Black, *Chicago Tribune* began "Erin Merryn has a tough story to tell. Not everyone wants to hear it, but those who do often cry as they slip her notes or share their own experiences in guarded whispers." As a child she was sexually molested and endured years of emotional and psychological distress. For years Black continued "Merryn had angry outbursts in school early on, then struggled with eating disorders as a teenager, she said." In this story we observe that disability follows CAN. This story also represents a combined information and personal story. Black begins:

> Beginning at age 11, Merryn was sexually molested by an older teenage cousin over an 18-month period. She began to speak out after her younger sister confided that she, too, was being groped and coerced into sexual acts by the same cousin – often while family members celebrated holidays in the next room.

Merryn is speaking up, addressing audiences, and writing about the effects of sexual abuse in her own life and in the lives of children everywhere. Black goes on:

> "People are more afraid of stranger danger," said Merryn, now 24, of Schaumburg, who has written two books on sexual abuse. She uses her pen name to avoid identifying family members.
> "If they took a good look, they would be shocked at how many times this is somebody people trusted with their kids."
> Sexual crimes are difficult enough to report, but as Merryn has found, incest remains even more socially taboo and is often minimized or brushed aside by family members. Even after her cousin, then age 15, confessed to police, was put on juvenile court supervision for 6 months and completed a treatment program, family members "took sides" and do not speak, she said.

Merryn goes on with her life now and "recently started a job as a youth and family therapist at OMNI Youth Services in Buffalo Grove, had finished her first book about her experience when she shocked her parents 2 years ago with another bombshell." Her first experience with sexual abuse was when "... she was raped by a friend's uncle during a 1st-grade sleep-over, a trauma she has described in her new book, 'Living for Today.'"

Exercise 3.11: Reflection
Do you believe that we need more people like Erin Merryn who are willing to talk about the impact of physical and sexual abuse, emotional and psychological abuse,

and neglect in their lives? *Why or why not? Write six statements to support your rationale.*

Implications for Research and Practice

What can researchers and practitioners do to prevent abuse and neglect in the lives of children with and without disabilities? CAN and ANCD will continue as long as we remain unaware of the facts associated with childhood exposure to trauma and as long as we are unwilling to get involved as researchers and practitioners. In this section, we will begin with a set of recommendations for researchers and conclude with a set of recommendations for practitioners.

Recommendations for Researchers

Researchers and practitioners who are aware of the disproportionate ANCD are poised to recognize the signals of child trauma. Arrival at this awareness is complicated by the lack of consensus around what constitutes CAN. Is it possible for parents, caregivers, and the professional community to develop a shared definition of what constitutes the physical abuse of children? Is it possible to establish that hitting children constitutes child physical abuse? We believe that shared and strict definitions of child physical abuse, sexual abuse, emotional abuse, and neglect are essential for parents, caregivers, and professionals in order to stop the exposure of children with and without disabilities the trauma of CAN. Therefore, we recommend that professionals across disciplines:

Recommendation 1:   Build interdisciplinary consensus around shared definitions of child physical, emotional, and sexual abuse as well as of child neglect.

***

The prevention of CAN and ANCD will remain a platitude as long as we fail to realize the magnitude of this egregious social scourge. More compelling and ongoing data need to be generated on abuse and neglect in the lives of children with and without disabilities. Researchers across disciplines and across disability areas have a long way to go in order to articulate the immediate, latent, and long-term impact of CAN. How do children with disabilities differentially experience neglect? Is it possible that a child with an anxiety disorder will be traumatized by being left alone whereas a child with autism will be traumatized by insufficient time alone? Does abuse and neglect manifest differently across disability areas?

Mattison (2014) observed that children who are labeled with psychiatric disorders, such as schizophrenia, depression, or obsessive compulsive disorders, are frequently traumatized by some form of abuse and neglect. How do children who are deaf manifest the impact of their exposure to trauma? What are the immediate signals of this exposure? What are the latent signals? What are the life-long signals? What can be done to modify the immediate, latent, and long-term effects of CAN and ANCD? We observe the need to provide:

Recommendation 2: Private and public funding and interagency collaboration in ongoing and intense basic and applied research on abuse and neglect in the lives of children with and without disabilities.

***

We may dream of a world that is so safe that children with and without disabilities grow and mature to adulthood unscathed by the trauma of CAN. Such a world will remain a dream. We may dream, more realistically, of a world that is safer and more assuring that children are well cared for, live in safety and with appropriate assistance and care as they mature to adulthood. The more we know about the intersection of abuse and neglect and childhood disability the better prepared we are to negotiate its impact when it occurs.

What variables contribute most to children's recovery when they are exposed to trauma in their lives? What differences exist across males and females that contribute to increased vulnerability or increased resilience? What is the contribution of mild, moderate, and severe disability? Are there cultural differences across children with disabilities that increase their vulnerability or resilience during traumatic events? Are there specific protective factors that make a positive difference in children's recovery from exposure to abuse and neglect? We advocate for an organized compilation of research data that guides our in-depth understanding of abuse and neglect in the lives of children across disability areas. We support research efforts to:

Recommendation 3: Conduct comparative, comprehensive, and ongoing research programs to determine the differential impact of abuse and neglect among males and females across age, disability, cultural, and socioeconomic groups.

***

Resources are finite. Too often we experience the unavailability of professional and support personnel to meet the individual needs of children with disabilities. We experience limited and at times no financial support for programming to meet the individual needs of these children. It is therefore essential that we both use the resources we have as wisely as possible and advocate for the needs of these children whenever possible and in the most effective ways. What do we know about the match between recovery from trauma exposure in childhood and the essential features of effective intervention programming? What else do we need to know?

Adult caregivers and professionals who work with children with disabilities who have been abused and neglected are often unaware of the signals of children's trauma exposure (Kenny, 2004; Lusk, Zibulsky, & Viezel, 2015). Some might suspect but are so unsure about their observations that they do nothing. Children are in the best position to recover from abuse and neglect exposure when they are engaged in effective intervention programming.

What do we know about effective interventions and programs to meet the needs of these children? What are the essential characteristics of the most effective programs that mediate trauma exposure among children across an assortment of disabilities? What indicators do children provide to inform us that specific interventions and programs promote their recovery? Are there biological indicators of increased adjustment following trauma exposure? What ongoing data may be generated to indicate enhanced recovery following abuse and neglect in the lives of children with disabilities? Are there specific interventions and programmatic variables that contribute especially to short-term recovery of children of trauma exposure? Are there aspects of ongoing interventions and programs that need to be in place in order to maintain recovery over time? For example, what is the role of peer buddy systems? What is the role of play, rest, and nutrition in these children's lives? Are there characteristics of counseling sessions that are particularly significant in the recovery of these children from traumatic events? What is the role of nontraditional therapeutic interventions including animal therapy, art therapy, dance therapy, and music therapy? Is it possible that involvement in outdoor adventure programming and participation in wilderness programming are particularly significant in children's recovery from traumatic events in childhood? We recommend research on interventions in order to:

Recommendation 4:   Characterize the essential variables of effective interventions and programs that address the recovery of children with and without disabilities who were exposed to traumatic abuse and neglect.

***

Technological advances hold unique promise in the dissemination of research findings. The dissemination of data based findings on CAN and ANCD to multiple audiences, in multiple formats and through multiple outlets is essential. How can technology assist in developing public awareness about the particular vulnerability of children with disabilities to abuse and neglect? How can we use technology to disseminate data based findings on disability as outcome of abuse and neglect in children's lives? What innovative social media might be employed to share facts that would increase general and specific social awareness about CAN and ANCD? We believe that social media can be used to prevent childhood exposure to the trauma of abuse and neglect, therefore:

Recommendation 5: Disseminate the data based findings on abuse and neglect in the lives of children with disabilities to multiple audiences, in multiple formats, and through multiple outlets.

***

Recommendations for Practitioners

How can technology assist in the real-time reporting of child exposure to the trauma of abuse and neglect? Data in this chapter indicate that children who are exposed to traumatic abuse and neglect events are the likely targets of repeated episodes. Children who are repeatedly traumatized are at increased risk for greater medical, educational, social, and emotional morbidity. There are no positive outcomes for repeated exposure to CAN or ANCD. We believe that individualized immediate short-term or long-term supports for a child, family, and caregivers need to be put in place, even before the report of CAN or ANCD is confirmed. We observe the need to:

Recommendation 6: Use technology in real-time reporting of CAN and ANCD and provide immediate supports prior to the confirmation of actual child abuse and neglect.

***

Exercise 3.12: Reflection
Do you believe that immediate and individualized supports need to be put in place for children, families, and caregivers even when CAN and ANCD reports remain unconfirmed? *Write five supporting statements for the provision of immediate individualized supports. Write five statements of risk that might be associated with the provision of immediate supports. Do you believe that the advantages of immediate supports far outweigh the risks that might be associated with them? Provide a rationale to support your conclusions.*

The belief that parents, caregivers, teachers, and others involved in children's lives may use corporal punishment is most troubling. What is the difference between corporal punishment and physical abuse? Under the guise of discipline, corporal punishment is sanctioned in 19 states throughout the United States and in many countries all over the world. Clearly, policy changes need to be made in order to stop the corporal punishment of children. However, this cannot be done without public outcry that recognizes that corporal punishment is a serious issue with far-ranging negative consequences. Practitioners and professionals who work with children are well situated to build relationships with families and advocate on behalf of children. It is ultimately up to us to break through the barriers of ignorance that allow corporal punishment of children with and without disabilities in homes, and in public and private schools and institutions under the veil of "discipline." Parents, caregivers, professionals, and child advocates must work together to:

Recommendation 7: Stop the corporal punishment of children and thereby protect the most vulnearble members of our society.

***

Exercise 3.13: Analysis
Does your school or workplace have a formal CAN prevention program that is supported by the administration and embraced by the staff? If not, what would it take to implement such a program at your school or workplace? *Write five initial steps that need to be taken in order to formalize such a program.*

The practice of accusing caregivers and professionals as perpetrators of CAN and ANCD and relying solely on a law enforcement solution must stop. Calling in law enforcement and accusing perpetrators represents an *all systems failure* to engage in appropriate care and protection of children from traumatic events. An educational approach differs from a punitive approach to CAN and ANCD. An educational approach regards the potential exposure of children to the trauma of abuse and neglect as an opportunity to teach and learn. Child abuse and neglect is anticipated in an educational model and naively unanticipated and punished profoundly, at times, when observed in a law enforcement model.

CAN and ANCD are human phenomenon. We can anticipate their occurrence. What policies and procedures guide caregivers who are at-risk to abuse and neglect their children with and without disabilities? Can we not anticipate that some children with and without disabilities uniquely challenge the social, emotional, and intellectual resources of some especially vulnerable caregivers? Can we not embrace the fact that when caregivers do not understand their children's needs; when they do not have the resources to meet their needs; or when they live in circumstances which prevent them from fulfilling their caregiving roles they are at-risk to abuse and neglect their children? Can we move beyond stigmatizing child abuse, child disability, and the people associated with them? Instead, we recommend that we move toward:

Recommendation 8: A proactive approach that requires the education of parents, caregivers, affirm and professionals on the risks associated with CAN and ANCD and thereby affirm the importance of engaging in prosocial child behavior management.

***

Once interdisciplinary consensus is built around the definition of physical, emotional, sexual abuse, and neglect, the long road of educating the public begins. Professionals across disciplines such as those in medicine, law, and education and related fields have a role in educating the community on the care and treatment of children with and without disabilities. Child maltreatment is one of the most serious threats to public health and its costs to society are immeasurable. We provide more detail on the costs of CAN in Chap. 4. CAN is a preventable public health hazard. The way we manage the behavior of children with and without disabilities is a public concern that requires those who interact with children to have the knowledge and skills to do so without risk to their safety. Therefore we recommend that we:

Recommendation 9: Conduct extensive, intense, and ongoing public programs on child-centered behavior magagement.

***

Once we have established the boundaries of CAN and the appropriate care and treatment of children, we turn our attention to the development of public programs designed to educate parents, professionals, and community members about the characteristics of disability in childhood. The medical community is in an ideal position to engage parents in prenatal programs that promote appropriate care and treatment of children. When parents know prenatally that their child may have a disability they are in an ideal position to maximize their own potential as caregivers and their children's potential as human beings. It is in the parents' best interest to recognize and acknowledge child behaviors of concern at any age. Caregivers are positioned to learn about how to provide appropriate care and protection for their children following their acknowledgement of a child's unique and individualized behavior management needs. Thereby, they prevent potential CAN and avoid potential accusations of child maltreatment.

Exercise 3.14: Reflection
Consider your professional preparation thus far and describe how much you have learned about the forms of abuse and neglect to which children with disabilities are exposed. *Are you convinced that knowing this information is important to your professional preparation? Support your rationale with at least three observations?*

Ignorance of the characteristics of childhood disability promotes the risk of CAN. For example, parents will be well served to know that consistent daily routines will go a long way to provide children with disabilities the care and protection they need. Consistent daily routines are even more essential for children with anxiety disorders, autism, attention deficit disorders, and those with fragile medical conditions. Clearly communicated behavioral expectations are particularly essential for children with intellectual disabilities, emotional and behavioral disorders among others. Parents and caregivers who have a shared understanding of the behavior management needs of children with disabilities are positioned to maximize their own and their children's potential. We observe the need to:

Recommendation 10: Conduct extensive, intense, and ongoing public health care programming on the unique behavior management needs of children across disability areas.

***

Exercise 3.15: Analysis

Do you believe that children with attention deficit disorders might be more at-risk for physical abuse than children with intellectual disabilities? *Consider the different disability conditions under which children are at increased risk of physical, emotional, and sexual abuse? How might these conditions differ from those under which neglect of children with disabilities occurs?*

Data in Chap. 6 indicate that biological parents expose children to abuse and neglect more frequently than any other individuals in their children's lives. These data suggest that biological parents need to be educated about the potential challenges of parenting their children, particularly those with unique needs resulting from their disabilities. Parents will be well served when they are aware that support is available for them when they need it. Parents of very young children are in particular need of support as they adjust to their parenting roles. Prenatal and postnatal medical care providers are in an ideal position to show new parents the resources that are available to them in such organizations as National Down Syndrome Society. Some hospitals have supports in place, such as a new mom's hotline that is available 24 h per day.

The new parents of children with disabilities chart new frontiers and they need time to assimilate new information. There is a unique role for respite care programs in their lives. The administration of medicine, the use of medical supports, such as respiratory machines and sleep apnea machines tumble some new parents into a new world. Their children with disabilities may need medical support 24 h per day. Professionals from pediatricians to feeding specialists, from physical therapists to mobility instructors and early interventionists spin into their world such that their old lives are gone and now they stumble to establish their feet in a new world. They may need financial support, intellectual guidance, or emotional counsel in order to navigate their new world. We observe the need to:

Recommendation 11: Increase the availability of such supports for new parents as crisis nurseries, respite care, hotlines, and parent and caregiver crisis intervention centers.

***

Kenny (2004) found that most teachers report being unaware of the signs and symptoms of the different types of CAN, as well as of reporting procedures despite the fact that they are mandated reporters. Teachers were more likely to recognize the signs of sexual abuse than to recognize the signs of physical abuse. Those who were exposed to child abuse information in their preservice teacher training programs were less likely to recognize the signs of abuse and neglect. They were also less likely to report CAN to the authorities than were teachers who had no preservice exposure to this information. Mathews (2011) suggests that teachers with training, either at the preservice or in-service levels, have higher confidence in their ability to identify the indicators of CAN. They also have higher self-rated knowledge of CAN indicators than those without training. Physicians were significantly more likely to recognize and report CAN than were teachers, even though they described minimal training in their preservice programs (Kenny, 2001). Lusk et al. (2015) found that school psychologists who had knowledge of their roles as mandated reporters accurately recognized the signals of CAN. The findings of these studies illustrate the need for:

Recommendation 12: Ongoing professional development programming to inform professionals about their roles as mandated reporters of abuse and neglect in the lives of children with and without disabilities.

***

Summary

In this chapter, we defined the four most common forms of CAN as physical abuse, sexual abuse, psychological or emotional abuse, and neglect. We also examined the data available in large federal and state databases, and on the research that focuses directly on abuse and neglect in the lives of children with disabilities. From this we explored how the data at an aggregate level informs our knowledge of the scope of the problem, and what abuse types are most common. We presented the data from the findings of an analysis of the newspaper coverage in the *Chicago Tribune* and illustrated these findings with stories of children whose lives remain forever changed because of the abuse and neglect to which they had been exposed. Throughout the chapter, we provided critical thinking and reflection exercises to promote a deeper understanding of the content, to hone our powers of observation, and to brainstorm strategies that we can employ to intervene on behalf of children who are exposed to one type of abuse or another. We concluded this chapter with a set of implications for researchers and practitioners.

References

Black, L. (2009, November 8). Vocal victim fights against a silent crime. *Chicago Tribune*. Retrieved from http://articles.chicagotribune.com/2009-11-08/news/0911070272_1_sexual-abuse-silent-crime-offenders

Caldas, S. J., & Bensy, M. L. (2014). The sexual maltreatment of students with disabilities in American school settings. *Journal of Child Sexual Abuse, 23*(4), 345–366. doi:10.1080/10538712.2014.906530

Chicago Tribune. (2007, August 31). Teen gets 11 years for sex assaults of boy, 4 girls. *Chicago Tribune*. Retrieved from http://articles.chicagotribune.com/2007-08-31/news/0708300920_1_assaulting-molesting-offender

Chicago Tribune. (2013, October 21). Is 'shaken baby syndrome' shaky science? *Chicago Tribune*. Retrieved from http://articles.chicagotribune.com/2013-10-21/opinion/ct-edit-baby-1021-jm-20131021_1_shaken-baby-syndrome-shaking-infants-injured-infants

Child Abuse Prevention and Treatment Reauthorization Act. (2010). CAPTA Reauthorization Act (2010). P.L. 111–320. Retrieved from https://www.childwelfare.gov/systemwide/laws_policies/federal/index.cfm?event=federalLegislation.viewLegis&id=142

Farrell, C. (2015). *Corporal punishment in U.S. schools*. Retrieved from http://www.corpun.com/counuss.htm#stats

Global Initiative to End All Corporal Punishment of Children. (2014, June). End all corporal punishment of children. *Newsletter*, 27. Retrieved from http://www.endcorporalpunishment.org/pages/frame.html

Healy, M. (2012, August 15). Study links spanking to mental health problems. *Chicago Tribune*, 5. http://search.proquest.com/chicagotribune/docview/1033473494/C39CA52EFC0340D5PQ/1?accountid=11578

Holden, G. W., Williamson, P. A., & Holland, G. W. (2014). Eavesdropping on the family: A pilot investigation of corporal punishment in the home. *Journal of Family Psychology, 28*(3), 401–406. doi:10.1037/a0036370

Jones, L., Bellis, M. A., Wood, S., Hughes, K., McCoy, E., ... Officer, A. (2012). Prevalence and risk of violence against children with disabilities: A systematic review and meta-analysis of observational studies. *Lancet, 380*(9845), 899–907. doi:10.1016/S0140-6736(12)60692-8

Kenny, M. (2004). Teachers' attitudes toward and knowledge of child maltreatment. *Child Abuse and Neglect, 28*, 1311–1319. doi:10.1016/j.chiabu.2004.06.010

Kenny, M. C. (2001). Child abuse reporting: Teachers' perceived deterrents. *Child Abuse & Neglect, 25*(1), 81–92.

Lusk, V. L., Zibulsky, J., & Viezel, K. (2015). Child maltreatment identification and reporting behavior of school psychologists. *Psychology in the Schools, 52*(1), 61–76. doi:10.1002/pits.21810

Mandell, D. S., Walrath, C. M., Manteuffel, B., Sgro, G., & Pinto-Martin, J. A. (2005). The prevalence and correlates of abuse among children with autism served in comprehensive community-based mental health settings. *Child Abuse & Neglect, 29*(12), 1359–1372. doi:10.1016/j.chiabu.2005.06.006

Mathews, B. (2011). Teacher education to meet the challenges posed by child sexual abuse. *Australian Journal of Teacher Education, 36*(11), 13–32. Retrieved from http://dx.doi.org/10.14221/ajte.2011v36n11.4

Mattison, R. E. (2014). The interface between child psychiatry and special education in the treatment of students with emotional/behavioral disorders in school settings. In H. M. Walker & F. M. Gresham (Eds.), *Handbook of evidence-based practices for emotional and behavioral disorders* (pp. 104–126). New York, NY: Guilford.

Mueller-Johnson, K., Eisner, M. P., & Obsuth, I. (2014). Sexual victimization of youth with a physical disability: An examination of prevalence rates, and risk and protective factors. *Journal of Interpersonal Violence, 29*(17), 3180–3206. doi:10.1177/0886260514534529

Rose, C. A., Espelage, D. L., & Monda-Amaya, L. E. (2009). Bullying and victimisation rates among students in general and special education: A comparative analysis. *Educational Psychology, 29*(7), 761–776. doi:10.1080/01443410903254864

Sandgrund, H., Gaines, R., & Green, A. (1974). Child abuse and mental retardation: A problem of cause and effect. *American Journal of Mental Deficiency, 79*, 327–330. Retrieved from http://psycnet.apa.org/psycinfo/1975-09726-001

Scheier, L. (2005, June 12). Shaken baby syndrome: A search for truth. *Chicago Tribune*. Retrieved from http://articles.chicagotribune.com/2005-06-12/features/0506120513_1_child-abuse-syndrome-shaken

Sevlever, M., Roth, M., & Gillis, J. (2013). Sexual abuse and offending in autism spectrum disorders. *Sexuality & Disability, 31*(2), 189–200. doi:10.1007/s11195-013-9286-8

Sobsey, D. (1994). *Violence and abuse in the lives of people with disabilities: The end of silent acceptance?* Toronto, ON: Brooks.

Sobsey, D. (2002). Exceptionality, education, and maltreatment. *Exceptionality, 10*(1), 29–46. doi:10.1207/S15327035EX1001_3

Sommarin, C., Kilbane, T., Mercy, J. A., Maloney-Kitts, M., & Ligiero, D. P. (2014). Preventing sexual violence and HIV in children. *Journal of Acquired Immune Deficiency Syndrome, 66*(2), 217–223. doi:10.1097/QAI.0000000000000183

Soylu, N., Alpaslan, A. H., Ayaz, M., Esenyel, S., & Oruc, M. (2013). Psychiatric disorders and characteristics of abuse in sexually abused children and adolescents with and without intellectual disabilities. *Research in Developmental Disabilities, 34*(12), 4334–4342. doi:10.1016/j.ridd.2013.09.01

Sparrow, S. S., Cicchetti, D. V., & Balla, D. A. (2005). Vineland adaptive behavior scales. In *Survey forms manual* (2nd ed.). Circle Pines, MN: American Guidance Service.

U.S. Department of Health and Human Services, Administration for Children and Families, Administration on Children, Youth and Families, Children's Bureau. (2013). *Child maltreatment 2012*. Retrieved from http://www.acf.hhs.gov/programs/cb/research-data-technology/statistics-research/child-maltreatment

Viezel, K. D., Lowell, A., Davis, A. S., & Castillo, J. (2014). Differential profiles of adaptive behavior of maltreated children. *Psychological Trauma: Theory, Research, Practice, and Policy, 6*(5), 574–579. doi:10.1037/a0036718

Weiner, M. T., Day, S. J., & Galvan, D. (2013). Deaf and hard of hearing students' perspectives on bullying and school climate. *American Annals of the Deaf, 158*(3), 324–343. doi:10.1353/aad.2013.0029

Wells, M., & Mitchell, K. J. (2014). Patterns of internet use and risk of online victimization for youth with and without disabilities. *The Journal of Special Education, 48*(3), 204–213. doi:10.1177/0022466913479141

World Health Organization (WHO). (2014). *World report on violence and health*. Retrieved from http://www.who.int/violence_injury_prevention/violence/world_report/chapters/en

Zeedyk, S. M., Rodriguez, G., Tipton, L. A., Baker, B. L., & Blacher, J. (2014). Bullying of youth with autism spectrum disorder, intellectual disability, or typical development: Victim and parent perspectives. *Research in Autism Spectrum Disorders, 8*(9), 1173–1183. doi:10.1016/j.rasd.2014.06.001

Zirpoli, T. J. (1990). Physical abuse: Are children with disabilities at greater risk? A look at the facts. *Intervention in School and Clinic, 26*(6), 6–11. http://eric.ed.gov/?id=EJ421409

Helpful Resources for Further Study

Child Welfare Information Gateway. (2012). *The risk and prevention of maltreatment of children with disabilities*. Washington, DC: U.S. Department of Health and Human Services, Children's Bureau.

Individuals with Disabilities Education Improvement Act (IDEA). (2004). (20 U.S.C. §§ 1400 et seq). S. 2781–111th Congress: Rosa's Law. (2009). In www.GovTrack.us. Retrieved from http://www.govtrack.us/congress/bills/111/s2781

Shaken baby syndrome http://www.mayoclinic.com/health/shaken-baby-syndrome/DS01157 National Center on Shaken Baby Syndrome http://www.dontshake.org/sbs.php? topNavID=3&subNavID=22

Southern Poverty Law Center (SPLC). http://www.splcenter.org/what-we-do/teaching-tolerance Education, litigation, and advocacy are the primary tools used by SPLC to teach tolerance and seek justice and develop equal opportunity in the United States for its most vulnerable members, including those with disabilities. SPLD provides educators with free resources designed to teach school children "to reject hate, embrace diversity and respect differences.

Chapter 4
The Outcomes of Abuse and Neglect in the Lives of Children with Disabilities

Be the change that you want to see in the world.
(Mohandas Gandhi, lawyer, political and spiritual leader in India, 1869–1948.)

Abstract The negative outcomes of abuse and neglect in the lives of children with and without disabilities are immeasurable. These outcomes are observable in negative physical, emotional, and psychological short- and long-term effects. Child fatality is the result of abuse and neglect in the lives of some children with and without disabilities. In this chapter we examine the data on the outcomes of abuse and neglect (CAN) and abuse and neglect of children with disabilities (ANCD) provided by the U.S. DHHS. We analyze the literature in this area and present the findings of a study on the newspaper coverage that focused specifically on abuse and neglect in the lives of children with disabilities. We present stories from the *Chicago Tribune* from 2004 to 2010 that illustrate the prevailing trends in these data. We conclude this chapter with a set of recommendations for researchers and practitioners. Throughout the chapter we provide reflections and critical thinking exercises.

The immediate, short- and long-term outcomes of the abuse and neglect of children with and without disabilities are devastating. These outcomes are often well hidden and frequently underestimated (Akbas et al., 2009). The physical, intellectual, and emotional traumas that children with and without disabilities endure in such aversive circumstances often mark the entire lifespan of each child.

The immediate marks of CAN and ANCD are observed in emergency rooms and among children assigned to hospital beds. Still, many outcomes remain unidentified. In the long-term, such outcomes as, psychiatric disorders and addictions remain unconnected to the original traumas sustained by children due to their abuse and neglect. Traumatized children continue to live their lives, albeit hurt and injured, and some do not survive. Some children with disabilities who have sustained such traumas acquire added disabilities that frequently go unrecognized. Regardless of their disabilities and with appropriate and intensive intervention, it is possible for some children to live long, strong, and fulfilled lives.

© Springer International Publishing Switzerland 2016   83
E.P. Crowley, *Preventing Abuse and Neglect in the Lives of Children with Disabilities*, DOI 10.1007/978-3-319-30442-7_4

Exercise 4.1: Reflection

List as many predictable and immediately observable short- and long-term effects of

CAN as you can. These effects may be observed into adulthood or they may never be observed directly during the life-span. *Are you surprised by either how few or how many effects you listed?*

What exactly do we know about the outcomes of abuse and neglect in the lives of children with disabilities? How do they fare following their abuse and neglect? What information do we have? What national databases might lead the way in the development of our understanding and thereby assist us in our attempts to reclaim and recover the lives of as many children as possible? Too often, those who have been abused and neglected are retargeted for future abuse and neglect. Rather than prevention in the first place, this chapter focuses on after-the-fact information that is essential to data based intervention and prevention. Chapter 10 provides an examination of and recommendations for intervention and prevention programming. According to the World Health Organization (WHO), violence against children happens on a daily basis in every country all over the world (2014). The WHO provides a list of the long-term disabilities that are often associated with the outcomes of violence against children. These include such injury-related disabilities as:

- Physical and/or cognitive limitations due to neurotrauma
- Paralysis due to spinal cord trauma
- Partial or complete amputation of limbs
- Physical limb deformation resulting in mobility impairments
- Psychological trauma
- Sensory disability such as blindness and deafness

Child maltreatment has observable and measurable effects on children's growth and development. The traumatic effects of CAN globally are summarized in the United Nations (UN) *Secretary-General's Study on Violence Against Children* (2006). According to the UN the top six effects are:

1. physical health problems such as changes in the development of the brain, injuries, bruises, and fractures
2. difficulties in dealing with other people
3. learning problems
4. finding it hard to express feelings in a way that other people can understand
5. emotional health problems including anxiety, depression, aggression directed toward self or others
6. being more likely to do dangerous things like using drugs or having sex at a very young age

In this chapter we will examine what the U.S. DHHS (2013) database tells us about the outcomes of ANCD. We will then examine the data based findings in the professional literature as well as in the newspaper coverage. Finally, we will get behind the numbers and provide case examples of the outcomes of abuse and neglect in the lives of real children with real disabilities from birth to 18 years of age.

The Outcomes of Child Abuse and Neglect at the National Level

The U.S. DHHS, Children's Bureau publishes a report on child maltreatment in the United States annually. Data are provided on the child disability category designation relative to CAN (see Chap. 2). No data in this report focus directly on the outcomes of abuse and neglect in the lives of children with disabilities per se. Therefore, we do not have data on how children with disabilities fare following their abuse and neglect. For example, we do not know how many children with disabilities were diagnosed with additional disabilities following their abuse and neglect. We do not know how many children with disabilities actually survived the abuse and neglect to which they were subjected. Furthermore, we do not know how many children with disabilities were removed from their homes, schools, or from their residential placements following their abuse and neglect.

Data from the U.S. DHHS indicate that between 2008 and 2012, an average of 1610 children died every year following their abuse and neglect. In 2012, 1593 children died as a result of abuse and neglect. Among 100,000 children an estimate of 2.2 children die as a result of their exposure to abuse and neglect in the United States annually. We may wonder how many of these children have disabilities.

The data on child fatality due to abuse and neglect underestimates the extent of this problem due to some very obvious reasons and to other less obvious ones. For example, the U.S. DHHS reports the total child fatality data from two sources. The total number is the sum of the data from state child files and state agency files. In 2012, only 44 out of 50 (88 %) of the states reported data on state child fatalities resulting from CAN in child files and only 41 out of 50 (82 %) states reported data on child fatalities resulting from CAN in state agency files. In Idaho, Maine, and Massachusetts no data (blank entries) were entered on child fatalities in either the state child files or the state agency files. Further analysis of the statistics indicates a wide range in the number of child deaths resulting from child maltreatment in 2012. For example, Vermont reported zero child fatalities resulting from CAN in both the state child files and the state agency files in 2012. Table 4.1 provides a closer look at the states with the lowest child fatality rate per 100,000 children resulting from CAN in the United States in 2012.

Arkansas reported the highest child death rate per 100,000 children in 2012 (see Table 4.2). No data from the U.S. DHHS indicate an estimate of how many of these children had disabilities but based on the prevailing evidence, that we discussed in Chap. 1, up 25 % of these children and perhaps more had disabilities. Texas and Florida reported the highest number of unique children who died as a result of CAN in 2012. In Texas – a total of 215 child fatalities were reported (213 reported in state child files and 2 from state agency files) in Florida – a total of 179 child deaths were reported (179 reported in state child files and 0 in state agency files).

In addition, the U.S. DHHS (2013) reports that from 2008 to 2012, a total of 8052 died as a result of abuse and neglect in the United States. We may be confident that this number represents an underestimation of the scope of deaths resulting from

Table 4.1 Child fatality among states reporting lowest rates[a] per 100,000 children

State	n	Child fatality rate per 100,000 children
Vermont	0	.00
New Hampshire	1	.36
Rhode Island	1	.46
North Dakota	1	.65
Connecticut	6	.76
Minnesota	10	.78

Data from the U.S. DHHS, *Child Maltreatment Report*, 2013
[a]Absent from the U.S. DHHS *Child Maltreatment Report*, 2013 are child fatality statistics in agency and child files from Idaho, Maine, and Massachusetts

Table 4.2 Child fatality in the six highest states[a] reporting per 100,000 children, 2012

State	n	Child fatality rate per 100,000 children
Arkansas	33	4.6
Florida	179	4.5
Louisiana	42	3.8
Colorado	40	3.3
Illinois	108	3.5
New Mexico	16	3.1

Data from the U.S. DHHS, *Child Maltreatment Report*, 2013
[a]Absent from the U.S. DHHS *Child Maltreatment Report* are statistics from Idaho, Maine, and Massachusetts

CAN. For example, in 2008 and 2009 no data were provided by North Carolina, in 2011 no data were provided by Massachusetts and as stated above, Idaho, Maine, and Massachusetts, neither state nor state agency statistics on child fatality were provided in 2012. Though incomplete, these data provide at least a conservative estimate of the potential scope of the CAN that result in child fatalities in the United States. Based on data from the U.S. DHHS report in 2013, during the last 5 years on average 1610, and most probably more, children died each year as a result of injuries sustained from CAN. Furthermore, we may safely conclude that children with disabilities were indeed disproportionately represented among these children.

What Else Do We Know About the Outcomes of CAN and ANCD?

The statistics provided by the U.S. DHHS do not differentiate the outcomes of abuse and neglect in the lives of children with and without disabilities. We examine these statistics in order to get a foothold for a deeper understanding of the CAN and potentially of ANCD. For example, once abuse and neglect of children is confirmed, what happens next? Do they return home? If not, where do they go?

Table 4.3 Child victims of CAN who received foster care and only in-home services in 2012

Type of child maltreatment	% in foster care	n	% in-home services	n
Neglect	66.6	(97,219)	60.6	(140,865)
Two of more types of maltreatment	18.3	(26,666)	13.8	(32,137)
Physical abuse	7.7	(11,291)	12.5	(29,118)
Other maltreatment	2.7	(3,949)	0.7	(1,695)
Sexual abuse	2.4	(3,545)	6.3	(14,631)
Psychological maltreatment	1.5	(2,256)	5.0	(11,663)
Medical neglect	0.8	(1,150)	1.0	(2,403)
Unknown	0.0	(7)	0.0	(5)
Total	100.0	146,083	100.00	232,517

Data from the U.S. DHHS, *Child Maltreatment Report*, 2013

Data from the U.S. DHHS (2013) indicate that 38.6 % of the children with and without disabilities who were confirmed victims of CAN were placed in foster care in 2012 and 61.4 % received only in-home services. In-home services are defined as any service provided to the family while the child remains in their homes. Children who received foster care services were removed from their families and also might have received in-home services. The most children to receive these services were those who were neglected. The second largest group of children who received these services experienced two or more types of abuse and neglect. See Table 4.3 for details on the types of abuse and neglect experienced by children who were subsequently placed in foster care or who received in-home care.

In 2012, it took an average of 47 days to initiate services for children who were abused and neglected. Over 20 % (21.4 %) of them became involved in court actions and 17.1 % received court-appointed representatives (U.S. DHHS, 2013). These data also indicate that during the previous 5 years, 14.7 % of these children received family preservation services and 5.2 % had been reunited with their families. We may wonder about the assortment – the quality and extent of the institutional responses to the needs of children with and without disabilities who are victimized by abuse and neglect on a daily basis.

Exercise 4.2: Critical Thinking

How might we derive focused data on the potentially different outcomes of abuse and neglect of children with disabilities? In what ways might the outcomes of abuse and neglect of children with and without disabilities differ? *Select one of these questions and consider how making this information available might increase our potential to protect children with and without disabilities from the, too often, deadly abuse and neglect to which they are exposed.*

The Outcomes of CAN and ANCD for Perpetrators

We might well wonder whether the outcomes of CAN and ANCD differ for the perpetrators? How frequently are perpetrators actually found guilty of CAN and ANCD? What financial burdens are incurred by immediate families and local communities due to CAN and ANCD? Do the state, regional, and national level financial burdens incurred following the abuse and neglect of children with and without disabilities differ? These and other questions go on and on and failure to address them perpetuates violence against the most vulnerable among us.

The social burden of CAN is immeasurable. To what extent are we aware of the real cost of CAN of children with and without disabilities in our own communities, as well as at the state and at national levels? How many children reappear in the next year's statistics? How might we calculate the actual projected costs of the abuse and neglect of children with and without disabilities on a year-by-year basis?

Exercise 4.3: Reflection
Now it is your turn! Make a list of questions you would like to ask about the abuse and neglect of children with disabilities? Think of every possible question of interest to you. *Pick the most compelling questions and consider who could possibly provide the answers you seek? What challenges get in the way? Can you think of ways to overcome these challenges?*

Now we turn to the findings of researchers who have examined compelling questions about the outcomes of abuse and neglect in the lives of children with disabilities.

What Do Researchers Say About the Outcomes of Child Abuse and Neglect?

Researchers affirm that abuse and neglect in childhood is associated with a host of negative disabling short- and long-term outcomes (Lu et al., 2013; Norman et al., 2012; Sobsey, 1994, 2002; Stalker & McArthur, 2012; Wier, Hao, Owens, & Washington, 2013). These outcomes vary widely and are determined by such variables as a child's age and developmental status at the time the abuse or neglect occurred (Child Welfare Information Gateway Children's Bureau, 2013). Physical abuse, neglect, and sexual abuse or a combination of these differentially impact child outcomes. The severity and the frequency of exposure to CAN as well as the relationship of the perpetrator affect child outcomes.

In the short-term, emergency room medical staff may be the first to encounter children who have been abused and neglected. Weir and her colleagues (2013) found that injuries and poisonings, which are potentially both preventable and disabling, most frequently bring children to emergency rooms. Respiratory disorders and nervous system disorders take second and third places. Weir and her colleagues also found that children wind up in emergency rooms due to mental and behavioral health conditions. In the short-term, children with and without disabilities who are abused and neglected may exhibit bruises, cuts, or burns. They may exhibit broken bones, seizures, hemorrhages, and even death.

Researchers link a multitude of long-term disabling effects with CAN. Norman et al. (2012) identified the link between abuse and neglect with delinquency, childhood depression, and bipolar disorders. Data indicate that children who have been abused and neglected exhibit a host of self-destructive behaviors including alcoholism and drug use. More than a third of adolescents who have a record of abuse or neglect have a substance use disorder before their 18th birthdays (Wilson, Dolan, Smith, Casanueva, & Ringeisen, 2012). Furthermore, these children are three times more likely to have these problems than are their peers who do not have a report of abuse or neglect.

Other long-term disabling effects of CAN have been identified by researchers. These include mental illnesses which are manifested in a range of emotionally disabling internalizing and externalizing behaviors (Cohen, Berliner, & Mannarino, 2010; Liu, 2010; Mallett, Dare, & Seck, 2009); hyporesponsivity (Ford, Fraleigh, Albert, & Connor, 2010); schizophrenia (Gil et al., 2009); chronic fatigue syndrome, eating disorders, and a range of psychiatric and somatic manifestations (Fuemmeler, Dedert, McClernon, & Beckham, 2009; Reinberg, 2010; Ross, 2009; Scott, 2007; Wilson, 2010).

Lu and colleagues (2013) found that among 851 individuals with long-term severe mental illnesses and probable posttraumatic stress disorders in adulthood, sexual abuse in childhood loomed large. Among the most common traumatic childhood events reported by both adult males and females were witnessing and experiencing domestic violence, warfare, robberies, and stranger assaults. The most traumatic of all events self-reported were exposure to the sudden death of a loved one and exposure to childhood sexual abuse by adults and peers. Lu and colleagues found that 28.8 % of these adults exhibited major depressive disorders and 18.3 % exhibited other mood disorders. Schizophrenia and schizoaffective disorders were observed 14.5 % of the participants in this study. Bipolar, anxiety, posttraumatic stress, and adjustment disorders, acute stress, and eating disorders were among the clinical characteristics of these participants.

The cycle of abuse and neglect often goes on and on from one generation to the next. For some adults the exposure to abuse and neglect in childhood is associated with an increased probability of disorganized and punitive parenting and consequent, negative effects across family generations (Avery, Hutchinson, & Whittaker, 2002; Dilillo, Tremblay, & Peterson, 2000; Kim, Noll, Putnam, & Trickett, 2007; Kim, Trickett, & Putnam, 2010; Roberts, O'Connor, Dunn, & Golding, 2004; Ruscio, 2001).

Self-Perpetuating Abuse and Neglect

Bones (2013) argues that the prevailing social perceptions of their vulnerability uniquely dispose children with disabilities to be the targets of abuse and neglect. Bones adds that children with disabilities who have been abused and neglected are more vulnerable to repeated abuse and neglect throughout their life spans. Lu and colleagues (2013) found that the participants in their study experienced an average of seven different traumatic events in childhood and sexual abuse was the most commonly reexperienced traumatic event.

Exercise 4.4: Critical Thinking
Researchers observe that once children with disabilities have been abused physically, sexually, or emotionally or once they have experienced neglect they are at heightened risk of repeated victimization. *Have you ever considered the impact of repeated abuse and neglect? Does it surprise you that children with disabilities may be exposed to repeated acts of abuse and neglect? Write three reasons why you think that repeated acts of abuse and neglect would affect a child with a disability differently than would a singular episode of abuse and neglect?*

The High Cost and Low Awareness of CAN and ANCD

It is not possible to overestimate the high cost of short- and long-term negative outcomes resulting from the CAN (Fang, Brown, Curtis, & Mercy, 2012). The physical health effects alone bring about a host of negative outcomes. These include, but are not limited to, head trauma, impaired brain development, poor physical health, difficulties during infancy, poor mental, and emotional health. Additionally, cognitive and social difficulties, juvenile delinquency and adult criminality, alcohol and other drug abuse and the continued cycle of abusive behaviors that go on and on into future generations (Child Welfare Information Gateway Children's Bureau, 2013).

The negative outcomes of abuse and neglect in childhood do not stop at the individual and family levels. These outcomes ripple outwards to unfathomable societal losses. According to the U.S. Centers for Disease Control (CDC) (2013) the lifetime direct cost of CAN and ANCD and related fatalities for 1 year alone is $124 billion. Together these negative outcomes cost more than the combined cost of stroke and Type 2 diabetes (CDC, 2013). The long-term indirect negative outcomes of abuse and neglect in childhood are indeed immeasurable. Examples of these losses include the social, emotional, and economic instability of individuals and families, their increased use of the health care system, the high cost of juvenile and adult crime, mental illness, substance abuse, and the ongoing cycle of domestic violence.

Despite the evidence about the high physical, emotional, and intellectual costs of CAN and ANCD, Corso, Ingels, and Roldos (2013) found that among randomly selected adults in the United States, there is little awareness of these facts. Only 25 % of respondents in the United States indicated that they had personal experience with CAN. In Ecuador, only 50 % of the respondents indicated such personal experience with CAN. However, when asked, respondents in Ecuador were more willing than respondents in the United States to spend money in order to prevent the occurrence of CAN.

In the next section we will focus directly on the outcomes data based on the findings of the newspaper coverage of abuse and neglect in the lives of children with disabilities. We will describe these findings and illustrate them with stories of real children with disabilities who were exposed to abuse and neglect.

Newspaper Coverage and Outcomes

An in-depth analysis of the newspaper stories provides a lens through which we may see the outcomes of ANCD more clearly. First, we analyze the types of articles used to cover these stories, and then we analyze the outcomes as described in these articles.

Most of the newspaper coverage of the ANCD are stories about criminal cases in which specific instances of ANCD were detailed. The second most frequent stories focused on providing information to readers. These stories focused on such topics as the impact of head injuries or falls on children. The third most frequent stories were those in which individuals recounted their own personal memories and experiences with CAN. For more details on the types of stories in the newspaper coverage of ANCD, see Chap. 3.

Outcomes of ANCD Up Close

The newspaper coverage of the ANCD provides readers with information about the outcomes of the abuse and neglect. Outcomes include continued investigation of the circumstances of the abuse and neglect, death, disability, and removal of the child from the environment in which the abuse and neglect occurred. The most frequent outcome described in stories about the ANCD was law enforcement involvement (see Table 4.4). The second and third most frequent outcome were under investigation and the death of a child with a disability following his/her abuse and neglect. The fourth most frequent outcome was an acquired disability following CAN. The removal of the child with a disability from his/her family/home was the outcome described in 15 % of the stories. A cluster of assorted outcomes described included incarceration of the perpetrator, assignment to a rehabilitation program, and recommended reforms of the legal system.

Table 4.4 The outcomes of abuse and neglect of children with disabilities (n = 113)

Outcome type	n	%
Law enforcement involvement	45	39.8
Under investigation	36	31.9
Death	33	29.2
Acquired disability	31	27.4
Removed from family/setting	17	15.0

Data from a study of the newspaper coverage in the *Chicago Tribune*

Percentages can be over 100 % due to multiple categories present in each story

More Up-Close Outcomes

Acquired child disability perpetrated by biological parents was the most common outcome described in stories of ANCD. This outcome was described in 15 out of 113 stories (13.3 %) (see Table 4.5). Involvement with law enforcement personnel described the outcomes following ANCD by an assortment of perpetrators including doctors, police officers, and juvenile detention staff. This outcome was described in 39.8 % of the stories. Deaths of children with disabilities perpetrated by biological parents were the outcomes described in 9.7 % of the stories. Other common outcomes of ANCD described in the newspaper coverage included the removal of children from their homes and cases that were under investigation.

The most frequently occurring overall outcome of ANCD was the involvement of law enforcement personnel. The second most frequent overall outcome was under investigation.

Investigations of ANCD were conducted by supervising hospital or care facility personnel, education or service agency personnel, or other family service personnel. The deaths of children with disabilities following their abuse and neglect were the third most prevailing outcome. The fourth most prevailing overall outcome was child disability resulting from abuse and neglect. For more specific details on the overall outcomes see Table 4.5.

Exercise 4.5: Critical Analysis

What information on Tables 4.4 and 4.5 surprises you most? Do you expect that this coverage is similar to the newspaper coverage of similar stories in any part of the United States? *Review your own local newspaper coverage of ANCD during the last month and consider the similarities and differences in your findings across these two data sources.*

Table 4.5 Prevailing outcomes of ANCD (n = 113 stories)[a]

Perpetrators	n	Child disability	Removed from family	Death	Under investigation	Law enforcement
Mother/father	33	15	9	11	9	7
Others i.e. peers, babysitters, roommates etc.	27	2	2	9	11	13
School personnel	14	0	0	1	7	7
Missing/unknown	11	3	2	1	1	4
Priest/minister	6	0	2	1	1	5
Stranger	6	2	0	4	2	4
Legal guardian	5	0	2	3	2	2
Relative	4	2	0	1	1	1
Multiple perpetrators	3	6	0	1	1	1
Family friend	2	1	0	1	0	1
Foster parent	2	0	0	0	1	0
Total	113	27.4	15.0	29.2	31.9	39.8

Data from a study of the newspaper coverage in the *Chicago Tribune*
[a]n of specific story outcomes exceeds number of stories due to multiple outcomes

The Lives of Children and Adults Represented in the Statistics

Chicago Tribune reporter, Christy Gutowski described the following case of neglect of a child with a disability that was under investigation and involved potential criminal perpetrator behavior. The story was published in the *Chicago Tribune* on June 8, 2012:

> When teenager Darlene Armstrong arrived at the emergency room curled on a stretcher, she weighed a skeletal 23 pounds. In serious condition, the 16-year-old had cerebral palsy and couldn't walk or talk, but the stunned medical staff also focused on her shriveled 3-foot-10-inch frame, her sunken cheeks and protruding ribs.

Continued efforts to understand the predicament of this child are illustrated in the following excerpt:

> When questioned by hospital staff in March, Harris said Darlene has lost about 10 pounds in the last three weeks but appeared healthy. Authorities were incredulous at the mother's story.
> "There is no way that this child eats what mom is describing," wrote a social worker at Comer Children's Hospital. It is unclear if mom is intentionally fabricating the history for fear of 'getting in trouble' or if mom truly believes she had been feeding her as described."
> The records show police found that Harris got various benefits, including Social Security, to help with Darlene's care.
> The woman's oldest daughter, Delichia Armstrong, 23, said her mother would never harm her children.
> "My mom does the best she can, that's the truth," she said.

Darlene and her younger sister were taken into protective custody while their mother was placed on probation for 18 months and ordered to attend parenting classes.

The death of a child with a disability was indicated as the outcome of the abuse and neglect in almost one third of the stories. In an excerpt from a story on September 23, 2012, once again Christy Gutowski wrote:

> Jay'Meon Wyatt, 21 months, Chicago. Died July 18, 2010. Two months before Jay'Meon died, the child abuse hotline received an urgent call. A nurse said she had just left a Bronzeville apartment and was worried about the disabled toddler who weighed 13 pounds. She said his mother, Doulesha Wyatt, refused to go to the hospital because her husband "doesn't like people in their business."
> The investigator was at the door within hours of the call. She determined the home was safe enough for Jay'Meon and his two sisters even though the mother had a bloody wound and might have been stabbed, according to records.

As in the literature, the link between CAN and disability as outcome is clearly apparent in the newspaper coverage. Stories that describe disability, medical complications, and eventual death resulting from CAN are illustrated in a story by Lee, Schlikerman and Gorner (March 9, 2011):

> On Monday, Oyeyinka, 17, died at Rush University Medical Center. After an autopsy Tuesday, the Cook County medical examiner's office ruled her death was a homicide – due in part from lack of oxygen to the brain from blunt head trauma years ago as well as pneumonia and complications from diabetes.

Acquired disabilities following CAN documented in the newspaper in 2012 alone included such conditions as, posttraumatic stress disorder, severe depression, anxiety, mania, drug and alcohol dependency, mental health issues, and personality disorders. For example, in the case of a 47 year old male, while recalling his personal experiences with CAN stated that he had been diagnosed with attention deficit hyperactivity disorder and bipolar disorder.

Other Outcomes of the Abuse and Neglect of Children with Disabilities

The newspaper coverage indicated other outcomes of ANCD including the jail and prison sentences of perpetrators, assignment to drug rehabilitation programs, parenting classes, not guilty verdicts, adoptions denied, and the recommendation of medical and psychological treatments. Legal reforms, new procedures pending, and stiffer fines were also observed in these data. The prison sentence outcome is described in the following excerpt from "20 years for drugging son" (Ward, 2012, September 25):

> An Elmhurst woman, who drugged her young son, reportedly in an attempt to kill him, was sentenced Monday to 20 years in prison by a DuPage County judge who said he found her actions almost inconceivable. Cheryl Luchetta, 42, had pleaded guilty earlier this year to aggravated battery of a child for feeding her 7-year-old son up to 18 pills – a mixture of

Tylenol and prescription sedatives – before cutting her own throat at the apartment they shared.

The judge said a pre-sentence report indicated that Luchetta had mental health issues. There was testimony that the boy has attention deficit hyperactivity disorder and was used to receiving medication from his mother.

Abuse and neglect disrupt the school life of many children with disabilities. Placements in special schools, home-based programs and simply absenteeism result. Yajaira Rivera missed 68 days of school in 1 year due to medical, emotional, and psychological disorders (Jackson & Marx, 2012). We will discuss her story in more detail in Chap. 9.

Law enforcement, child protection agencies, and service organizations have been overwhelmed by the number of reports of CAN in recent years. This is due in part to reduced personnel and budgetary limitations. The procedures of the most recent Department of Children and Family Services (DCFS), 2010) indicate that following an investigation:

> By law, the decision must be made within 60 days, but usually the decision is announced within 30 days. The investigator can make one of two findings: a report can be "unfounded" when there is no credible evidence that the child was abused or neglected or a report can be "indicated" when there is credible evidence that the child was abused or neglected. Credible evidence means that the facts gathered by the investigator would lead a reasonable person to believe that a child has been abused or neglected.

Outcomes are not known for many cases of reported CAN. The Illinois Department of Children and Family Services (DCFS) reported on alleged victims of CAN from July 1 to August 31, 2014. Only 1754 of the alleged 17,003 child victims of abuse and neglect were indicated. In July 1, 2013–2014 only 32,898 of the 109,769 children who were alleged victims of CAN in Illinois Department of Children and Family Services (2014) were indicated. For many children, including those with disabilities, reports of abuse and neglect often drag on for months, all the while, the children remain at-risk for further harm.

Information Articles

Informative articles focus on such topics as legal protections, the relationship between substance abuse and disability, and the proposed or actual procedural changes in organizations following accusations of the abuse and neglect. Other information articles focus on the development of parent and caregiver knowledge about the potential link between disability and CAN. Melissa Healy (August 15, 2012) provides parents with information on the dangers of spanking their children. She wrote:

> A child who is spanked, slapped, grabbed or shoved as a form of punishment runs a higher risk of becoming an adult who suffers from a wide range of mental and personality disorders, even when that harsh physical punishment was occasional and when the child

experienced no more extreme form of violence or abuse at the hands of a parent or caregiver, says a new study.

This article informs readers about the very clear connection between the potential injuries to children following physical abuse.

In another information article, by Stuart Kaplan (June 29, 2011), "Mommy, Daddy, am I really bipolar?: Hundreds of thousands of children in the U.S. have been wrongly diagnosed with the trendy disorder, argues a noted psychiatrist. And the results can be tragic." Readers learn about the professional challenges inherent in the effort to differentiate between psychiatric disorders and CAN. The author:

> ... identified Rebecca as suffering from pediatric bipolar disorder at the age of 2. (The psychiatrist concluded that Rebecca's two siblings were bipolar as well). In addition to diverting the psychiatrist from the very real problem in Rebecca's family – a well-chronicled history of child abuse – the diagnosis led to the prescription of a common cocktail of medications. Rebecca's parents misused one of these medications – clonidine, prescribed to treat high blood pressure in adults but also given to children because of its sedative effects – to quiet their child. Forever. "There was no waking her up," Rebecca's mother stated on "60 Minutes." (The psychiatrist later settled the malpractice suit for $2.5 million).

Information stories provide readers with knowledge that potentially prevents disability. An example of such newspaper coverage is in an article titled, "Maternal drinking and its effects on children" by Bonnie Miller Rubin, September 26, 2012. The information provided in this article has potential to prevent CAN and subsequent disability. The following excerpt illustrates this potential:

> The Centers for Disease Control and Prevention, U.S. surgeon general, American Academy of Pediatrics, American Congress of Obstetricians Gynecologists and others advise women who are pregnant or could be pregnant to abstain from alcohol because of the risk of birth defects. There is no known safe type or amount of alcohol during pregnancy. Leading authorities like Dr. Ira Chasnoff here in Chicago are expanding practitioner training nationally so doctors are comfortable addressing maternal alcohol use and can diagnose FASD and turn to intervention strategies when necessary.

Personal Stories

Eleven percent of the newspaper coverage of the abuse and neglect of children with disabilities describes personal stories of abuse and neglect. In the article "Putting bin Laden and pain behind me" Hovitz (May 3, 2011) began by stating "Osama bin Laden is dead and I'm finally beginning to understand the phrase, "fear tends to age you." I am Helaina, 21, daughter of Denise and Paul, granddaughter of Lucy and Charles . . .." This article makes it clear that the impact of current events change the lives of some children forever. This author went on to say:

I was 12 years old.

My grandparents were too frail to be relocated. We remained in Southbridge Towers along with hundreds, maybe thousands of others, without water, phones, elevators, electricity or anybody to help us.

Whirlwinds of ash blew into my grandparents' apartment as the fiery remains of the twin towers burned into ashes.

My life was overtaken by panic, fear, paranoia, insomnia, feelings of detachment and alienation, apprehension, shame, despair, difficulty controlling impulsivity and emotions, self-destructive behavior, substance abuse, severe mood changes, fear of abandonment, and the loss of a sense of safety, trust and self-worth.

This is what governed my journey from childhood to adulthood in the aftermath of the attacks.

I contemplated suicide most days between the ages of 14 and 19.

This author describes the memoir she is preparing and shows clearly that unless provided the appropriate intervention, there is no end to the potential destruction of emotional and psychological trauma she might have experienced. She writes:

In 2009, I finally found a doctor who saved my life and helped me begin to heal. I learned to overcome many of my fears. I learned to be self-sufficient, to stop caring what others said or did. I learned to let go of my desire to control what I could not. I am well on my way to recovery, cultivating a healthy and fulfilling life. My wounds of 9/11 may reopen, but now, when I step outside my front door, I see a structure on its way to standing tall, filling what's been missing for 10 years.

Overall, stories that refer to the outcomes of the abuse and neglect of children with disabilities most frequently focus on criminality and the ongoing investigation that ensues. Death of the child with disability was a common outcome of ANCD. Disability that resulted from CAN and the removal of the child from the family were other common outcomes. Informational stories accounted for close to 40 % of the articles and personal stories accounted for 11 % of the coverage. To what extent do the data from an analysis of the newspaper coverage corroborate with the interdisciplinary data generated on the abuse and neglect of children with disabilities?

Implications for Research and Practice

Researchers and practitioners must be aware that abuse and neglect are manifested unpredictably in childhood. Children who have been denied appropriate care and protection may be physically ill and exhibit an assortment of physical symptoms including respiratory disorders, eating and sleeping disorders among others discussed in this chapter. They may seem angry and generally unhappy. They may exhibit aggression in their acting-out behaviors or they may withdraw and isolate themselves in depression and anxiety disorders. Much remains unknown in our understanding of the outcomes of abuse and neglect in the lives of children with and without disabilities. Here we will consider recommendations for researchers and practitioners that focus on the potential important contributions of basic and applied research and public awareness programming about the abuse and neglect of children with and without disabilities.

The Crucial Role of Basic and Applied Research

Basic and applied researchers have the potential to innovate this field such that the impact of trauma might be understood and potentially reversed. Initial observations indicate that the exposure of children's lives to abuse and neglect has life-long traumatizing effects. Physical, emotional and sexual abuse and neglect of any kind change human beings at the most fundamental levels. Biological and neurological changes occur that forever alter the lives of these children. The changes following traumatic events may be observed in detrimental effects on children's health, education, social, and emotional well-being. We know little about the specifics of the biological and neurological effects of such trauma. We know even less about its effects relative to disability in childhood. For example, does abuse and neglect affect children with intellectual disabilities differently than their nondisabled peers? Does exposure to trauma effect children with sensory impairments, autism, cerebral palsy, or any other disability, differently than it does their nondisabled peers? We use the word disability with little consideration of its epistemological roots. These roots have potentially profound implications for children's education and treatment.

How might the effects of abuse and neglect be differentiated and ameliorated in childhood? Is there potential for biological reversal of these effects? Is there potential for neurological renewal for those who have been exposed to traumatic events? These are among the questions that mark the frontiers of our knowledge base on the effects of abuse and neglect in childhood. Therefore, we need to:

Recommendation 4.1: Develop a focused research agenda to examine the potential reversal of the effects of abuse and neglect in the lives of children with and without disabilities.

***

Researchers in a variety of disciplines have crucial contributions to make in understanding the outcomes of abuse and neglect in children's lives. Researchers in the forensic sciences have much to contribute to this area by unveiling and chronicling the biological and neurological changes brought about by varied forms of abuse and neglect in childhood. When these changes are understood, researchers in an assortment of disciplines, including the biological and social sciences as well as in psychology, education, and related fields might unveil and chronical potential effective interventions. For example, Pasqualone and Michel (2015) make it very clear that innovative nursing programs include professional preparation of nurses such that they, more readily, observe the impact of trauma in their patients' lives and make therapeutic professional decisions based on their own behavioral observations of their patients. Thus, the work of researchers in a variety of disciplines is essential for an increased understanding of the outcomes of abuse and neglect in childhood. This increased understanding will potentially lead to more effective intervention and prevention. We advocate for increased:

Recommendation 4.2: Interdisciplinary research that focuses on unveiling and observing the effects of abuse and neglect in the lives of children with and without disabilities.

***

Public Awareness Programming on Violence – Abuse and Neglect in Children's Lives

To what extent are we comfortable talking about abuse and neglect in children's lives? Do we so want to avoid difficult and disturbing topics that we quickly steer the conversation to the latest sports' news, the newest movie, or the beautiful weather? Abuse and neglect in the lives of children with disabilities adds a new shudder to the subject. The stigma of disability remains to this day (Chiu, Yang, Wong, & Li, 2015; Viezel & Davis, 2015). Who wants to talk about disability in children's lives? We often ignore the disability, as long as possible, with the belief that ignoring it will somehow manage to make it go away. Abuse and neglect will not go away just because we wish that it would and neither will disability, thus we are left with the challenge of acknowledging and embracing reality. This implies that we:

Recommendation 4.3: Work to reduce the stigma associated with abuse and neglect in children's lives as well as the stigma associated with disability.

***

Violence is one of the leading human hazards in modern society and children's lives are overexposed to it. To what extent are people aware of violence in the lives of children with and without disabilities? Are fathers, mothers, extended family members, neighbors, teachers, and others who have access to children's daily routines aware that children are exposed to violence on a daily basis? Are they aware that the lives of some of these children are at risk of injury and death? To what extent are people aware that children die as a result of exposure to violence – abuse and neglect on a daily basis in countries all over the world? An estimated average of 1,500 children die each year as a result of child abuse and neglect in the United States alone and 80 % of these children are under 4 years old. The average documented cost of child abuse and neglect in the United States is an estimated $124,000,000,000.00 per year (Children's Bureau, 2014).

To what extent do we have a mythical understanding of the violence that is perpetrated in children's lives? Do we believe that child physical, emotional and sexual abuse, as well as child physical and emotional neglect occurs, but only among children who live far away, in some distant and nameless countries that are devoid of the infrastructure that is necessary to provide for their basic human provisions? To what extent are people aware that this violence begins in their own homes, in their own families, in the homes of their extended families and in their local neighborhoods? From there, the impact of violence expands outwards and limitlessly beyond the reaches of our imaginations and into generations after generations. Thus, we:

Recommendation 4.4: Promote and support public awareness programs that expose the truth about violence – abuse and neglect; its deadly and life-long impact on the lives of children and for generations to come.

*** *

Childhood disability both precedes and follows abuse and neglect. Children with a variety of disabilities, including intellectual disabilities, autism, physical disabilities, low incidence disabilities, such as blindness and deafness, exhibit a host of characteristics that challenge caregivers and members of their families and communities. When the characteristics of their disabilities are not understood, children are at increased risk for abuse and neglect. To what extent are family members prepared to care for infants and toddlers with disabilities? Do they know what to expect of their children with disabilities as they grow older? Do they know where to turn when they need help? To what extent are there supports in place that provide them with the information, resources, and services that they need as they care for their children with disabilities? It is essential that:

Recommendation 4.5: Upon diagnosis, the child with a disability and the child's immediate family must be provided with needed ongoing information, support, services, and resources in order to meet the unique needs of the child and those of the family of which they are part.

*** *

The American Humane Association (2013) explains that in the area of emotional abuse:

> ... some parents may emotionally and psychologically harm their children because of stress, poor parenting skills, social isolation, lack of available resources or inappropriate expectations of their children. They may emotionally abuse their children because the parents or caregivers were emotionally abused themselves as children.

The Butler Institute for Families (2014a, 2014b) provides participants with the knowledge and skills they need to support families and members of their own local community during times of particular need. They provide training for local community members to participate in *Communities Now*. The families of children with disabilities are empowered by the support that their own families, neighbors, and members of the communities provide. When their needs and the needs of their children with disabilities are understood clearly, they are in a better position to protect their children from every form of abuse and neglect. Support, such as a few hours of child care, can provide a parent with needed respite and it can also provide a child with a disability with an opportunity to experience a supportive and inclusive community. Thus we encourage:

Recommendation 4.6: Providing support to families at the local level in order to protect them from overwhelming stress, isolation, and lack of resources.

***

Exercise 4.6: Reflection
Are there programs in your community that are designed to support families during particularly challenging circumstances such as child care challenges, job loss, bereavement, financial stress, work related stress, or illness? *Identify a list of at least five such programs. If you note any particularly glaring community needs, consider what you can do to address them?*

During intake procedures, doctors, nurses, dentists, education, law enforcement, and other service professionals will serve children more effectively when they are aware of the emotional and physical markers of abuse and neglect. Their protocols will reflect reality more reliably when questions about abuse and neglect are included in essential information before treatment. Hiding abuse and neglect of children with and without disabilities does a disservice to everyone including the child and the professionals involved. Children's lives are changed following abuse and neglect and what might otherwise constitute effective treatment, falls short for children who have been exposed to traumatic experiences of abuse of any kind. We encourage professionals to uncover any trace of abuse and neglect in the children in their care and upon doing so, proceed with awareness and sensitivity to the unique needs that may result from this exposure. It is essential to:

Recommendation 4.7: Include questions about exposure to child abuse and neglect in intake forms at schools, hospitals and in other health, education, law enforcement and related professional service settings in order to match the child and service needs.

***

How well-versed are law enforcement personnel on the manifestation of abuse and neglect among children with disabilities? Is it possible that a police officer who observes the cries of a child who has autism would dismiss such cries? Is it possible that a child with a communication disorder would dial 911 and be unable to communicate information about an emergency? Is it possible that a nurse would delay responding to the call button of a child with cerebral palsy, such that, upon arrival the child had already died following a choking episode? Parents and professionals have unique roles when they are providing services to children with disabilities. We encourage:

Recommendation 4.8: Service delivery personnel to be alert to disability characteristics and their contribution to increased vulnerability in children's lives.

***

Exercise 4.7: Analysis
The markers of abuse and neglect of children with and without disabilities are numerous
and diverse. *Why might the markers of abuse and neglect of children with disabilities be even more numerous and diverse? List at least five reasons why professionals might miss these markers among children with intellectual disabilities, communication disorders, and physical disabilities and among those with emotional and behavioral disorders?*

Observe the lives of children in your community. When you look around at your local community do you see that children with disabilities comprise an integral part? Do they participate in children's programs, or community activities such as picnics, fairs, and exhibits? Are they engaging in the life of the community in age appropriate ways? Are they accepted? Are their mobility needs met? Do they have access to every possible age appropriate aspect of the community? Community members who engage in such observation will go a long way to meeting the needs of children with disabilities and develop the kind of inclusive settings that maximize the potential of children with disabilities. Inclusive communities promote the safety and well-being of children with disabilities. Children in inclusive communities are poised to become participating members of their communities and will, more likely find their place as contributing members of society. In such circumstances, everyone wins!

On the other hand, upon looking around our community do you observe that accidents occur more frequently in specific playgrounds? Are children engaged in frequent automobile accidents? Do you observe newspaper coverage of stories about child abuse and neglect that illustrate common themes such as children who are home alone? Are the homeless shelters in your community particularly crowded? Have you observed children begging for food or shelter? Have you observed children unattended? Have you thought about the fact that homeless children are at higher risk of abuse and neglect? Community statistics illustrate community needs. Therefore:

Recommendation 4.9: Examine the data on child care and treatment at local, state and national levels in order to identify gaps in supports and services for children with and without disabilities.

***

Once a report of child abuse and neglect is substantiated the immediate initiation of intense and ongoing services is warranted. Currently, this is not happening in the United States. Data from the U.S. DHHS (2013) *Child Maltreatment* report indicates that on average, it takes 47 days before services are initiated for children who have substantiated cases of abuse and neglect in the United States. Specifically, in Illinois – 37 days pass before child services are initiated following the confirmation that a child was abused and neglected. It takes longest to initiate such services in Alabama; there it takes 133 days to initiate services for children who are traumatized by abuse and neglect. In the District of Columbia, it takes only 4 days to initiate such services to children with substantiated cases of abuse and neglect.

Long durations before the initiation of services for 20 % of substantiated cases are especially serious in the context of the 80 % of the reported cases of child abuse and neglect that are not substantiated (U.S. DHHS, 2013). We might well wonder what services might be needed by those children whose reports were unsubstantiated? Might we need to provide support, perhaps less formal and less intense for the 80 % of those who, for some reason, came to the attention of someone who was concerned about their health and safety? Children who are abused and neglected need to be provided with intense and ongoing support when their abuse and neglect in substantiated and therefore it is necessary to:

Recommendation 4.10: Reduce the duration between the initial report and the initiation of services for children with substantiated trauma exposure and consider the services that might be needed by children whose abuse and neglect is unsubstantiated.

***

Focused attention to the egregious outcomes of abuse and neglect are increasing with every passing year. In 2009, and from the White House Briefing Room, President Barack Obama declared April as National Child Abuse Prevention Month and in his letter to the public he stated:

> As we recognize that we all suffer when our children are abused, that we all benefit from mutual concern and care, and that we all have a responsibility to help, more American children will grow up healthy, happy, and with unlimited potential for success.
>
> NOW, THEREFORE, I, BARACK OBAMA, President of the United States of America, by virtue of the authority vested in me by the Constitution and laws of the United States, do more hereby proclaim April 2009, as National Child Abuse Prevention Month. I encourage all citizens to help prevent and respond to child abuse by strengthening families and contributing to all children's physical, emotional, and developmental needs.
>
> IN WITNESS WHEREOF, I have hereunto set my hand this first day of April, in the year of our Lord two thousand nine, and of the Independence of the United States of America the two hundred and thirty-third.

Prevent Child Abuse America and its state Chapters deserve our support. The International Society for the Prevention of Child Abuse and Neglect deserves our support. The American Humane Association (2014) and countless organizations that focus their missions on the health and safety of children deserve our support. Government personnel and agencies that are dedicated to data generation about vital statistics on child abuse and neglect deserve our support and cooperation at every possible juncture. The abuse and neglect of children is an emergency and we must:

Recommendation 4.11: Provide increased support to people and organizations that are dedicated to preventing abuse and neglect. We must also increase our support to people and organizations that provide resources and services to children and families already traumatized by abuse and neglect.

***

The effects of abuse and neglect in the lives of children with disabilities are so harmful that the only sensible solution is to engage in every effort possible to prevent it from occurring in the first place. The participation of every member of society is needed in order to ensure that the human dignity of every child is acknowledged and their every need is taken seriously. There is no defense for exposing children to trauma that is perpetrated by deliberate abusive and neglectful behaviors. The high costs associated with intervention far exceed any calculation of prevention costs. Become an advocate for child health and safety and:

Recommendation 4.12: Above all, participate in every effort to prevent the abuse and neglect of children with and without disabilities.

***

Reflection

Which of the recommendations above seems more significant to you? *How might you participate in addressing the outcomes of abuse and neglect in your own personal or professional endeavors?*

Chapter Summary

Beyond the numbers, percentages, and disability category data, there is surprisingly little information in the national databases about the ANCD. Data from research in this area indicate the immeasurably harmful short- and long-term effects of CAN and ANCD. The newspaper coverage indicates that most stories about the ANCD focus on the criminality and on the ongoing effort to investigate the specific details of what happened. The next most common outcome was that of the death of the child with a disability. The newspaper coverage makes a very clear connection between the disability outcome as a consequence of child abuse and neglect. Finally, we may be optimistic about the information articles that focus specifically on providing coverage of critical – prevention and intervention – information about the ANCD.

References

Akbaş, S., Turla, A., Karabekiroğlu, K., Pazvantoğlu, O., Keskin, T., & Böke, O. (2009). Characteristics of sexual abuse in a sample of Turkish children with and without mental retardation, referred for legal appraisal of the psychological repercussions. *Sexuality & Disability, 27*, 205–213. doi:10.1007/s11195-009-9139-7

American Humane Association. (2013). *Emotional abuse.* Retrieved from http://www. americanhumane.org/children/stop-child-abuse/fact-sheets/emotional-abuse.html

American Humane Association. (2014). *Child abuse and neglect: Together we can help families and children.* Retrieved from http://www.americanhumane.org/children/programs/child-abuse-neglect-prevention/

Avery, L., Hutchinson, K. D., & Whitaker, K. (2002). Domestic violence and intergenerational rates of child sexual abuse: A case record analysis. *Child and Adolescent Social Work Journal, 19*(1), 77–90. Retrieved from http://link.springer.com/article/10.1023/A:1014007507349#page-1

Bones, P. D. C. (2013). Perceptions of vulnerability: A target characteristics approach to disability, gender, and victimization. *Deviant Behavior, 34*(9), 727–750. doi:10.1080/01639625.2013.766511

Butler Institute for Families. (2014a). *Strong systems, strong communities, strong families.* Retrieved from http://thebutlerinstitute.net/

Butler Institute for Families. (2014b). *Communities now: Connecting for kids.* Retrieved from http://www.thebutlerinstitute.org/why-do-we-need-communities-now/

Child Welfare Information Gateway Children's Bureau. (2013). *Long-term consequences of child abuse and neglect* (Factsheet). Retrieved from https://www.childwelfare.gov

Children's Bureau. (2014). Child abuse statistics. *National Children's Alliance, Child Help.* Retrieved from http://www.statisticbrain.com/child-abuse-statistics/

Chiu, M. Y. L., Yang, X., Wong, H. T., & Li, J. H. (2015). The mediating effect of affective stigma between face concern and general mental health–The case of Chinese caregivers of children with intellectual disability. *Research in Developmental Disabilities, 36*, 437–446. doi:10.1016/j.ridd.2014.10.024

Cohen, J. A., Berliner, L., & Mannarino, A. (2010). Trauma focused CBT for children with co-occurring trauma and behavior problems. *Child Abuse & Neglect, 34*(4), 215–224. doi:10.1016/j.chiabu.2009.12.003

Corso, P. S., Ingels, J. B., & Roldos, M. I. (2013). A comparison of willingness to pay to prevent child maltreatment deaths in Ecuador and the United States. *International Journal of Environmental and Research and Public Health, 10*(4), 1342–1355. doi:10.3390/ijerph10041342

Department of Children and Family Services (DCFS). (2010). *Reports of child abuse and neglect.* http://www.state.il.us/dcfs/docs/ocfp/procedure/Procedures_300.pdf

Dilillo, D., Tremblay, G. C., & Peterson, L. (2000). Linking childhood sexual abuse and abusive parenting: The mediating role of maternal anger. *Child Abuse & Neglect, 24*(6), 767–779. doi:10.1016/S0145-2134(00)00138-1

Fang, X., Brown, D., Curtis, F. S., & Mercy, J. A. (2012). The economic burden of child maltreatment in the United States and implications for prevention. *Child Abuse & Neglect, 36*(2), 156–165. doi: 10.1016/j.chiabu.2011.10.006

Ford, J. D., Fraleigh, L. A., Albert, D. D., & Connor, D. F. (2010). Child abuse and autonomic nervous system hyporesponsivity among psychiatrically impaired children. *Child Abuse & Neglect, 34*(7), 507–515. doi:10.1016/j.chiabu.2009.11.005

Fuemmeler, B. F., Dedert, E., McClernon, F. J., & Beckham, J. C. (2009). Adverse childhood events are associated with obesity and disordered eating: Results from a US population- based survey of young adults. *Journal of Traumatic Stress, 22*(4), 329–333. doi:10.1002/jts.20421

Gil, A., Gama, C. S., deJesus, D. R., Lobato, M. I., Zimmer, M., & Belmonte-de-Abreu, P. (2009). The association of child abuse and neglect with adult disutility in schizophrenia and the prominent role of physical neglect. *Child Abuse & Neglect, 33*(9), 618–624. doi:10.1016/j.chiabu.2009.02.006

Gutowski, C. (2012a, June 8). DCFS failed 23-pound teen girl. *Chicago Tribune*. Retrieved from http://articles.chicagotribune.com/2012-06-08/news/ct-met-dcfs-starved-girl-20120606_1_dcfs-data-kendall-marlowe-neglect

Gutowski, C. (2012b, September 23). How DCFS failed these kids. *Chicago Tribune*. Retrieved from http://search.proquest.com/docview/1058488235?accountid=11578

Healy, M. (2012, August 15). Study links spanking to mental health problems. *Chicago Tribune*. Retrieved from http://search.proquest.com/docview/1033473494?accountid=11578

Hovitz, H. (2011, May 3). Putting bin laden and pain behind me. *Chicago Tribune*. Retrieved from http://articles.chicagotribune.com/2011-05-03/opinion/ct-oped-0502-recovery-20110503_1_panic-attacks-bin-childhood

Illinois Department of Children and Family Services. (2014, August 31). *Child abuse and neglect statistics*. Retrieved from http://www.state.il.us/dcfs/docs/canstat.pdf

Jackson, D., & Marx, G. (2012, November 13). A challenge unmet. *Chicago Tribune*. Retrieved from http://search.proquest.com/docview/1151262036?accountid=11578

Kaplan, S. L. (2011, June 29). Mommy, daddy, am I really bipolar? *Chicago Tribune*. Retrieved from http://articles.chicagotribune.com/2011-06-29/opinion/ct-oped-0629-bipolar-20110629_1_bipolar-disorder-psychiatrist-diagnosis

Kim, K., Noll, J. C., Putnam, F. W., & Trickett, P. K. (2007). Psychosocial characteristics of nonoffending mothers of sexually abused girls: Findings from a prospective, multigenerational study. *Child Maltreatment, 12*(4), 338–351. doi:10.1177/1077559507305997

Kim, K., Trickett, P. K., & Putnam, F. W. (2010). Childhood experiences of sexual abuse and later parenting practices among non-offending mothers of sexually abused and comparison girls. *Child Abuse & Neglect, 34*(10), 610–622. doi:10.1016/j.chiabu.2010.01.007

Lee, W., Schlikerman, B., & Gorner, J. (2011, March 9). Teen dies of shaken baby syndrome. *Chicago Tribune*. Retrieved from http://articles.chicagotribune.com/2011-03-09/news/ct-met-shaken-baby-death-20110308_1_baby-syndrome-autopsy-rules-child-abuse-deaths

Liu, R. T. (2010). Early life stressors and genetic influences on the development of bipolar disorder: The roles of childhood abuse and brain-derived neurotrophic factor. *Child Abuse and Neglect, 34*(7), 516–522. doi:10.1016/j.chiabu.2009.10.009

Lu, W., Yanos, P. T., Silverstein, S. M., Mueser, K. T., Rosenberg, S. D., Gottlieb, J. D., ...Giacobbe, G. (2013). Public mental health clients with severe mental illness and probable posttraumatic stress disorder: Trauma exposure and correlates of symptom severity. *Journal of Traumatic Stress, 26*, 266–273. doi:10.1002/jts.21791

Mallett, C. A., Dare, P. S., & Seck, M. M. (2009). Predicting juvenile delinquency: The nexus of childhood maltreatment, depression and bipolar disorder. *Criminal Behavior and Mental Health, 19*(4), 235–246. doi:10.1002/cbm.737

Norman, R. E., Byambaa, M., De, R., Butchart, A., Scott, J., & Vos, T. (2012). The long-term health consequences of child physical abuse, emotional abuse, and neglect: A systematic review and meta-analysis. *PLoS Medicine, 9*(11), e1001349. doi:10.1371/journal.pmed.1001349

Obama, B. (2009). *National child abuse prevention month, 2009*. Retrieved from http://www.whitehouse.gov/the_press_office/Presidential-Proclamation-Marking-National-Child-Abuse-Prevention-Month/

Pasqualone, G., & Michel, C. (2015). Forensic patients hiding in full view. *Critical Care Nursing Quarterly, 38*(1), 3–16. doi:10.1097/CNQ.0000000000000043

Reinberg, S. (2010). Childhood trauma tied to chronic fatigue syndrome. *Health Day Reporter*, Tuesday, January 6, 2010. http://www.cfids.org

Roberts, R., O'Connor, T., Dunn, J., & Golding, J. (2004). The effects of child sexual abuse in later family life: Mental health, parenting and adjustment of offspring. *Child Abuse & Neglect, 28*(5), 525–545. doi:10.1016/j.chiabu.2003.07.006

Ross, C. A. (2009). Psychodynamics of eating disorder behavior in sexual abuse survivors. *American Journal of Psychotherapy, 63*(3), 211–226. http://psycnet.apa.org/psycinfo/2009-24391-001

Rubin, B. M. (2012, September 26). Maternal drinking and its effects on children. *Chicago Tribune*. Retrieved from http://articles.chicagotribune.com/2012-09-26/news/xt-x-0926- expert-donaldson-20120926_1_fetal-alcohol-spectrum-disorders-fasd-prenatal-alcohol-exposure

Ruscio, A. M. (2001). Predicting the childrearing practices of mothers sexually abused in childhood. *Child Abuse & Neglect, 25*(3), 369–387. doi:10.1016/S0145-2134(00)00252-0

Scott, S. T. (2007). Multiple traumatic experiences and the development of posttraumatic stress disorder. *Journal of Interpersonal Violence, 22*(7), 932–938. doi:10.1177/0886260507301226

Sobsey, D. (1994). *Violence and abuse in the lives of people with disabilities: The end of silent acceptance?* Toronto, Canada: Brooks.

Sobsey, D. (2002). Exceptionality, Education, and Maltreatment, *Exceptionality, 10*(1), 29–46. Retrieved from http://dx.doi.org/10.1207/S15327035EX1001_3

Stalker, K., & MacArthur, K. (2012). Child abuse, child protection and disabled children: A review of recent research. *Child Abuse Review, 21*(1), 24–40. doi:10.1002/car.1154

U.S. Centers for Disease Control and Prevention. (2013). *Injury prevention & control: Traumatic brain injury*. Retrieved from http://www.cdc.gov/TraumaticBrainInjury/index.html

U.S. Department of Health and Human Services, Administration for Children and Families, Administration on Children, Youth and Families, Children's Bureau. (2013). *Child maltreatment 2012*. Retrieved from http://www.acf.hhs.gov/programs/cb/research-data-technology/statistics-research/child-maltreatment

United Nations. (2006, August). *United Nations Secretary-General's study on violence against children adapted for children and young people*. Retrieved from http://www.unicef.org/violencestudy/pdf/Study%20on%20Violence_Child-friendly.pdf

Viezel, K. D., & Davis, A. S. (2015). Child maltreatment and the school psychologist. *Psychology in the Schools, 52*(1), 1–8. doi:10.1002/pits.21807

Ward, C. (2012, September 25). 20 years for drugging son. *Chicago Tribune*. Retrieved from http://articles.chicagotribune.com/2012-09-24/news/chi-elmhurst-mom-gets-20-years-for-drugging-7yearold-son-20120924_1_cheryl-luchetta-drug-dealer-elmhurst-mom

Wier, L. M., Hao, Y., Owens, P., & Washington, R. (2013, June). *Overview of children in the emergency department, 2010* (HCUP Statistical Brief #157). Rockville, MD: Agency for Healthcare Research and Quality. Retrieved from http://www.hcup-us.ahrq.gov/reports/statbriefs/sb157.pdf

Wilson, D. R. (2010). Health consequences of childhood sexual abuse. *Perspectives in Psychiatric Care, 46*(1), 56–65. doi:10.1111/j.1744-6163.2009.00238.x

Wilson, E., Dolan, M., Smith, K., Casanueva, C., & Ringeisen, H. (2012). *NSCAW child well-being spotlight: Adolescents with a history of maltreatment have unique service needs that may affect their transition to adulthood* (OPRE Report #2012-49) Washington, DC: Office of Planning, Research and Evaluation, Administration for Children and Families,

U.S. Department of Health and Human Services. Retrieved from http://www.acf.hhs.gov/sites/default/files/opre/youth_spotlight_v7.pdf

World Health Organization. (2014). *Injury-related disability and rehabilitation*. Retrieved from http://www.who.int/violence_injury_prevention/disability/en/

Helpful Resources for Further Study

"The Risk and Prevention of Maltreatment of Children with Disabilities." The bulletin Highlights some additional sources of national data for these children, including the National Incidence Study of Child Abuse and Neglect (NIS). Retrieved from https://www.childwelfare.gov/pubs/prevenres/focus/focus.pdf

American Academy of Pediatrics website was recommended in the August 15, 2012 article and specific reference was made to the negative outcomes associated with spanking. www.aap.org

Child Welfare Information Gateway: "Statistics on abuse and neglect of children with disabilities." Retrieved from http://www.acf.hhs.gov/sites/default/files/cb/cm2012.pdf#page=56

Child Welfare Information Gateway: The risk and prevention of maltreatment of children with disabilities (2012, March). https://www.childwelfare.gov/pubs/prevenres/focus/focus.pdf

National Survey of Child and Adolescent Well-Being (NSCAW) Project. (1997–2013). NSCAW is a national representative, longitudinal survey of children and families who have been the subjects of investigation by child protective services agencies. Retrieved from http://www.acf.hhs.gov/programs/opre/research/project/national-survey-of-child-and adolescent-well-being-nscaw-1

Wilson, E., Dolan, M., Smith, K., Casanueva, C., & Ringeisen, H. (2012). *NSCAW child well-being spotlight: Adolescents with a history of maltreatment have unique service needs that may affect their transition to adulthood* (OPRE Report #2012-49). Washington, DC: Office of Planning, Research and Evaluation, Administration for Children and Families, U.S. Department of Health and Human Services. Retrieved from http://www.acf.hhs.gov/sites/default/files/opre/youth_spotlight_v7.pdf

World Health Organization. (2014). *Injury-related disability and rehabilitation*. Retrieved from http://www.who.int/violence_injury_prevention/disability/en/

Part II
What Do We Know About the Perpetrators of Abuse and Neglect of Children with Disabilities?

Chapter 5
The Age and Sex of the Perpetrators of Abuse and Neglect in the Lives of Children with Disabilities

*If a country is to be corruption free ... three key societal members make a difference. They are the father, the mother and the teacher. (*A. P. J. Abdul Kalam, Former President of India, b. 1931)

Abstract Who perpetrates the ANCD? If we can anticipate the perpetrators of abuse and neglect in the lives of children with disabilities we have a greater chance of anticipating it and interrupting it. In this chapter and in the next two chapters, we focus on getting to know the characteristics of the perpetrators of child abuse and neglect (CAN) and abuse and neglect of children with disabilities (ANCD). We begin with a focus on the chronological age characteristics of these people. We might wonder whether perpetrators are young, middle-aged, or old. We might also wonder whether there are inherent patterns across perpetrator ages. Then we will focus on the prevailing patterns across the sex of perpetrators. Are there patterns we might recognize across males and females? We examine the research findings and present data from and analysis of newspaper coverage of ANCD. We illustrate our findings from stories from the newspaper coverage and conclude the chapter with a set of recommendations for researchers and practitioners.

Few people stop long enough to think about who might be the perpetrators of CAN and ANCD. The assumption among many is that this topic is remote and affects the lives of only few people (Corso, Ingels, & Roldos, 2013). We believe that the development of awareness and the provision of readily available information about abuse and neglect in the lives of children with and without disabilities are essential for effective intervention and prevention programming. In this chapter we will focus on getting to know the perpetrators.

What do we know about the characteristics of the perpetrators of ANCD? Who are these people? How old are they? Are they males or females? More specifically, what patterns distinguish the age and sex characteristics of the perpetrators of the ANCD? Caregivers, professionals and program developers who know this information have a higher chance of developing relevant abuse and neglect intervention and prevention programs for children with and without disabilities. Children with disabilities will be better served when they and those who care about their health,

© Springer International Publishing Switzerland 2016
E.P. Crowley, *Preventing Abuse and Neglect in the Lives of Children with Disabilities*, DOI 10.1007/978-3-319-30442-7_5

safety and welfare can anticipate the prevailing characteristics of their potential perpetrators.

First, we will analyze what the data in the most recent U.S. DHHS, *Child Maltreatment* report (2013) tell us about the age and sex characteristics of the perpetrators of abuse and neglect in the lives of children with and without disabilities? Then we will analyze the findings in the professional literature which addresses the age and sex patterns of perpetrators of ANCD. We present an analysis of the data on the newspaper coverage of ANCD in the *Chicago Tribune* in the 10-year span from January 2004 to December 2013. We will conclude by getting behind the numbers and illustrate our findings with focused case examples of people who exhibit the prevailing characteristics of the perpetrators of abuse and neglect in the lives of children with disabilities.

Exercise 5.1: Reflection

ANCD is preventable. The more we know about and understand the intersection of child disability, abuse, and neglect the greater the possibility of preventing it as well as developing targeted and effective intervention programs. Let us now focus on finding out all we can about the perpetrators of ANCD. *Do you expect that the perpetrators of ANCD are young or old? Are they primarily males or females? What other expectations do you have about their characteristics?*

National Level Trends in Perpetrator Age and Sex Characteristics: What Do we Know?

The authors of the *Child Maltreatment* (U.S. DHHS, 2013) report combine perpetrator statistics for children with and without disabilities. This is a loss for those who want to know specific information on the perpetrators of ANCD. We hypothesize that the perpetrators of CAN and ANCD share some age and sex characteristics. However, it is quite conceivable that the perpetrators of ANCD have unique characteristics.

The data from the U.S. DHHS provide us with a starting place in our efforts to understand the characteristics of the perpetrators of CAN in general. We will examine these data with the data based awareness that an estimated 25.0–30.0 % of these perpetrators abused and neglected children with disabilities (see Chap. 1 of this text).

The U.S. DHHS provides data on the number of unique perpetrators as well as on the number of their child victims. Some perpetrators victimized more than one child. In the United States there were an estimated 528,000 unique perpetrators and 686,000 unique victims of CAN in 2012. The National average of child victims per perpetrator in 2012 alone was estimated at 1.3 children. For example, for every 10 children who were confirmed cases of CAN there are 7.7 perpetrators. Furthermore, national level statistics are not available on how many of these unique perpetrators were identified as perpetrators of CAN in years prior and how many were newly identified in 2012.

How Old Are the Perpetrators of Child Abuse and Neglect?

We analyzed the data in the U.S. DHHS (2013) *Child Maltreatment* report using the hypothesis that prevention and intervention program development personnel must learn as much as they can about the age and sex characteristics of the perpetrators of CAN. These data represent a beginning point in our quest to know who abuses and neglects children with disabilities. From the outset, we are at a loss because these data are not disaggregated. Researchers noted that for decades that children with disabilities have been at increased risk for abuse and neglect and this finding is confirmed once again by Mueller-Johnson, Eisner, and Obsuth (2014). The current estimate is that among every 10 children who are abused and neglected, among them are 2.5-3 children with disabilities. We now turn our attention to examining what we know about the age and gender characteristics of the perpetrators of ANCD.

The U.S. DHHS (2013) estimates that the perpetrators of CAN, including those who perpetrate the ANCD, are between 6 and 75 years old. This age group represents an estimated 97.8 % of all unique perpetrators. Most of these individuals are between 25 and 44 years old (63.0 %) (see Table 5.1). Child perpetrators between 6 and 17 years comprise an estimated 2.4 % of the perpetrators of CAN and ANCD. Perpetrators between 45 and 54 years comprise an estimated 9.4 % of all CAN and ANCD perpetrators. The remaining estimated 3.7 % of the perpetrators of CAN and ANCD are between 55 and 75 years old. The ages of an estimated 2.2 % of unique perpetrators are unknown.

These numbers underestimate the actual perpetrator statistics in each age group for many reasons which include incomplete reporting from states. An average of 48.3 states reported perpetrator age statistics across the nine age groups in 2012 and these included data from the District of Columbia and Puerto Rico. Data were not reported from the remaining territories such as the Virgin Islands, Guam, and American Samoa. Only 47 states reported on the unknown age category and 38 reported statistics on perpetrators aged 6–11 years of age.

Table 5.1 The age of the perpetrators of CAN in the United States in 2012

# of states reporting	Ages	n	% of total
38	6–11	1,153	0.2
50	12–17	11,287	2.2
50	18–24	98,478	19.2
50	25–34	202,632	39.6
50	35–44	119,597	23.4
50	45–54	48,370	9.4
50	55–64	12,979	2.5
50	65–75	6,090	1.2
47	Unknown	11,454	2.2
Average 48.3	Total	512,040	99.9

Data from the U.S. DHHS, *Child Maltreatment Report*, 2013

Are Perpetrators Males or Females?

Would you be surprised to find that in the United States most perpetrators of CAN of children with and without disabilities are female? In 2012 the U.S. DHHS estimated that 53.5 % of the perpetrators of CAN were females and an estimated 45.3 % were males. The sex of 1.1 % of the perpetrators was unknown in 2012. A more in-depth state-by-state analysis indicated that California, New York, Texas, Florida, Ohio, and Michigan reported the highest numbers of female perpetrators in 2012 (see Table 5.2). Females were consistently the most frequent perpetrators and in these states the rate of CAN per 1,000 children was far above the national average. For example, in California, New York, Texas, Florida, Ohio, and Michigan an estimated 12.0 children per 1000 were abused and neglected in 2012 versus 9.2 children per 1,000 were abused and neglected nationally.

Clearly females outnumber male perpetrators at the national level; a closer analysis shows that male perpetrators outnumber female perpetrators in 12 states (U.S. DHHS, 2013). Among these are six states where male perpetrators outnumber females by the largest margins. These include Pennsylvania, Vermont, Kansas, Utah, Delaware, and Missouri (see Table 5.3).

Exercise 5.2: Reflection
Do you expect that the age and gender characteristics of the perpetrators of children with and without disabilities differ from the overall National trends reflected in the U.S. DHHS (2013) data? *Provide a rationale for your observations.*

Conversely, female perpetrators outnumber male perpetrators by a large margin in Washington D.C., Puerto Rico, Mississippi, Louisiana, South Carolina, and South Dakota (see Table 5.4). It is also notable that the rate of CAN per 1000 children is highest in states where female perpetrators prevail. In states where females outnumber male perpetrators, the average rate of CAN is 10.6 children per 1000 children. This rate exceeds the 2012 national average of 9.2 children per 1000 and overall national average of 9.3 children per 1,000 from 2008 to 2012 (U.S. DHHS, 2013).

Table 5.2 Male and female perpetrators of CAN per six highest states, 2012

States	Male	Female	% Male	% Female	% Female increase	Rate of CAN per 1000 children
California	26,561	32,996	44.4	55.2	+10.8	8.2
New York	24,180	30,807	44.0	56.0	+12.0	16.0
Texas	21,607	28,130	43.4	56.5	+13.1	9.0
Florida	19,225	20,200	48.7	51.2	+2.5	13.3
Ohio	11,549	11,654	48.1	48.5	+0.4	11.0
Michigan	11,106	16,231	40.6	59.4	+18.8	14.7
		Average	*44.9*	*54.5*	*+9.6*	*12.0*
		National average	*45.3*	*53.5*	*+8.2*	*9.2*

Data from the U.S. DHHS, *Child Maltreatment Report*, 2013

Table 5.3 A comparison of male and female perpetrators – males prevailing, 2012

State	Male	Female	% Male	% Female	% Male increase	Rate of CAN per 1,000 Children
Pennsylvania	2,496	939	72.7	27.3	+45.4	1.2
Vermont	381	154	71.2	28.8	+42.4	5.2
Kansas	952	573	62.2	37.5	+24.7	2.6
Utah	3,972	3,075	56.3	43.6	+12.7	10.6
Delaware	1,006	823	54.9	44.9	+10.4	11.4
Missouri	2,181	1,794	53.7	44.2	+9.5	3.3
		Average	*61.8*	*37.6*	*+24.2*	*5.7*
		National average	*45.3*	*53.5*	*−8.2*	*9.2*

Data from the U.S. DHHS, *Child Maltreatment Report*, 2013

Table 5.4 A comparison of male and female perpetrators – females prevailing, 2012

State	Male	Female	% Male	% Female	% Female increase	Rate of CAN per 1,000 children
Washington DC	508	1,127	30.2	67.0	+36.8	19.6
Louisiana	2,129	4,072	34.3	65.5	+31.2	7.6
Puerto Rico	1,816	3,471	34.3	65.5	+31.2	10.0
Mississippi	2,167	3,796	36.3	63.6	+27.3	10.2
South Dakota	315	518	37.5	61.7	+24.2	6.0
South Carolina	3,286	5,383	37.9	62.0	+24.1	10.6
		Average	*35.0*	*64.2*	*+29.1*	*10.6*
		National average	*45.3*	*53.5*	*+8.2*	*9.2*

Data from the U.S. DHHS, *Child Maltreatment Report*, 2013

We do not know the sex of 5,828 unique perpetrators (1.1 %) in the United States (U.S. DHHS, 2013). Notable differences may be observed in how states report "unknown" sex designation statistics. For example, in North Carolina the sex of 1291 perpetrators (27.6 %) was unknown and in Wisconsin the sex of 539 (13.8 %) of perpetrators was unknown. In contrast, the sex of 100 % of the identified perpetrators was known in Minnesota, Nevada, Pennsylvania, and Vermont.

What Else Do We Know About Perpetrators?

Perpetrators come from every race and ethnicity in the United States (U.S. DHHS, 2013). DHHS reports that Whites, African Americans, and Hispanics together comprise 87.7 % of perpetrators. The race and ethnicity of the remaining 12.3 %

Table 5.5 The race and ethnicity of perpetrators of CAN in the United States, 2012

Race and ethnicity	n	% of CAN	% of U.S. Population Census (2010)
White	246,166	48.9	72.4
African American	100,112	19.9	12.6
Hispanic	95,189	18.9	16.3
Unknown	43,762	8.7	*
Multiple race	5,988	1.2	2.9
Native American	5,799	1.2	0.9
Asian	5,146	1.0	4.8
Pacific Islander	1,147	0.2	0.2
Total perpetrators	503,309		

*missing data
Data from the U.S. DHHS, *Child Maltreatment Report*, 2013

of perpetrators are scattered among Native American, Asian, Pacific Islander, Multiple Race, and Unknown race and ethnicity (see Table 5.5). These data are not provided across sex designation though they may provide important information for the development of intervention and prevention programs.

Exercise 5.3: Critical Thinking

Does knowing the sex of perpetrators matter? Why? Or why not? Do you believe that the varying male and female data from state-to-state has implications for increasing our understanding of the abuse and neglect of children with and without disabilities? Do you believe that male and female perpetrator trends are different for children with and without disabilities?

White males and females comprise almost half of the identified unique perpetrators of CAN in 2012 though they comprise almost 75 % of the population in the United States. African American and Hispanic males and females comprise almost 40.0 % of unique perpetrators (19.9 % and 18.9 %) respectively and they comprise 12.6 % and 16.3 % of the population respectively.

Perpetrators come from all races and ethnic backgrounds. Focused attention on the prevailing race and ethnicity will serve to guide effective intervention and prevention program decision-making. Available resources will be well spent by first analyzing the data that reflects what is known about perpetrators at the local, state, and regional levels. Moreover, resources will be more wisely spent when program developers focus on males and females from White, African American, and Hispanic backgrounds, who are primarily between 25 and 34 years old. Data indicate that males and females who are between 18 and 44 years old warrant specific and focused CAN intervention and prevention programming. The relevance of these programs will be enhanced when developers focus on data based targeted topics that are designed for targeted and data based populations.

The Age and Gender and the Abuse and Neglect of Children with Disabilities in the Literature

Children with disabilities are exposed to abuse and neglect, such that, at times it is so severe that it is fatal (Coorg & Tournay, 2013; Douglas & Mohn 2014; Esernio-Jenssen, Tai, & Kodsi, 2011). Coorg and Tournay generated data from an analysis of newspaper coverage of filicide-suicide involving children with disabilities from 1982 to 2010. They analyzed the age, gender, and disability characteristics of both the perpetrators and victims. In addition, they analyzed the cause of death, attempts and marital status of the perpetrators.

Coorg and Tournay found that the perpetrators of filicide-suicide were 21 parents and one grandfather of children with disabilities – 50 % (11) were mothers and 50 % (11) were fathers (including one grandfather). The children involved in this study ranged from 2 to 17 years old and 57 % (12 out of 21) of them had autism while 43 % (9 out of 21) had medical conditions such as epilepsy, mitochondrial disease, attention deficit hyperactivity disorder and one child was in a coma.

The average age of the parent and grandparent perpetrators was 42.7 years old. The ages of eight mothers ranged from 29 to 49 years old. The ages of nine fathers ranged from 34 to 54 years old. The grandfather who engaged in filicide-suicide was 75 years old. The ages of three females were unknown. Coorg and Tournay found that on average the males who engaged in filicide-suicide were slightly older than females (42.6 years versus 38.8 years).

Fathers and mothers used different methods when they engaged in filicide-suicide. Fathers completed these acts, in that the child actually died, more often than mothers. The children of 54.5 % of the mothers who engaged in the act of filicide-suicide died. The children of 58.8 % of the fathers died. Mothers attempted but did not complete filicide-suicide more often than fathers. Among mothers, 83.3 % attempted to kill their children but their children did not die. Only 16.7 % of the fathers attempted but did not kill their children.

There are differences in the way mothers and fathers initiated filicide-suicide. Mothers used passive methods, such as prescription overdose (80.0 %), more frequently than did fathers (20.0 %). Fathers and mothers both used active methods, such as gunshots, but fathers did so more frequently than did mothers (55.6 % versus 44.4 %). Fathers used poisonings, such as carbon monoxide, more frequently than did mothers (75.0 % versus 25.0 %). One father stabbed his child and one father used fire to cause the deaths of his children with disabilities. One mother engaged in suffocation and another engaged in falling from a bridge to cause the deaths of their children. No father engaged in suffocation or falling from a bridge and no mother engaged in fire or stabbing as methods to bring about the deaths of their children with disabilities.

Exercise 5.4: Critical Thinking
Are you surprised to read that mothers and fathers, grandfathers and grandmothers might engage in filicide-suicide? Under what circumstances might this happen?

Write at least five scenarios in which you might expect that parents and grandparents might engage in filicide-suicide. What can be done to prevent the occurrence of filicide-suicide involving children with disabilities?

What else do we know about the age and gender of the perpetrators of CAN and more specifically the perpetrators of ANCD? Yampolskaya, Greenbaum, and Berson (2009) examined the records of 196 perpetrators who were involved in fatal (n = 126) and nonfatal (n = 70) cases of child abuse and neglect in Florida from 1999 to 2002. Though they did not disaggregate for disability characteristics, consistent with the findings of Coorg and Tournay, they found that male perpetrators were slightly older than females and that males engaged in child fatality more frequently than females. More specifically, Yampolskaya et al. found that the median age of female perpetrators was 29 years old and the median age of males was 33 years old. Males had a higher probability (.89) of perpetrating child fatality than females (.82). Consistent with the findings, we will discuss in Chap. 8, males with added risk factors such as a history of domestic violence were 12 times more likely to perpetrate child fatality than females with behavioral health conditions, such as anxiety and depression.

Yampolskaya et al. also found that age and gender coupled with substance abuse, physical and psychological symptomology and criminal history increased the probability of perpetrator behaviors. These findings are also consistent with the findings in Chap. 8 of this text in which we found that contexts in which disposing variables, such as domestic violence, substance abuse, and poverty, converge and increase the probability of the abuse and neglect of children with and without disabilities.

Gender and Allegations of Abuse and Neglect of Children with Disabilities

Gender matters in predicting physical abuse and in responding to the abuse when it happens (Rodriguez & Tucker, 2015; Tucker & Rodriguez, 2014). Gender also matters among the observers of the abuse and neglect of children with and without disabilities (Bottoms, Kalder, Stevenson, Oudeker, Wiley, & Perona 2011; Devine & Caughlin 2014; Rogers, Lowe, & Boardman, 2014). That is, males and females respond differently to the abuse and neglect of male and female children. They also respond differently to the abuse and neglect of children with and without disabilities.

Bottoms et al. (2011) examined the perceptions of male and female jurors. They found differences across the perceptions of jurors when they evaluated cases involving the abuse and neglect of children with and without disabilities.

The gender of perpetrators and the disabilities of their child victims influenced the perceptions of male and female jurors who are deciding the outcomes of abuse and neglect allegations (Bottoms et al., 2011). These researchers used a mock trial format which involved cases of alleged infanticide involving fathers of children with and without disabilities. The jurors read cases which described infants as severely mentally disabled or as not having a disability. They made a series of judgments about the guilt of the perpetrators, the proposed length of prison sentences, their empathy, sympathy, and feelings of similarity toward the defendants and the victims.

Bottoms et al. found that male jurors were more sympathetic than were female jurors toward the perpetrators of infanticide involving children with and without disabilities. Female jurors rendered more guilty verdicts and they perceived greater culpability by the fathers in the scenarios describing infanticide. Females were less sympathetic, as well as, less empathetic toward alleged offending fathers than male jurors. Both male and female jurors proposed less severe sentences for the alleged perpetrators of infanticide when an infant was portrayed as having a severe disability versus for an infant who was portrayed as typically developing. They were less likely to view the perpetrator as mentally ill when the child had a disability. Finally, they felt less empathy toward infant victims with disabilities.

Children with Disabilities as Perpetrators

Male and female adolescents with and without disabilities perpetrate abuse and neglect of their peers and of younger children with and without disabilities (Martinello, 2014). Adolescent males appear more frequently in sexual abuse statistics than do females (Banks, 2014). This might be associated with cultural bias as females are more associated with sexuality and are perceived as less dangerous than males. Adolescent males and females with disabilities are more frequently represented in perpetrator statistics than are their nondisabled peers (Bladon, Vizard, French, & Tranah, 2005; Martinello, 2014).

The Newspaper Coverage of the Abuse and Neglect of Children with Disabilities

Females prevailed among the perpetrators of ANCD in the stories that appeared in the *Chicago Tribune* from January 2004 to December 2013. Fifty seven females and 52 males perpetrated some form of abuse and neglect in the lives of children with disabilities during that time. The ages of 46 females were included in the stories and their ages were not included in 11 stories. The ages of 39 males were included in the stories and the ages of 13 were not included. The youngest perpetrator was a 9 year old male and the oldest perpetrator was a 69 year old male – a 60 year age range. The youngest female perpetrator was 15 years old and the oldest female perpetrator was 67 years old – a 52 year age range.

Table 5.6 Male and female perpetrators of ANCD, 2004–2013

Age range	Male	Female	% Male	% Female
Teens	13	4	33.3	8.7
20–29	6	5	15.4	11.0
30–39	12	18	30.7	39.1
40–49	1	11	2.6	23.9
50–59	1	7	2.6	15.2
60–69	6	1	15.4	2.1
70–79	0	0	0	0
80–89	0	0	0	0
Unknown	13	11	25.0	19.3

Data from a study of the newspaper coverage in the *Chicago Tribune*

The largest percentage of male perpetrators of abuse and neglect in the lives of children with disabilities were in their teens and the largest percentage of female perpetrators were in their 30s (see Table 5.6) for more precise details. Females in their 30s and 40s comprised 63.0 % of female perpetrators. Males in their 60s perpetrated 7.3 times more abuse and neglect in the lives of children with disabilities than did females in the same age range.

These findings have implications for intervention and prevention program planning. How can these data inform program, processes, and procedures so that more children with disabilities will be protected from abuse and neglect? What intervention and intervention programming would it take to stop the abusive and neglectful behaviors toward children with disabilities by male and female perpetrators across the age span?

Exercise 5.5: Critical Thinking

Review Table 5.6 and observe the age trends of the perpetrators of ANCD. Note that one third of the males perpetrators of abuse and neglect in the lives of children with disabilities were in their teens. Both males and females in their 30s are highly represented. Why? *What other observations did you make based on the data on Table 5.6? Write at least three implications of your observations for the prevention of abuse and neglect of children with disabilities. Additionally, write three implications of your observations for the prevention of perpetrator abuse and neglect behavior in the first place?*

The People Behind the Numbers: The Age and Gender of the Perpetrators of ANCD

A teenaged mother was associated with the abuse and neglect of a newborn baby boy. The baby was born in July 2008. At that time, the baby's mother, "Scared her parents would be angered by her pregnancy, the teen decided to hide the newborn outside." This young mother was later accused of attempted murder of her infant. Williams-Harris report (September 10, 2008):

> A 15-year-old girl admitted in front of her parents at the Belmont Area Detective Division to abandoning the newborn, police said.
>
> The case started in the early hours of July 8, when Brandon Shepard, a resident of the building where the infant was found, heard strange noises as he returned home from a date. He went to investigate and found a baby inside a plastic grocery bag with its umbilical cord still attached, he said.
>
> Shepard took the baby to a nearby fire station, where paramedics were called. The baby was rushed to Advocate Illinois Masonic Medical Center and later listed in serious condition. He was named Wilson after the street on which the fire station is located.

The medical examiners found that a CT scan indicated that the infant had a skull fracture. He had bruising on his body and a cut on his lip and these injuries indicated intended rather than accidental trauma. He was placed in a temporary facility for children with special needs. According to Williams-Harris, due to the condition of his health, "... He will need long-term care."

There is legal support for a much different story here. Illinois Law provides protection for mothers about which this young mother seemed unaware. Williams-Harris reminds readers that "... the 2001 Illinois law ... extends protection to parents who drop off children up to 7 days after birth to havens, which include hospitals, police and fire stations, and emergency medical facilities, no questions asked." The author continued this story by discussing the need for education about the legal supports that do exist and which remain unexercised. She concluded the story by discussing the quest to identify the father of the child and the ongoing human toll on the child, and on the people directly, as well as, on those indirectly involved. Stories of children like that of Baby Wilson burden the legal system, the medical system, and social service, education systems and family systems. There are no winners here.

Exercise 5.6: Critical Thinking

Read the entire story referenced here. *Make a list of what contextual variables set the stage for this story? How might this story have a positive outcome from the outset?*

Males less than 20 years old were the most commonly identified male perpetrators of ANCD. This is illustrated in a story that Houde (2013) broke involving Robert Sobczak, 19 who was charged with aggravated criminal sexual abuse of a boy with special needs. At the time of the abuse allegations, Sobczak was a volunteer at the Willow Creek Community Church in South Barrington. "He served as an aide helping children with disabilities and special needs on weekends while their parent attended church services" (Houde, 2013, May 15).

Sobczak was accused of fondling the boy after leading him to an isolated area of the large church. Though he denied these accusations, he was arrested and then released on a $10,000 cash bond. The director of the church's family services said there were no other allegations of abuse by Sobczak. In preparation for his volunteer position, Sobczak even passed a thorough background check.

On the day of the alleged abuse, the child was having unspecified difficulties. Sobczak removed him from the classroom and was alone with him for a short period of time. The boy told his mother that "something happened, and she [mother] told the church volunteers." The volunteers notified the Illinois DCFS promptly, who notified the police. Sobczak was denied any future volunteer work with children in the church. The church officials reviewed their standards for protecting children and ensured that their volunteers knew of the policy to never leave a child alone with an adult. In addition, they installed additional surveillance cameras.

Males in their 30s were also frequent perpetrators noted in the newspaper coverage of ANCD. This is illustrated in a story about Andy Gabel, a three-time Olympic speed skater, who grew up in the Chicago suburbs. He apologized in March 2013 for sexual misconduct with a 15-year-old teammate and speed skater, Bridie Farrell when he was in his 30s. Her subsequent depression and eating disorders were linked to her sexual abuse. Gabel acknowledged:

> Almost two decades ago I displayed poor judgment in a brief, inappropriate relationship with a female teammate, "Gabel told the Tribune. "It did not include sex, however, I know what happened was wrong, and I make no excuses for my behavior. I apologize to her, and I am sorry for bringing negative attention to the sport that I love." Hersh (2013, March 2)

Gabel engaged in improper sexual contact with her in 1997 and 1998. The two spent much time together in training and Gabel was a family friend. The girl finally told her story in order to make young athletes who are exposed to sexual abuse aware of the resources that are available to protect them. In the years following the relationship, Farrell endured physical and emotional trauma. No charges were filed. Hersh concluded:

> We are glad that Ms. Farrell chose to tell her story, because it will make others who have been abused aware that they are not alone and hopefully shine a light on the resources that are available to administrators, coaches, parents and athletes to help protect our young athletes.

Exercise 5.7: Reflection
These stories illustrate that disability precedes and follows the abuse and neglect perpetrated by young males in trusted roles. *What can be done? Make a list of five ways that you suggest to increase awareness of child maltreatment and its relation to childhood disability?*

A story by Working and Rodriguez published in the *Chicago Tribune* on May 21, 2004 illustrated how a couple, Irma and Dino Pavis, fared when they adopted two children with disabilities:

> Alexei Geiko needed rescuing. At 20 months, he had been removed from alcoholic parents in Russia who underfed him and made him sleep on the floor of their roach- infested apartment. He then spent nearly 5 years in an orphanage.

Irma and Dino Pavlis "...hoped to start a family last fall by adopting two needy children: Alexei, 6, and his sister, 5."

Working and Rodriguez reported that this couple was not aware that they were working with "...an orphanage for special-needs children ... six weeks after the family arrived in the United States in November, Alex Pavlis – as he became known – was dead and his new mother jailed on charges of murdering him." On April 16, 2005, *Chicago Tribune* reporter Mary Ann Fergus stated:

> A tearful, remorseful Irma Pavlis, on trial for first-degree murder, took the stand Friday in her own defense and said she was only trying to discipline her son, 6-year-old Alex, when she slapped and punched him one morning in December 2003.

The adoptive parents "completed the required pre-adoption training. ... this training consisted of reading two books and writing essays about them ...." Did they have the skills to parent children with disabilities? Fergus stated:

> ... Alexei suffered from a central nervous system disability that severely handicapped his motor functions. He also was badly malnourished and suffered from anemia and rickets. Physicians who reviewed photographs at the request of the *Tribune* say Alexei's facial features indicate his mother drank while he was in the womb.

Working and Rodriguez (May 21, 2004) stated:

> Both children showed troubling behavior: When the girl was told to stand in her room, she clawed at her face and drew blood, Dino Pavlis said. Alex began copying her.
>
> But the girl was doing well in her home schooling, learning the alphabet and repeating English words. Alex, who was unable to learn to read, was jealous. He would react if his parents told him to stand still for some quiet time, Dino Pavlis said. Sometimes he would throw himself on the floor.
>
> "He began to urinate and defecate on himself as an act of defiance," Dino Pavlis said. "He urinated on himself once after we complimented his sister on reciting the ABC's."
>
> ... In an interrogation, Irma Pavlis stated that her son had been wetting his bed, running into walls and playing aggressively, thus bruising himself. But on Dec. 20, Irma Pavlis allegedly admitted her involvement in the death, a police report states.
>
> ...Irma Pavlis, 32, admitted to striking the child and slamming him into a closet when he threw a tantrum Dec. 18. He died in a hospital the next day ... Alexei had had severe behavior issues and would throw himself onto the ground and scream. Additionally, he would urinate and defecate on himself "as an act of defiance." Police say Irma admitted to the death by shaking, slapping, and twisting the neck of Alexei.

Irma Pavlis admitted:

> "I hit him in the head. It was hard," she told police and Assistant State's Atty. Cathy Nauheimer, who conducted the interview. "I slapped him again in the face. I punched him in the stomach," and closed her fist to demonstrate the punch. (Fergus & Slivinski, April 15, 2005)

Further Mary Ann Fergus and Krystyna Slivinski reported that Irma and Dino Pavlis:

> ... acknowledged that the couple never took Alex to a doctor. They had scheduled a doctor's appointment for Alex in November, but the child did not see a doctor until Dec. 18, when Schaumburg firefighters responded to Irma Pavlis' 911 call that her son was not breathing.

On April 16, 2005 Fergus reported that the Cook County jury concluded their report. A jury comprising eight women and four men:

… gave her the benefit of the doubt Friday afternoon, convicting Pavlis of involuntary manslaughter. The Schaumburg woman now faces a sentence as lenient as probation rather than the minimum 45-year sentence for first-degree murder.

Fergus reported the outcome of the legal deliberations on May 5, 2005:

Saying Irma Pavlis cannot blame anyone but herself for the beating death of the 6-year- old boy she adopted from a Russian orphanage, a judge sentenced the Schaumburg woman Wednesday to 12 years in prison.

"It's time we as a nation and we as individuals take responsibility for what we do," Cook County Circuit Judge Thomas Fecarotta said. "The evidence is clear: Irma Pavlis beat Alex Pavlis to death. Period."

The sentence for involuntary manslaughter was shorter than the maximum 14 years, but Pavlis also could have received probation. Last month, she avoided a first-degree murder conviction that could have brought a 45-year sentence.

Working and Rodriguez (May 21, 2004) reminded readers that the Irma and Dino Pavis are not alone. They reported that "… At least 12 adoptive parents have been accused of killing their Russian children since 1996."

Exercise 5.8: Reflection

Read the entire story using the references at the end of this chapter. *Are you surprised to read a story like this? What did or did not surprise you? What other reflections do you have as you think about this story?*

The stories of male and female perpetrators of ANCD cross the age spectrum. In a story in the *Chicago Tribune* on August 18, 2004 John Hartzell reported that a 46 year old church elder, Ray Hemphill:

… was sentenced to 2 1/2 years in prison Tuesday for abusing an 8-year-old autistic boy who died in what prosecutors called an exorcism at a storefront church. … [he] laid on Terrance Cottrell's chest while trying to release "demons" from him before the boy died Aug. 22, 2003.

Hartzell reported that "… The youngster died at the Faith Temple Church of the Apostolic Faith in Milwaukee of what the medical examiner ruled was suffocation." Hemphill had no experience working with children with autism. He was charged with physical abuse of a child and recklessly causing bodily harm. The boy's mother, Pat Cooper, was a member of Hemphill's church "… said after Tuesday's hearing that she regretted ever taking her son to the church and was glad Hemphill was given a prison sentence."

Adoptive parents Michael Gravelle was 56 years old when he and his wife Sharen, 57 years old, were sentenced to 2 years in prison for their abuse of 11 children with a variety of disabilities (*Chicago Tribune*, February 16, 2007). On December 23, 2005 Mabin reported that:

A couple who adopted 11 children with a host of health and behavioral problems abused some of the youngsters by making them sleep in wooden cages without pillows or mattresses, a judge ruled Thursday.

… The children, ages 1 to 15, have problems such as fetal alcohol syndrome and a disorder that involves eating dirt. The judge said their psychological, behavioral and health problems became too much for the couple.

Kropko (September 14, 2005) reported that the couple "...said a psychiatrist recommended they make the children sleep in the cages... some who had mental disorders, needed to be protected from each other ..." One of the children testified that "... the couple forced him to stay in his 'box' for up to two weeks for taking peanut butter, bread and cereal from the kitchen." And another child testified that "... he was forced to live in the bathroom for nearly 3 months for urinating in his enclosed bed." The couple assured their attorney, Ken Myers "... We love our children very much and we will continue to do everything possible to get them home..." The children remained in foster care and awaited the custody decision of the courts.

Exercise 5.9: Reflection
In each of these stories there are clues to intervention and prevention programming. Review the details of each story using the references provided at the end of this chapter. *What are your observations about the intervention and prevention of abuse and neglect in the lives of children with and without disabilities?*

Implications for Research and Practice

What do we know about the perpetrators of abuse and neglect in the lives of children with and without disabilities? In this chapter we learned that most perpetrators of CAN and ANCD are between the ages of 18–34. Males and females perpetrate CAN differently. Adult males are more likely to engage in physical abuse and females are more likely to engage in neglect.

Exercise 5.10: Reflection
Beyond the age and sex differences of perpetrators and the type of abuse perpetrated, what perpetrator characteristics do we need to know in order to position ourselves to prevent CAN and the ANCD? *How might knowing perpetrator characteristics matter in our professional practice? Write as many arguments as you can think of to support the need for increased awareness of perpetrator characteristics?*

This section contains a set of recommendations for researchers and practitioners based on what we know and need to know about the perpetrators of CAN and ANCD. First, we make recommendations for researchers in order to inform perpetrator prevention programming, then we make recommendations for research on public perception and bias relative to ANCD, and we provide recommendations for the enhancement of children, families and service providers.

Research on Perpetrator Characteristics to Inform Perpetrator Prevention Programming

At this time we do not know the unique characteristics of those who perpetrate ANCD. The U.S. DHHS is in an ideal position to provide these data in the annual *Child Maltreatment* report. The data on the perpetrators of CAN do not differentiate between those who abuse and neglect children without disabilities and those who abuse and neglect children with disabilities. It is conceivable that perpetrators of children with disabilities do not know how to provide care for these children and therefore wind up accused of maltreatment. Such perpetrators need information about caring for their children with disabilities. Justice is not served by law enforcement alone.

Is it sufficient to identify the perpetrators of CAN and ANCD as quickly as possible and do everything to make sure that their contact with children is severed? Surely not. Increasing the number of individuals in jails and prisons solves superficial problems and generates new ones such as absorbing the high costs associated with incarceration and inestimable toll on family and community life. Does our work end when perpetrators of CAN and ANCD are incarnated for as long as possible and as far away as possible? We believe that the identification of perpetrators and potential perpetrators is an important beginning – a first step towards understanding the characteristics of the perpetrators of ANCD. Are they males or females? What are their roles and relationships relative to children with and without disabilities? We recommend that researchers:

Recommendation 5.1: Disaggregate the data in order to differentiate the characteristics of the perpetrators of abuse and neglect in the lives of children with disabilities.

***

We believe that the perpetrators of abuse and neglect of children with and without disabilities have unique characteristics. At this time we do not know how the characteristics of these groups of perpetrators are similar and/or how they differ. It is insufficient to know that biological mothers are the most frequent perpetrators. We need to know more about these women. Likewise, it is insufficient to know that males perpetrate physical abuse more frequently than females. Research is needed on their attitudes toward their children with and without disabilities. Do they perceive that they have the knowledge, resources, and supports they need to raise their children with and without disabilities? What disposing variables might predict their perpetrator behaviors? We recommend that researchers:

Recommendation 5.2: Differentiate the primary, secondary, and tertiary characteristics of perpetrators who abuse and neglect children with and without disabilities.

***

Perpetrator prevention programming for those who engage in ANCD will not be possible unless we know more about perpetrators' attitudes and dispositions toward their children with disabilities. What are their attitudes toward children in general? Do they regard male and female children differently? Are they particularly vulnerable to engage in perpetrator behaviors in the presence of very young male or female children? How do they regard children with disabilities? Are there specific child behaviors that challenge them as caregivers? If so, it is predictable that they are particularly vulnerable as potential perpetrators of children with disabilities who are associated with these behaviors. We recommend that researchers on the perpetrators of ANCD:

Recommendation 5.3: Provide data on the child disability characteristics that increase perpetrators' vulnerability to engage more readily in abusive and neglectful behaviors.

***

Are children with disabilities more frequently neglected by their mothers than are children without disabilities? Is it possible that specific perpetrators, such as biological mothers, are uniquely poised to abuse and neglect males and females with specific disability characteristics? What perpetrator attitudes and behaviors do those who perpetrate abuse and neglect among children with a variety of disabilities exhibit? Is it possible to predict perpetrator risk factors among caregivers of children who are medically fragile, deaf or blind, or among those who have intellectual disabilities or learning disabilities? At this time we do not know. We recommend that researchers identify:

Recommendation 5.4: The predictable perpetrator risk behaviors that are associated with specific child disability characteristics.

***

Exercise 5.11: Analysis
Do you believe that single mothers are particularly vulnerable to perpetrator behaviors? Or, do you believe that this is an unfair stereotype and not at all an indicator of potential perpetrator behaviors? *List five reasons that support your observations.*

Knowing perpetrator characteristics will guide the development of programs that have potential to prevent the development of perpetrator behaviors in the first place. Perpetrator prevention programming is comparable to the work of health educators who teach participants how to care for their health. Participants in health education programs learn how to make food choices to meet their dietary needs and to engage in appropriate physical exercise programs. In such programs participants learn how to care for their health and thereby avoid potential health problems. Likewise, perpetrator prevention programming may be designed to inform audiences about the care and treatment of children with disabilities. Focused perpetrator prevention programming will be possible when we find out the knowledge and skills that are needed by male and female perpetrators of ANCD. We need:

Recommendation 5.5: Data on specific caregiver knowledge and skills that reduce the incidence of abuse and neglect in the lives of children with disabilities.

***

Researchers and practitioners have a great deal to learn from the perpetrators of abuse and neglect in the lives of children with disabilities. We will increase our potential to conduct more relevant research and more targeted intervention and prevention programs when we know more about who these people are and how they perceive the children they abuse and neglect. Understanding perpetrators' perspectives and behaviors requires us to ask research and intervention questions differently. Is it possible that perpetrators could inform us about what would have prevented them from engaging in ANCD? Viewing perpetrators as informants would require us to listen to them, hear their perspectives, and analyze the data on what they tell us, thus understanding their perspectives at a foundational level (Denzin & Lincoln, 2011). We recommend qualitative research in order to:

Recommendation 5.6: Develop our understanding of the perspectives of those who perpetrate abuse and neglect in the lives of children with disabilities.

***

The Influence of Public Perception

What do public perceptions have to do with perpetrator research and effective professional practice? Public perceptions of perpetrators matter when evaluating CAN and ANCD. The perception that males are more likely to engage in physical abuse and females are more likely to engage in neglect may lead to false assumptions in specific instances.

Perceptions guide our research hypotheses and our willingness to investigate a case of CAN or ANCD based on the available facts. When considering the age of the perpetrator, would you believe a 7-year old boy with a communication disorder if he told you that he was sexually abused by another 7-year old boy in the school bathroom? Or, would you believe a 7 year old girl who reported that she was physically abused by a peer with a communication disorder? In what ways do you perceive these scenarios differently?

Perpetrator characteristics and abuse type influence public perception. For example, sexual abuse perpetrated by males was seen as more abusive and more severe than sexual abuse perpetrated by females (Davies & Rogers, 2009). The accounts of sexual abuse by victims of males were seen as more credible than the accounts of sexual abuse by female victims. In addition, opposite-sex interactions were seen as less abusive than same-sex interactions. We encourage researchers to:

Recommendation 5.7: Examine the prevailing public perceptions at the intersection of CAN and ANCD and public perception of perpetrator culpability.

***

Public perception associates females as victims of sexual abuse and males as perpetrators. Cashmore and Shackel (2014) found that males perpetrate sexual abuse more frequently but that males are more likely to be sexually abused by female perpetrators. The authors observe that:

> The social construction of gender identity for adolescent boys carries a different meaning for abuse by both male and female perpetrators. Where the perpetrator is female, it may be seen as a 'rite of passage', rather than abuse... Where the perpetrator is male, the same-sex element of the abuse carries significant meaning for boys, and a body of research indicates that boys may be deeply troubled by the perceived homosexual dimension of same-sex molestation, which may manifest in feelings of guilt, shame and confusion about their sexuality. (p. 77)

These findings have implications for research and practice. For example, are males less willing to report their abuse due to fears about the impact of disclosure? Are they fearful of being labeled "homosexual," or of stigmatization? Or are they fearful of further victimization, or of becoming sexual predators themselves (Cashmore & Shackel, 2014; Giglio, Wolfteich, Gabrenya, & Sohn, 2011). As researchers and practitioners it is important to be aware that:

Recommendation 5.8: Prevailing public perception of male and female stereotypes impact the accurate reporting of and intervention in CAN and ANCD.

***

Exercise 5.12: Analysis
Are you surprised to find that boys may be less willing to disclose sexual abuse than girls? Why or why not? *What are the implications of these findings for your work?*

Confronting bias about age and gender is pivotal when a child discloses that he or she has been abused or neglected. Educators tend to believe children when they report a case of abuse, regardless of the age or gender of the perpetrator. Davies and Rogers (2009) found that teachers were overwhelmingly provictim in cases of child reported abuse and neglect. They believed what the child said and they were willing to take action. Females were slightly more willing to believe the victim than males. Davies and Rogers examined the role of male family friends and found that sexual abuse perpetrated by a father was perceived as a more severe crime than sexual abuse perpetrated by a family friend. Yet, a father who sexually abuses his own child was seen as less culpable than a stranger who sexually abuses someone else's child. Additionally, a female who was sexually abused by her father was deemed less honest than a female who was sexually abused by a stranger. These data indicate the need for:

Recommendation 5.9: Dissemination of research findings on bias in public perceptions in order to inform the work of researchers and practitioners.

***

Exercise 5.13: Reflection

Imagine yourself as a teacher of a 7-year-old child with autism who came to you and reported that she was sexually abused by the school principal in the bathroom. *What would you do? Would you believe the child's report? What public perceptions put you at risk of ignoring the child's report? How would this scenario be different if the child was nonverbal and unable to tell you about the incident? Consider the potential differences in your responses across disability areas.*

Children with and without disabilities have imperative rights (United Nations General Assembly, 1989). They have a right to live free from all forms of violence, to be educated, participate in their communities, and be heard. Child protection is more assured in communities of care that provide individualized and intensive services to children with their disabilities and their families (Fiorvanti & Brassard, 2014). They state that "coordinated, comprehensive and individualized services" (p. 360) are essential and in such environments:

> (a) the child receives the services that he or she needs, (b) the services are as helpful as possible, (c) the child and family do not receive services that are competing with one another or working at cross purposes, and (d) the child's needs are being honored and addressed. (p. 361)

Communities of care provide families with the supports they need, thus reducing their vulnerability and strengthening their resilience. ANCD will be reduced when we:

Recommendation 5.10: Build communities of care for children with disabilities and their families.

***

What can be done to enhance the capacity of child protection staff members to recognize, intervene, and interrupt CAN and ANCD more rapidly? Data from the U.S. DHHS (2013) indicate that in some states it takes an average of 47 days to initiate services to children who are victimized by perpetrators of abuse and neglect. In the meantime many children are reexposed to their perpetrators. What can be done to enhance service delivery to children in need? What interagency collaboration might make a difference in reducing the determination of child need and the initiation of services? We believe that we must:

Recommendation 5.11: Increase the capacity of child protection agency staff to interrupt, more quickly, abuse and neglect in the lives of children with and without disabilities.

***

The study of the ANCD does not fit neatly into one discipline. Child protection agency staff members, sociologists, special educators, physicians, school psychologists, among others know this field uniquely. How can we increase opportunities for more professional exchanges among diverse professionals who are involved in this area? Those who engage in the study of child disability in medical sciences have few opportunities to engage with professionals who are involved in the education and treatment of these children. Child protection agency staff members engage in daily experiences that uniquely exhibit the clinical needs of children with disabilities who are abused and neglected. They encounter the perpetrators of ANCD and their observations have critical implications for research and practice. We need to:

Recommendation 5.12: Engage in interdisciplinary scholarly inquiry in order to understand, anticipate, and interrupt the behaviors of the perpetrators of ANCD.

***

Chapter Summary

The focus of this chapter was an analysis of the age and sex of the perpetrators of abuse and neglect in the lives of children with disabilities. We examined the data in the U.S. DHHS *Maltreatment Report* (2013) that indicate that males and females, young and old perpetrate the abuse and neglect of children with and without disabilities. These data do not analyze the age and sex characteristics of the perpetrators of ANCD separately. Children with disabilities are disproportionately victimized by these perpetrators. Perpetrators of CAN are most frequently between 25 and 34 years old and they are represented across ethnic groups. We presented the findings of an analysis of the newspaper coverage that indicate females in their 30s are among the most frequent perpetrators of ANCD. Male teens are the second most frequent perpetrators of ANCD. Males in their 30s are the third most frequent perpetrators of ANCD. We illustrated these findings with stories from the newspaper coverage of children with disabilities who were abused and neglected. We concluded the chapter with a set of recommendations for researchers and practitioners.

References

Banks, N. (2014). Sexually harmful behaviour in adolescents in a context of gender and intellectual disability: Implications for child psychologists. *Educational & Child Psychology, 31*(3), 9–21. Retrieved from http://eds.a.ebscohost.com/eds/pdfviewer/pdfviewer?sid=cb3c045e-c276-4455-a0e0-37f83da32e34%40sessionmgr4003&vid=6&hid=4108

Bladon, E. M., Vizard, E., French, L., & Tranah, T. (2005). Young sexual abusers: A descriptive study of a UK sample of children showing sexually harmful behaviours. *Journal of Forensic Psychiatry & Psychology, 16*(1), 109–126. doi:10.1080/1478994042000270265abc

Bottoms, B., Kalder, A., Stevenson, M., Oudeker, B., Wiley, T., & Perona, A. (2011). Gender differences in jurors' perceptions of infanticide involving disabled and non-disabled infant victims. *Child Abuse & Neglect, 35*(2), 127–141. doi:10.1016/j.chiabu.2010.10.004

Cashmore, J., & Shackel, R. (2014). Gender differences in the context and consequences of child sexual abuse. *Current Issues in Criminal Justice, 26*(1), 75–104.

Chicago Tribune. (2007, February 16). Parents who caged kids are sentenced to 2 years. *Chicago Tribune*. Retrieved from http://search.proquest.com/docview/418006269?accountid=11578

Coorg, R., & Tournay, A. (2013). Filicide-suicide involving children with disabilities. *Journal of Child Neurology, 28*(6), 745–751. doi:10.1177/0883073812451777

Corso, P. S., Ingels, J. B., & Roldos, M. I. (2013). A comparison of willingness to pay to prevent child maltreatment deaths in Ecuador and the United States. *International Journal of Environmental and Research and Public Health, 10*(4), 1342–1355. doi:10.3390/ijerph10041342

Davies, M., & Rogers, P. (2009). Perceptions of blame and credibility toward victims of childhood sexual abuse: Differences across victim age, victim-perpetrator relationship, and respondent gender in a depicted case. *Journal of Child Sexual Abuse, 18*(1), 78–92. doi:10.1080/10538710802584668

Denzin, N. K., & Lincoln, Y. S. (2011). *The SAGE handbook of qualitative research*. Thousand Oaks, CA: Sage.

Devine, D. J., & Caughlin, D. E. (2014). Do they matter? A meta-analytic investigation of individual characteristics and guilt judgments. *Psychology, Public Policy, and Law, 20*(2), 109–134. doi:10.1037/law0000006

Douglas, E. M., & Mohn, B. L. (2014). Fatal and non-fatal child maltreatment in the US: An analysis of child, caregiver, and service utilization with the National Child Abuse and Neglect Data Set. *Child Abuse & Neglect, 38*(1), 42–51. doi:10.1016/j.chiabu.2013.10.022

Esernio-Jenssen, D., Tai, J., & Kodsi, S. (2011). Abusive head trauma in children: A comparison of male and female perpetrators. *Pediatrics, 4*, 649–657. doi:10.1542/peds.2010-1770

Fergus, M. A. (2005, May 05). Mom gets 12 years in killing; Adopted son was beaten to death. *Chicago Tribune*. Retrieved from http://search.proquest.com/docview/420327393?accountid=11578

Fergus, M. A., & Slivinski. K. (2005, April 15). Adoptive father testifies about boy's tantrums; he says he only saw his wife spank son. *Chicago Tribune*. Retrieved from http://articles.chicagotribune.com/2005-04-15/news/0504150129_1_adoptive-fetal-alcohol-syndrome-russia

Fergus, M. A., & Working, R. (2005, April 16). Adoptive mom guilty in boy's slaying: Convicted of involuntary manslaughter. *Chicago Tribune*. Retrieved from http://search.proquest.com/docview/420276386?accountid=11578

Fiorvanti, C. M., & Brassard, M. R. (2014). Advancing child protection through respecting children's rights: A shifting emphasis for school psychology. *School Psychology Review, 43*(4), 349–366. Retrieved from http://eds.a.ebscohost.com/eds/pdfviewer/pdfviewer?vid=3&sid=bc948680-4ec8-40fd-94c6-4b2de7caa622%40sessionmgr4003&hid=4211

Giglio, J. J., Wolfteich, P. M., Gabrenya, W. K., & Sohn, M. L. (2011). Differences in perceptions of child sexual abuse based on perpetrator age and respondent gender. *Journal of Child Sexual Abuse, 20*(4), 396–412. doi:10.1080/10538712.2011.593255

Hartzell, J. (2004, August 18). Churchman gets prison in fatal abuse of boy, 8. *Chicago Tribune*. Retrieved from http://search.proquest.com/docview/420080390?accountid=11578

Hersh, P. (2013, March 2). Olympian sorry for misconduct. *Chicago Tribune*. Retrieved from http://articles.chicagotribune.com/2013-03-02/sports/chi-olympian-apologizes-for-alleged-sexual-misconduct-20130301_1_sexual-misconduct-andy-gabel-olympic-speedskater

Houde, G. (2013, May 15). Church volunteer charged with child sexual abuse. *Chicago Tribune*. Retrieved from http://articles.chicagotribune.com/2013-05-15/news/ct-met-willow-creek-church-fondling-charge-20130515_1_church-volunteers-willow-creek-community-church-church-officials

Kropko, M. R. (2005, September 14). Kids allegedly put in cases well-behaved, neighbors say. *Chicago Tribune*. Retrieved from http://search.proquest.com/docview/420490731?accountid=11578

Mabin, C. (2005, December 23). Judge rules caged kids were abused by parents. *Chicago Tribune* Retrieved from http://search.proquest.com/docview/420423024?accountid=11578

Martinello, E. (2014). Reviewing risks factors of individuals with intellectual disabilities as perpetrators of sexually abusive behaviors. *Sexuality and Disability*, 1–10. doi:10.1007/s11195-014-9365-5

Mueller-Johnson, K., Eisner, M. P., & Obsuth, I. (2014). Sexual victimization of youth with a physical disability: An examination of prevalence rates, and risk and protective factors. *Journal of Interpersonal Violence, 29*(17), 3180–3206. doi:10.1177/0886260514534529

Rodriguez, C. M., & Tucker, M. C. (2015). Predicting maternal physical child abuse risk beyond distress and social support: Additive role of cognitive processes. *Journal of Child and Family Studies, 24*(6), 1780–1790. doi:10.1007/s10826-014-9981-9

Rogers, P., Lowe, M., & Boardman, M. (2014). The roles of victim symptomology, victim resistance and respondent gender on perceptions of a hypothetical child sexual abuse case. *Journal of Forensic Practice, 16*(1), 18–31. Retrieved from http://dx.doi.org/10.1108/JFP-08-2012-0004

Tucker, M. C., & Rodriguez, C. M. (2014). Family dysfunction and social isolation as moderators between stress and child physical abuse risk. *Journal of Family Violence, 29*(2), 175–186. doi:10.1007/s10896-013-9567-0

U.S. Department of Health and Human Services, Administration for Children and Families, Administration on Children, Youth and Families, Children's Bureau. (2013). *Child maltreatment 2012*. Retrieved from http://www.acf.hhs.gov/programs/cb/research-data-technology/statistics-research/child-maltreatment

U.S. Census. (2010). *United States census 2010*. Retrieved from http://www.census.gov/2010census/

United Nations General Assembly. (1989). *Convention on the rights of the child*. Retrieved from http://digitalcommons.ilr.cornell.edu/child/8

Working, R., & Rodriguez, A. (2004, May 21). Rescue of boy ends in tragedy. *Chicago Tribune*. Retrieved from http://articles.chicagotribune.com/2004-05-21/news/0405210351_1_adoptive-parents-russian-children-foreign-children

Williams-Harris, D. (2008, September 10). Cop finds abandoned boy's mom sadder tale. *Chicago Tribune*. Retrieved from http://search.proquest.com/docview/420814645?accountid=11578

Yampolskaya, S., Greenbaum, P. E., & Berson, I. R. (2009). Profiles of child maltreatment perpetrators and risk for fatal assault: A latent class analysis. *Journal of Family Violence, 24*(5), 337–348. doi:10.1007/s10896-009-9233-8

Chapter 6
The Roles and Relationships of the Perpetrators of Abuse and Neglect in the Lives of Children with Disabilities

It is easier to build strong children than to repair broken men. (Frederick Douglass, American Author, 1817–1895)

Abstract In this chapter we analyze the data on the roles and relationships of the perpetrators of abuse and neglect in the lives of children with disabilities. We examine the data in large data bases as well as the literature in this area. We present the findings of a study of the newspaper coverage which focuses directly on abuse and neglect in the lives of children with disabilities. We illustrate these findings with stories that illustrate the roles and relationships of the perpetrators of abuse and neglect in the lives of children with disabilities. We conclude this chapter with a set of recommendations for researchers and practitioners.

Who perpetrates abuse and neglect in the lives of children with disabilities? What roles do they serve in their relationships to these children? Are the perpetrators aware of the harm they are doing in the lives of children with disabilities? We must find answers to these and so many more questions. A multidimensional understanding of this problem is essential in the development of effective intervention and prevention programming.

Perpetrators either actively or passively engage in the abuse and neglect of children with and without disabilities. Active perpetrators are those who engage directly in physical abuse, sexual abuse or emotional and psychological abuse or physical or emotional neglect. Passive perpetrators are those who stand by knowingly without intervening to stop or even to report an event they observed.

Establishing What We Know

The U.S. DHHS (2013) defines a perpetrator as an individual who was determined to have caused or knowingly allowed the abuse and neglect of a child. The National Child Abuse and Neglect Data System (NCANDS) collects and analyzes data on the unique or duplicate perpetrators voluntarily submitted from the states and

© Springer International Publishing Switzerland 2016

E.P. Crowley, *Preventing Abuse and Neglect in the Lives of Children with Disabilities*, DOI 10.1007/978-3-319-30442-7_6

territories that comprise the United States. Unique perpetrators are those who are counted only once regardless of the number of children they victimized. Duplicate perpetrators are those who are counted per child maltreatment incident. Investigators use the term substantiated when "the allegation of maltreatment or risk of maltreatment was supported or founded by state law or policy" (U.S. DHHS, 2013, p. 16). Indicated claims were those that could not be substantiated under state law or policy "but there was reason to suspect that at least one child may have been maltreated or was at-risk of maltreatment. This is applicable only to states that distinguish between substantiated and indicted dispositions" (U.S. DHHS, p. 16). Data in the most recent *Child Maltreatment Report* indicate that in 2012, 17.7 % of all alleged reports of child abuse and neglect (CAN) to which CPS staff members responded were *substantiated*. CAN was *indicated* in an additional 0.9 % cases (see Table 6.1).

More than 80 % (81.4 %) of all reports of CAN in the United States in 2012 were either unsubstantiated, responded to in an alternative manner, closed with no finding, or denied one way or another (see Table 6.2). The most common other responses to alleged reports included the recommendation for counseling or the provision of respite care or access to the services of a social service agency. In addition to the 58 % unsubstantiated reports, 23.4 % were investigated but unconfirmed. Since 2008 the number of children who receive the services of child protection agency has increased steadily. The U.S. DHHS (2012) estimated that among 1000 children, 42.7 unique children receive child protection services, this number increased from 40.8 in 2008.

Table 6.1 Duplicate victim responses of child protection services in 2012

CPS responses	Number of duplicate responses	% of duplicate responses
Substantiated victims	678,047	17.7
Indicated victims	35,938	0.9
Alternative response victims	18,333	0.5
Total	732,318	19.1

Data from the U.S. DHHS, *Child Maltreatment Report, 2013*

Table 6.2 Duplicate nonvictim responses of child protection services in 2012

Response type	Number of response per type	% by type of response
Unsubstantiated	2,226,858	58.0
Alternative responses to nonvictims	408,898	10.7
No alleged maltreatment	372,246	9.7
Closed with no finding	58,127	1.5
Other	26,457	0.7
Intentionally false	9,029	0.2
Unknown	4,419	0.1
Total	3,106,034	80.9

Data from the U.S. DHHS, *Child Maltreatment Report, 2013*

There were 1,820,892 screened-in reports of CAN from the 512,040 identified unique perpetrators in 2012 (U.S. DHHS, 2013). Each identified perpetrator in the United States was estimated to be associated with 3.6 screened-in reports. Though these numbers appear exorbitant they actually represent underestimates for several reasons. For example, no perpetrator statistics were submitted for Georgia and Idaho, and from the Commonwealths and Territories of American Samoa, Federated States of Micronesia, Guam, North Marianas, and the Virgin Islands.

Compelling Questions

We have the estimated numbers of perpetrators of CAN and abuse and neglect of children with disabilities (ANCD) in 2012 and for many years prior to this. We want to get behind these numbers in order to find out who are the perpetrators of abuse and neglect in the lives of children with and without disabilities? What can we learn about the perpetrators of CAN and ANCD in order to inform the development of more effective processes, procedures, and programs? Then, when ANCD happens, what can be done? Specifically, what can we learn about the perpetrators so that we can better predict, identify, and eventually understand and assist both perpetrators and their victims? Overall, how can we intervene and stop the needless and deadly abuse and neglect of all children, including children with disabilities?

Exercise 6.1: Reflection
At this point, what compelling questions come to your mind? Add as many as you can. *How would you go about finding the answers to these questions? Consider the contribution knowing the answers to these questions would make.*

In this chapter, we analyze the roles and relationships of the perpetrators. First, we examine the data on perpetrators roles and relationships in the 23rd *Child Maltreatment Report* by the U.S. DHHS (2013). Then we will analyze the professional literature and make data based observations about the roles and relationships of perpetrators relative to the children with disabilities they victimize. We conclude this chapter by presenting the findings of the newspaper study and provide specific case examples that illustrate the roles and relationships of the perpetrators of ANCD. Throughout the chapter we will provide exercises for reflection and analysis.

Roles and Relationships of Perpetrators: What We Learn for the National Database

Data from the U.S. DHHS (2013) describe the roles and relationships of perpetrators without disaggregating these data across children with and without disabilities. The data do not differentiate unique perpetrators' roles and relationship patterns in the ANCD. We can observe the overall perpetrator relationship patterns and

Table 6.3 Victims by perpetrator relationship, 2013[a]

Perpetrator	n	% of duplicate victims
Mother	250,553	36.6
Biological parents – mother and father	132,557	19.4
Father	127,654	18.7
Mother and other	40,495	5.9
Father and other	6,399	0.9
Nonparent – extended family and trusted others	81,816	12.0
Others, unknown	44,774	6.5
Total	684,248	100

[a]Based on data from only 47 States
Data from the U.S. DHHS, *Child Maltreatment Report, 2013*

consider how these might be the same or different for children with and without disabilities.

Are there notable trends in the statistics on whether children are more vulnerable to abuse and neglect in the homes of their biological families, stepparents, or adoptive parents? The U.S. DHHS (2013) data indicate that children with and without disabilities are abused and neglected most frequently by their biological parents. Additionally, data from the World Health Organization (2014) exposes biological parents as perpetrators of CAN internationally.

Biological parents are estimated to account for 81.5 % of the perpetrators of CAN (see Table 6.3). Biological parents, those in parenting roles, family, and extended family members, professionals, and others in trusted roles accounted for 93.5 % of duplicate child victims of abuse and neglect in the United States in 2012. Mothers acting alone are the most frequent perpetrators of CAN (36.6 %). Fathers acting alone perpetrated 18.7 % of CAN and 19.4 % of the child victims were maltreated by both biological parents acting together. Extended family members, those in such trusted roles as child day care providers, foster parents, friends, neighbors, professionals, and parent partners perpetrated 12.0 % of CAN. The relationships of 6.5 % of the perpetrators to their child victims were designated as unknown.

Among nonparent perpetrators, male relatives (3.0 %) were the most frequent perpetrators. Other frequent perpetrators included male partner of a parent (2.3 %), female relatives (1.5 %) and more than one nonparent perpetrator (1.0 %). Less frequent nonparent perpetrators were female partners of a parent (0.3 %) and friends and neighbors (0.3 %). Foster parents accounted for 0.1 % of perpetrators and daycare providers (.4 %), professionals (0.1 %), legal guardians (0.1 %), and group home residential staff (0.1 %) were among perpetrators in trusted but nonparent roles and were the perpetrators of abuse and neglect in the lives of children in the United States in 2012.

Exercise 6.2: Reflection
Are you surprised by the data from the U.S. DHHS (2013) that indicate that mothers and biological parents are the most frequent perpetrators of CAN? *Do you predict*

that the most frequent perpetrators of children with disabilities are also their mothers and their biological parents? Provide a rationale to support your prediction.

Perpetrators of Child Fatalities

Children die as a result of CAN in the United State every year (see Chap. 4). Biological parents, acting alone, together or with others were the perpetrators of 80.0 % of the child fatalities following abuse and neglect in 2012 (see Table 6.4). Mothers acting alone accounted for most of these fatalities. Children aged 5 and under accounted for 84.8 % of these child deaths and 44.4 % of these children were less than 1 year old (U.S. DHHS, 2013). Children from 5 to 17 years old accounted for 13.8 % of the children who died as a result of CAN and the remaining 1.4 % of these children were abused and neglected by unknown individuals. We do not know how many of these children had disabilities prior to their deaths.

Overall, our best statistics on CAN and ANCD are estimates. Less than 20 % (18.6 %) of all alleged reports of CAN are substantiated and indicated. Perpetrators of CAN most often occupy trusted caregiver roles including those of biological parents, family members, friends, neighbors, and professionals. Similar role and relationship patterns were observed in the data on the perpetrators of child fatalities that resulted from CAN.

Exercise 6.3: Reflection
Had you ever considered that children die as a result of abuse and neglect? Are you surprised to find that biological mothers and fathers are the most frequent perpetrators of abuse and neglect such that children die? *Write your thoughts on what you consider to be the implications of these data.*

Table 6.4 Child fatalities by perpetrator relationship, 2013

Perpetrator	n	% duplicate victims
Mother	318	27.1
Biological mother/father	248	21.2
Father	200	17.1
Mother and other	147	12.5
Father and other	25	2.1
Extended family and trusted others	108	9.3
Others, unknown and more than one perpetrator	126	10.7
Total	1,172	100

Data from the U.S. DHHS, *Child Maltreatment Report, 2013*

The Literature on Perpetrators' Relationships to Children with Disabilities

Over time and consistently across disciplines, researchers confirm the increased vulnerability of children with disabilities to abuse and neglect (Alriksson-Schmidt, Armour, & Thibadeau, 2010; Bones, 2013; Khalifeh, Howard, Osborn, Moran, & Johnson, 2013; Sobsey, Randall, & Parrila, 1997; Soylu, Alpaslan, Ayaz, Esenyel, & Oruc, 2013; Stalker & McArthur, 2012; Wells & Mitchell, 2013). Children with disabilities have unique care and educational needs that dispose them to increased vulnerability (Goldberg et al., 2009; Leeb, Bitsko, Merrick, & Armour, 2012; McDonald, Milne, Knight, & Webster, 2013).

What influences the decision to consider whether to report an incident of CAN in the first place? In the United States observers who have concerns about the welfare and safety of children with and without disabilities are mandated reporters and are obligated to report their observations. We might wonder why so many reports are unsubstantiated, closed or denied. Sinanan (2011) concluded that future research is necessary in order to understand the factors that influence reporting practices as well as substantiated and unsubstantiated decisions.

Mothers, Fathers, and Extended Family and CAN

The health and well-being of parents and grandparents is relevant to the health and well-being of their children (Emerson & Brigham, 2014; Fentiman, 2014). Parents' history of childhood abuse and neglect indicates a risk factor for intergenerational cycles of CAN – childhood abuse and neglect that is ongoing and predictable from generation to generation (Emerson & Brigham, 2014; Moehler, Biringen, & Poustka, 2007; Sidebotham & Golding, 2001). Family research requires a particularly complicated methodology due to the involvement of staff members in a variety of disciplines and settings. It requires the use of a variety of definitions to describe the disabilities of the parents and children. Researchers continue to study the role of family members as perpetrators of CAN despite the challenging methodological issues involved.

Children with disabilities fare best when their parents and extended family members accept them and their special needs. Acceptance of children and their disabilities requires specialized knowledge, understanding, skills, support, and resources.

Abuse and neglect of children with and without disabilities cycles through generations (Wigham, Taylor, & Hatton, 2014). Mothers with histories of personal traumas associated with childhood abuse and neglect are predictably poised to perpetuate the cycle of abuse into the next generation. Moehler et al. (2007) examined the emotional availability of a sample of mothers who self-selected either with or without a history of their own abuse and neglect in childhood. Mothers of full term, healthy babies with Apgar scores of 7 and above were included in this study. The mothers completed a Childhood Trauma Questionnaire and demographic information such as marital status, and educational level. The sample selected included 119 mothers, 58 of whom described themselves as having histories of abuse and 61 who had no history of abuse. The mothers in this study were regarded as low risk perpetrators because of their economic stability and the stability they derived from their intact social relationships.

Moehler and her colleagues found only slight differences in the emotional availability of mothers with and without histories of childhood abuse. The biggest difference they found was that mothers who were abused during childhood were more intrusive during their interactions with their babies. This finding is consistent with the findings of previous researchers. Mothers with childhood abuse histories were more hypervigilent and more hyperaroused than those with no histories of childhood abuse (Douglas, 2014).

The findings of this study suggest that mothers with and without histories of abuse are similarly emotionally available to their very young children. This is good news! Moehler and her colleagues provide us with a good starting place as well as several unanswered questions. What are the effects of maternal intrusiveness? As children grow older, do the interactions of mothers with and without personal histories of childhood abuse differ? In what contexts might the behaviors of these two groups of mothers differ? Might there be differences in their emotional availability across the genders and behaviors of their children? Is it possible that they would respond differently to children with and without disabilities? At what point do demographic variables become significant indicators of their emotional availability or lack thereof?

Rodriguez and Tucker (2015) found that mothers who engage in conflicted parent-child exchanges and who make negative attributions about the behaviors of their children are at increased risk to engage in physically abusive behaviors. Maternal risk factors increase when children engage in challenging behaviors which increase parental stress, family dysfunction and social isolation.

Exercise 6.4: Reflection
Do you expect that the perpetrators of sexual abuse are different from the perpetrators of physical abuse? Are the perpetrators of neglect different from the perpetrators of sexual abuse and physical abuse? *What do you think? Provide a rationale for your observations.*

Perpetrators of Sexual Abuse of Children with and Without Disabilities

Are there differences across the roles and relationships of perpetrators of children with and without disabilities? Soylu and her colleagues (2013) analyzed the sociodemographics of sexually abused children with and without disabilities.

The 6–16 year old children in this study were placed in a residential center for treatment and forensic evaluation following sexual abuse. More girls with and without disabilities were sexually abused than boys with and without disabilities. More boys with disabilities (32.4 %) were sexually abused than nondisabled boys (18.0 %). More girls without disabilities (81.8 %) were sexually abused than girls with disabilities (67.6 %).

In this population family members, extended family members and acquaintances together accounted for 71.8 % of the sexual abuse of children with disabilities and 87.3 % of children without disabilities (Soylu et al., 2013). They also found that strangers accounted for 32.4 % of the sexual abuse of children with disabilities and for 20.8 % of the sexual abuse of children without disabilities. The roles and relationships of 2.9 % of perpetrators of sexual abuse were unknown to children with disabilities while none were unknown to their peers without disabilities. Immediate family members, such as parents and siblings, sexually abused 14.7 % of the children with disabilities and 22.7 % of children without disabilities.

Soylu and colleagues found that among this unique population, the most frequent of all the perpetrators of sexual abuse of children with and without disabilities were their acquaintances – known individuals. Acquaintances sexually abused 49.0 % of the children with disabilities and 56.5 % on their peers without disabilities. Strangers – unknown individuals were the second most frequent perpetrators of sexual abuse of children with and without disabilities. Family members, including father, step-father, and older brother were the third most frequent perpetrators of sexual abuse and these individuals targeted children without disabilities more frequently (16.9 %) than their peers with disabilities (7.8 %).

Data indicate that girls with disabilities are sexually abused by more and different perpetrators and they come from outside of families more frequently (Soylu et al., 2013). They become pregnant more frequently than their nondisabled peers as a result of sexual abuse. These researchers found that children with disabilities are diagnosed with psychiatric disorders, such as PTSD, conduct disorders, encopresis, and panic disorders, more frequently than their nondisabled peers. Following sexual abuse, typically developing children are diagnosed with major depressive disorders more frequently than their peers with disabilities. We may conclude that perpetrators of sexual abuse undermine the emotional stability of all children with and without disabilities.

Caldas and Bensy (2014) studied the sexual abuse of 352 children with disabilities between 14 and 17 years old were abused in school settings in the United States. Their findings indicated that 51.7 % of the sexual abuse of children with disabilities was perpetrated by adults in school environments. "Another student" (48.3 %) was identified as the second most frequent perpetrator of sexual abuse in these settings. "Teaching personnel" which included "teachers, teacher assistants/paraprofessionals, and substitute teachers and teacher assistants/paraprofessionals" were identified as the perpetrators of 30.3 % of the sexual abuse to which children with disabilities were exposed to in schools in the United States. Related service personnel including physical therapists, occupational therapists, and speech therapists were implicated in 8.3 % of the incidents of sexual abuse of children with disabilities. Transportation personnel (5.1 %) and school administrators (2.1 %) were also identified as perpetrators of sexual abuse of children with disabilities in school settings.

Disability and Child Fatality Data

As indicated in Chap. 4, the literature in the areas of CAN substantiates the findings that some parents of children with disabilities intentionally put their children to death (Barone, Bramante, Lionetti, & Pastore, 2014; Coorg & Tournay, 2013; Douglas & Mohn, 2014). Coorg and Tournay found that among biological parents – mothers and fathers both engaged in filicide-suicide. They found that mothers of children with disabilities initiated but did not complete the child deaths as frequently as fathers. Douglas and Mohn found that biological parents were the most frequent perpetrators of fatal child maltreatment. Family relatives, unmarried parent partners, and step-parents also perpetrated fatal child maltreatment.

Findings from an Analysis of the Newspaper Coverage

The newspaper study focused directly on abuse and neglect in the lives of children with disabilities. Biological mothers and fathers of children with disabilities were the most frequently alleged and accused perpetrators of ANCD (see Table 6.5). The focus of 64.4 % of the stories was on ANCD perpetrated by individuals in trusted

Table 6.5 Abuser's relationship to victim (n = 113 stories)

Perpetrator relationship	n[a]	% of stories
Biological parents	35	30.9
School professionals (not special educators)	12	10.6
Legal guardians	7	6.2
Strangers	7	6.2
Priests and Ministers	6	5.3
Other relatives	4	3.5
Family friends	3	2.7
Special education teachers/Aides	3	2.7
Foster families	3	2.7

[a]Only stories that included information about perpetrator relationship
Data from a study of the newspaper coverage in the *Chicago Tribune*

relationships such as parents, legal guardians, foster families, relatives, family friends, priests and ministers, special education teachers, and other school staff members. School professionals, including special education teachers, and school staff were the accused or alleged perpetrators of the ANCD in 13.3 % of the articles. Children spend most of their time in home and school environments. It is no surprise that school personnel are implicated in the ANCD second only to immediate and extended family members. This information is critical to our intervention and prevention efforts.

Allegations and accusations of ANCD were directed toward strangers in 6.2 % of the stories. We used the category "stranger" to describe individuals who occupied an assortment of roles including residential center staff members and others with whom children with disabilities might be associated. These "strangers" included individuals who were trusted to provide medical treatment to children with disabilities and staff in an assortment of environments including juvenile detention centers and nursing homes.

Priests and ministers remain the focus of relentless efforts to seek justice following CAN in the United States. Among children with disabilities, 5.3 % of the stories reflected allegations or accusations of ANCD by priests and ministers.

Exercise 6.5: Reflection
Up to this point, what information surprises you about the findings from the newspaper coverage of the ANCD in the *Chicago Tribune*? *For example, are you surprised that once again biological parents top the list? Are you surprised that school professionals are among the next largest group represented in these findings? Are our fears of strangers warranted? Select any one of these questions and consider, why or why not?*

Taking a Closer Look – The Real People Behind the Numbers

We read number after number, statistic after statistic. We busily make sense of every minute detail – one after another. By the time we have figured out exactly what an author is telling us, little energy remains for our efforts to understand the real people the statistics represent. Newspapers cover the stories of real people who are associated with real places – often ones we know well. The story of one 17-year-old boy and his mother that is described in the next few paragraphs reminds us that behind every new statistic are the lives of real children like Seamus and his family.

The Crystal Lake, Illinois Police Chief, Howard Parth could not understand the deterioration in a single parent home where a mother and her seven children between the ages of three and 17 years old lived. He pondered, "I keep asking myself why? Why? Why? Why wouldn't somebody else do something here?" (Starks & Long, 2004, March 14). Starks and Long reported that Ms. Leonard's

15-year-old son Seamus had cerebral palsy and inside the living room the police found:

> Seamus Leonard's body curled up on a piece of cloth on the floor, surrounded by garbage, wearing only a diaper and weighing as little as an infant.
>
> Neighbors said they knew that in recent years the family of seven children was in a terrible tailspin, with allegations of domestic abuse swirling, a divorce pending and a mother working three jobs to keep the family afloat.
>
> But apparently no one knew that tiny Seamus, 4 feet tall and emaciated, suffering from [who had] cerebral palsy, was wasting away. He weighed 23 pounds when he died.

The police report indicated that Seamus "died of pneumonia brought on by malnutrition." On March 13, Long and Starks reported that his mother, Katharine, 44 years old at the time was charged with involuntary manslaughter in the death of her son. The next day Starks and Long report that according to the police "Leonard 'recklessly failed to provide proper health and medical care' to Seamus. She is in the McHenry County Jail in lieu of $1 million bail".

Exercise 6.6: Reflection

In the story above, who were the active and passive perpetrators of abuse and neglect in the life of Seamus Leonard? Make a list of those you consider to be the active perpetrators and of those you consider to be the passive perpetrators? *Do some of these perpetrators surprise you more than others? Do you have any other thoughts as you reflect on the active and passive perpetrators in Seamus Leonard's life? What aspects of this story surprise you most of all?*

Disability may either precede or follow abuse and neglect, and infants and young children are particularly vulnerable. This is poignantly illustrated in a story about a father who disabled his daughter permanently while responding to her infant cries (Chicago Tribune, 2013, April 15). The report indicated that:

> A Chicago infant is brain-dead and on life support after her father smothered her last week in an attempt to stop her crying, according to Cook County prosecutors and court documents.
>
> Rigoberto "Rico" Rodriguez, 29, and Angela Petrov, 21, parents of a 5-month-old girl, were each charged with aggravated battery to a child younger than 13 resulting in permanent disability after an incident that Thursday at the couple's home, according to court records.

The infant's brain swelled due to lack of oxygen and was placed on life support. The night of the incident, the parents were drinking when the child woke and began to cry. He offered a bottle to the infant and she refused it. Then Rodriguez covered the infant's mouth with his hand in order to stop her crying. After putting his hand over the infant's mouth a third time, the girl's body went limp. Petrov was allegedly present and did nothing. After a night of sleep, the couple found their infant unresponsive. In an attempt to revive her, they threw water in her face and administered cardiopulmonary resuscitation before calling 911. Spokesperson for the Illinois DCFS, Dave Clarkin, stated that the infants' two siblings were removed from their home and they were placed in a relative's home. Petrov and Rodriguez were investigated on changes of abuse and neglect and the investigation continues.

The stories of biological mothers and fathers who abuse and neglect their children with disabilities go on. Data indicate that parents and other trusted individuals abuse and neglect children with disabilities, and in many instances, their abuse and neglect permanently disable their children.

Exercise 6.7: Reflection

What are your thoughts upon reading stories like these? Are you surprised that children and families live lives as described in these stories? Are you sad? Are you angry? *Do stories like this inspire you to do something that will make a difference? What differences can you make?*

Stories in the *Chicago Tribune* substantiated the data on child fatality associated with CAN (see Chap. 4). Fergus and Working (2005, April 16) reported:

> A tearful, remorseful Irma Pavlis, on trial for first-degree murder, took the stand Friday in her own defense and said she was only trying to discipline her son, 6-year-old Alex, when she slapped and punched him one morning in December 2003.

She was convicted of involuntary manslaughter of her adopted son, Alex. Alex had been in the Pavlis' home for 45 days before the incident occurred. The mother slapped her son on the head and punched him in the stomach when she was "only trying to discipline her son." She admitted to being "overwhelmed with caring for two children whose behavior was often erratic." Fergus and Working further reported that Alex died "of blunt force trauma."

Fergus and Working (2005) reported that Pavlis told the court that:

> Alex's behavior problems, particularly wide mood swings and aggression, surfaced before the couple left Russia . . . She said she did not tell authorities in Russia because she did not want to jeopardize the adoption. Back in the United States, she did not notify the Illinois Department of Children and Family Services of the children's arrival.
>
> According to Pavlis and her husband, Dino, Alex/s behavior problems got much worse in Schaumburg. He banged his head on walls. He urinated and defecated throughout the house. He often flew into rages, waving his arms and screaming--sometimes for no apparent reason. A pediatrician and expert on international adoption who reviewed Alex's records said he showed the classic signs of fetal alcohol syndrome and post-traumatic stress disorder.

During her court appearance Pavlis showed remorse and stated that she "never intended to do harm." Assistant State's Attorney stated "I'm trying to comprehend what it is to treat any human being the way this woman brutalized and tortured this little boy." Alex's younger sister, also adopted by the Pavlis', was taken under DCFS custody and given to a foster home after Alex's death.

Exercise 6.8: Reflection

What aspects of this story do you find most surprising? Make a list of them. *What can be done to make sure that such deadly abuse and neglect does not occur?*

The reporters of a story published by the Associate Press on December 23, 2006 described the abuse and neglect perpetrated by Sharen and Michael Gravelle (see Chap. 4). This couple adopted 11 children with special needs. The children were from 1 to 14 years old and some of them were diagnosed with fetal alcohol syndrome and pica, a disorder involving eating nonfood items. The couple was accused of forcing some of their adopted children with special needs "to sleep in wood and wire cages." They couple were convicted of "four felony counts of child endangering and seven misdemeanor counts." The Associated Press (2006) reported that:

> The parents, who showed no reaction when the guilty verdicts were read, claimed during the three-week trial that they needed to keep some of the youngsters in enclosed beds rigged with alarms to protect them from their own dangerous behavior and to stop them from wandering at night.

We may wonder why stories like this happen. What is missing in an infrastructure that puts 11 children, some of them with diagnosed disabilities in the home of two people who do not know how to parent children with special needs and who do not know how to ask for the help and support they need? This lack of infrastructure comes at a high price. We could spend time thinking about the cost, in human toll, and in the actual costs incurred in scenarios such as those described in this story.

Rozas and Breslin (2005, November 3) reported on the sexual assaults of residents with intellectual disabilities in Bloomingdale, Illinois. An 18-year-old named Reynaldo Brucal Jr., was an aide at the health facility and had an undisclosed disability. He was charged with the rape of a resident who had an intellectual disability (ID) and cerebral palsy. She lived in a room with her twin sister and another woman. When the medical personnel examined her, due to health concerns, they found that she was more than 28 weeks pregnant. When Brucal's DNA was matched with the baby's, he was arrested immediately. DuPage County State's Attorney, Joseph Birkett reported that:

> Brucal took the woman to a secluded area of the facility while she was in his care and raped her. Brucal has been charged with four counts of aggravated criminal sexual assault. *The Tribune* is not naming the woman because she is a victim of sexual abuse.

An Illinois Department of Public Health investigation found that Alden Village staff failed to protect residents and were cited for 19 deficiencies. Police records show that "former employees told investigators that other workers had touched female patients inappropriately." Rozas and Breslin reported that the family of an 11-year-old girl with ID "was repeatedly sexually abused between July 2000 and May 2001." There were rumors of other sexual assaults at Alden Village "... and people seemed to take it in stride." After hearing that her daughter was pregnant, her mother Cheryl Hale-Crom moved both of her daughters to another health facility. The victim's mother is raising her new granddaughter and felt safer after Brucal's arrest.

Exercise 6.9: Reflection
What are your reactions to reading a story like this? Are you surprised that children with disabilities are abused and neglected by those who are trusted to care for them? *Make a list of the people who contributed to the abuse and neglected outlined in the story. Make a list of the infrastructural limitations which would permit the occurrence of the abuse and neglect described in this story.*

Alden Village North, 7464 North Sheridan Road, Chicago, IL was in the news during the first days of January, 2011. Roe and Hopkins (2011, January 11) reported that this facility for children and youth with disabilities was cited for a number of child deaths and that it had the worst safety record among facilities of its type in Illinois. Roe and Hopkins reported that Alden was cited for 21 additional violations such as neglect and for not letting the children leave the facility for months at a time.

Most recently a 14-month-old child who had "signs of a serious infection" died within hours of being hospitalized. Her death was the 14th at Alden Village since 2000. Prior to her death, the staff at Alden Village waited for 2 days before they contacted the child's doctor. Once her doctor was reached, the child was hospitalized. She had a 105.4° fever and she died of septic shock within hours. The child, who remained unnamed, had heart ailments and a seizure disorder. Eight of the 14 deaths occurred since the new president of Alden Management Services, Floyd Schlossberg, took over in 2008. The public health violations more than doubled in his watch. Several state monitors visit the facility several times a week to observe the interactions between residents and staff. This facility remains open in 2015.

Alden Village North continued to be in the news for months. By March 2011, at least five more deaths involving poor care have been reported by the group Equip for Equality. Roe (2011, March 29) stated that:

> Saying they wanted to avoid more casualties, state authorities took steps Thursday to shut down the troubled Alden Village North nursing home, where numerous disabled children have died in recent years.
>
> "We don't want another tragedy to occur," said Michael Gelder, the governor's senior health policy adviser.
>
> State officials said they notified Alden that they planned to revoke its license, which would effectively close the facility. An Alden spokesman said the facility would appeal and remain open. . . .
>
> The key questions, he said, are: Has the home violated important rules? Have people died or been injured? Has this happened repeatedly and over time?
>
> "Now we have the evidence that, indeed, you would answer yes to those questions," he said. "So this is the appropriate action for the state to take."

Governor of Illinois, Patrick Quinn, ordered a team of state monitors to be placed at the facility. The team observes how staff treats the children. State policymakers and advocates for children with disabilities have been meeting to draft legislation to protect the children at Alden Village and in other facilities for children with disabilities in Illinois.

Exercise 6.10: Critical Thinking

How would you describe your feelings now that you have read stories about real people and real places behind the numbers? *Write at least ten feelings that come to your mind. What do you propose as the most important work that can be done in order to stop the abuse and neglect of children with disabilities?*

The stories continue. Alex was a 14-year-old, 200-lb boy with severe autism who was also diagnosed with aggression and a sleep disorder. He required care 24 h per day and 7 days per week. His mother and caregiver were at his side except for when he slept for very short durations at any given time. Alex hardly left his home except to receive medical care. On seven occasions six to eight police officers were needed to assist ambulance personnel in strapping the boy to a stretcher during ambulance trips. Rosemary Sobol, reporter from the *Chicago Tribune* first broke this story on June 12, 2013. Two stories followed in the *Chicago Tribune*. On June 23, reporters Healy, Gutowski, and Walberg (2013) wrote "Autism and the Tragedy of Alex Spourdalakis" that provided such details as:

> The mother and the caregiver of a 14-year-old River Grove boy with severe autism were charged with first-degree murder Tuesday in the teen's fatal stabbing over the weekend, authorities said.
>
> The child's mother, Dorothy Spourdalakis, 50, and Jolanta Agata Skrodzka, 44, will appear in Maywood courthouse Wednesday morning, according to Cook County state's attorney's office spokeswoman Sally Daly.
>
> Alex Spourdalakis' father and uncle found him dead Sunday when they went to the apartment after failing to reach anyone by phone, River Grove police Chief Rodger Loni said.
>
> At the time, his mother and caregiver were in another room in a semiconscious state, police said.
>
> Authorities said Dorothy Spourdalakis and Skrodzka had been frustrated with the condition and care of the boy, including dealing with his autism.
>
> The two women were taken to a hospital and being questioned by police, Loni said.
>
> Department of Children and Family Services spokesman Dave Clarkin said the agency received an abuse allegation regarding the boy in January but determined the accusation to be unfounded.

In this story readers learned that Alex's death was the result of an attempted murder-suicide plan that went awry. In a suicide note the child's mother and godmother explained that they planned to kill Alex because they believed that he was receiving subpar medical treatment from his medical care providers and that in recent weeks his condition was deteriorating.

Foster parents, Frank and Marylynnette Barney of Lombard, Illinois stated that an incident that involved hitting a child constitutes "... necessary discipline, while prosecutors say it was a brutal, cowardly attack." The *Chicago Tribune* staff reporter, Art Barnum (2005, July 14) reported the story of the alleged physical abuse of a boy with intellectual disabilities when he was 15 years old. The Assistant State's Attorney, Alex McGimpsey said that ..." the youth has an IQ in the 40s."

Barnum's story began "The 17-year-old disabled youth whose foster father, Frank Barney was caught on videotape punching him in the face and hitting him with a paddle testified Wednesday that the beatings hurt "a lot" and "I felt blood." A neighbor's wireless security camera provided the evidence for the court. Barnum reported:

> The youth, who is mentally disabled and mildly retarded, glanced nervously at them [foster parents] as he entered the courtroom, then rarely looked at them again until he was asked by prosecutors to point them out. ...
>
> A series of incidents in which Frank Barney is seen striking the then-15-year-old youth eight times in the face and dozens of times in the buttocks with a wooden paddle in 2002 was videotaped by the Barneys' neighbor.

At the court hearing the now 17-year-old "... testified that he also remembered being hit by an extension cord by Marylynnette Barney." The Barneys attempted to cover up their abuse. Barnum reported that "...After he suffered a bruised eye, he said, the couple told him to claim the injury was from "a basketball accident in the back yard."

Exercise 6.11: Reflection
Are you surprised to read stories like this? Do you believe that as a professional who works with children with disabilities and their families you are well served to have considered the reality of child ANCD as indicated in the story above? *In what ways do you believe you are more prepared professionally now that you have considered this and other stories like it? How would you respond to someone who might argue that they prefer not to know this information? Instead they want to focus only on best practices as a future professional?*

Implications for Research and Practice

In this chapter we learned about the roles and relationships of the perpetrators of abuse and neglect in the lives of children with and without disabilities. Here, we outline 12 recommendations for researchers and practitioners. These recommendations focus on child protection, parent, and caregiver support, as well as community awareness and capacity building.

Child Protection

Children have essential rights and privileges. We begin our recommendations with the need to reaffirm the dignity of every child. Children have a right to safety and protection. They have a right to grow and learn in human environments that affirm their human dignity. In November 2014, Kirsten Sandberg, Chairperson of the Committee on the Rights of the Child addressed the 69th session of the General Assembly. She stated:

> November 1989 was historical in many ways, not least because it was the first time that children were recognized as rights holders in an international treaty. It marked a critical turning point in addressing serious human rights abuses against children not simply with acts of charity but with advocacy for systemic change because children had rights which were to be respected. The Convention was the culmination of several decades of work to promote the rights of the child and the creation of a child-specific convention. Today, the Convention is the most widely ratified UN human rights instrument, with 194 states parties, and its three Optional Protocols continue to draw support from states around the world, ever improving legal standards for the respect, protection and fulfilment of children's rights. Between these four treaties there are over 530 ratifications – a clear sign of commitment to ensuring that all children have their rights respected.

It is essential that we reaffirm our commitment and:

Recommendation 1: Show our profound ongoing respect for the human dignity and rights of every child.

***

Children with disabilities have unique physical, emotional, educational, and social needs. These needs put them at an increased risk for maltreatment (Wigham et al., 2014). Children with disabilities have added disabilities following episodes of their abuse and neglect. For example, a child with a communication disorder will be additionally vulnerable to repeated episodes of abuse and neglect due to deficits in expressive language and communication skills. Repeated trauma increases child vulnerability both as a victim and as a potential future perpetrator. Abuse and neglect becomes a way of life and the cycle continues. Some children with disabilities may learn that antisocial behavior is the norm. When the needs of children with disabilities are known and understood they will, more likely, be met by parents and caregivers, therefore we suggest the need for focused programming that would:

Recommendation 2: Promote understanding and appreciation of the physical, emotional, educational, and social needs of children with disabilities.

***

Exercise 6.12: Analysis
Consider the needs of a young child with autism. How would you explain this child's physical, emotional, educational, and social needs to someone who has not encountered a young child with autism? *Name at least one characteristic relative to the child's physical, emotional, education, and social needs.*

Is it possible that some parents are ideally suited to have a child with a particular disability? Do some parents have dispositions that match the unique care needs of their children with disabilities? For example, the unique care needs of children with physical disabilities require caregivers to engage in appropriate positioning and handling of their children. Children with autism need assistance when making transitions from one activity to another. Picture schedules will help them to go through their days more smoothly. Is it possible that parents and caregivers who do not understand, accept, and have dispositions to work with children with disabilities are more at-risk to become perpetrators?

Recommendation 3: Increase research on the match between disability demand and the knowledge, dispositions, and skills of biological parents and other caregivers across child disability characteristics.

***

Parent and Caregiver Support

Mothers, fathers, school personnel, baby sitters, Sunday school staff, professionals, immediate and extended family members, and anyone else who has access to a child with or without a disability is a potential perpetrator of abuse and neglect. Statistically, biological mothers need to be particularly alert to their abuse and neglect potential. They are responsible for most of the abuse and neglect perpetrated in children's lives.

Too often, consideration of the needs of mothers of children with disabilities' is lost in conversations about the ANCD. Their unique needs are largely unknown, frequently unacknowledged, and at worst they are dismissed or disregarded. The implications of this finding are far-reaching. Practical supports for mothers of children with disabilities would include, support groups, information sessions, online chatrooms, and resource sharing such as equipment and clothing used to assist their children or as supports for their children. Other practical supports include mothers' respite programs, such as Mother's Morning Out, that would include child care and time for mothers to establish emotional connections with others who share their experience. Data on the particular vulnerability of mothers to perpetrate CAN and ANCD indicate the need to:

Recommendation 4: Conduct needs assessment on the unique needs of mothers of children with disabilities.

***

Data indicate that biological fathers are also frequent perpetrators of abuse and neglect in children's lives. They perpetrate physical violence such that children are at higher risk of serious injury and death at the hands of their fathers. Without careful attention to the unique needs of fathers of these children, serious injury and death will continue, as well as lengthy incarcerations for paternal perpetrators. The resulting losses are unfathomable. These losses touch our lives in multiple ways including the loss of human civility. What can we do?

Exercise 6.13: Reflection
Do you believe that a support group for fathers might look different from a support group for mothers? What do you know about the research on male bonding? Is it stereotypic to consider that males attribute higher importance to action orientation and involvement in physical activity? *Write at least five considerations for meeting the needs of fathers of children with disabilities?*

Knowing that the fathers of children with disabilities have unique needs is certainly an important first step in stopping the ANCD. What practical supports do fathers of children with disabilities need? Let us begin with the awareness that:

Recommendation 5:
Fathers have unique support needs as they learn to assume their roles in parenting children with disabilities.

***

The innovations of modern scientists provide access to data on the effectiveness of prenatal and early intervention programming. Prenatally, we may know when a child is either at-risk to have a disability or will in fact have a disability. These data may be used to inform parents about disability risk, manifestations, and potential needs of the baby at birth and following. Babies with disabilities have unique physical and emotional needs. Parents who understand these needs, anticipate them, and accept them, put their babies in the best position to mediate the effects of disabilities. Thereby they maximize each child's potential.

Early intervention programming has come a long way in the last two or three decades, such that today early programming comprises a menu of choices that address a variation of parent and caregiver needs. Might a day dawn when participation in mandatory prenatal programming is a prerequisite for access to medical services? What hurdles might the mandatory participation of parents and caregivers in prenatal programming encounter? Can you imagine a day when parents and caregivers of babies and young children would require a permit prior to child contact? However implemented, we are convinced that we need to:

Recommendation 6: Increase and enhance prenatal and early intervention programming for the parents and caregivers of children with disabilities.

***

How many parents go into their roles with the expectation that they might not be successful as child caregivers? To what extent are parents aware that parenting might exceed their physical, emotional or financial resources? How much do they know about the unique demands of parenting a child with a disability? How many parents are aware that parenting a child with physical disabilities is entirely different from parenting a child with sensory disabilities? To what extent are parents aware of the legal, educational, and medical protections that are in place to meet the unique and ever changing needs of their children? The needs of babies and young children with disabilities require that we:

Recommendation 7: Provide ongoing needs assessment, intervention and support to families of children with disabilities.

***

Community Awareness and Capacity Building

We learned in this chapter that children are at-risk when they are associated with parents or other caregivers who make negative attributions about their behaviors or characteristics. Adults who blame children for relational stress, financial challenges, or issues at work are at increased risk as potential perpetrators of CAN and ANCD. When adults lack understanding of child needs, behaviors, or characteristics they must be provided support or else denied access to children. Data indicate that such false attribution and lack of knowledge of child behaviors paves the way to abuse and neglect in the lives of children with and without disabilities. Thus, we recommend the development of programs to:

Recommendation 8: Increase public awareness of the dangers associated with negative attributions of child behaviors or characteristics by parents and caregivers.

***

The perpetrators of abuse and neglect in childhood too often manage to avoid the attention of child protection services. When they are finally identified, many of them have victimized children repeatedly. What can be done to find perpetrators and identify them upon first contact? What new methods might child advocates use to ensure the protection of children? How might an interdisciplinary response to perpetrator identification be employed? What is the role of forensic sciences in this work? The protection of children with and without disabilities from abuse and neglect requires that we:

Recommendation 9: Increase the frequency with which perpetrators are identified accurately and on the first contact.

***

To what extent is disability in childhood understood, accepted, and embraced by the general public? Are some childhood disabilities more easily understood, graciously accepted, and readily embraced? Do the behavioral manifestations of some disabilities in childhood so disturb members of the public that the children are at increased risk of abuse and neglect? The study of disability acceptance and rejection indicates a pecking order – overt physical and sensory disabilities are more readily accepted by the general public. Covert disabilities, such as autism, emotional and behavioral disorders, and learning disabilities, are less readily accepted by members of the general public. We observe the need to:

Recommendation 10: Develop public programs to disseminate information on the behavioral manifestations of childhood disabilities and appropriate interventions.

***

The individualized needs of children with disabilities challenge their caregivers uniquely. For example, children with ADHD may be unable to stay seated for long periods of time. They may hold short conversations and seem to flit from one activity to another. Their energy, disorganization, and seemingly illogical behaviors challenge caregivers, particularly those who do not understand their characteristics and needs. The withdrawn behaviors of children with emotional and psychological disorders leave caregivers bewildered. For example, children with anxiety or depression may be reluctant to leave the house or engage in human interaction.

What attitudes, behaviors, dispositions, and resources help parents to cope with the needs of their children with disabilities? Are there parent qualities that uniquely match their child caregiving roles? For example, how do parents who are disorganized fair when parenting their children with ADHD? Do high-structured parents fair better than low-structured parents in this role? More research is needed on effective parenting across child disability characteristics. Therefore we observe the need to:

Recommendation 11: Develop parent support groups that meet regularly in order to exchange information and provide needed support to parents of children with disabilities.

***

To what extent do families of children with disabilities engage regularly in an analysis of the stressors in their lives? Do they stop regularly to consider the stressors that may be changed and the ones that are unchangeable? Are families of children with disabilities aware that coping strategies may be emotionally based or pragmatic problem-solving based? Turriff, Levy, and Biesecker (2015) found that families fair best when they reframe their observations about family stressors and thereby increase their perceived capacity to cope. Reframing involves the affirmation of self-esteem, spiritual and psychological well-being, and social integration. Turriff and colleagues also found that engaging in problem-solving increases effective coping with disability.

The assessment of family stressors and the identification of needed resources and services might be done privately by families or if needed this work may be done with the assistance of professionals such as pediatricians, educators, counselors, or social workers. Upon acknowledgement and recognition, some stressors can be planned for and potentially abated. This analysis might be completed on a day-by-day basis at particularly stressful times. A week-by-week analysis of anticipated potential stressors might be completed during less stressful times. Once potential stressors are mediated either by reframing or by needed resources, a month-by-month check-up might be sufficient. Eventually, a family stressors evaluation and amelioration plan might be completed on an annual basis. In this way families would have increased awareness of their unique and individualized needs.

Chapter 8 of this text makes it clear that children with disabilities are at-risk for abuse and neglect when family life stressors pile up. Stressors are unique across families and are determined by each family's past, present, and future. In families of children with disabilities, the characteristics of a child's disability presents unique family stressors and resolution may require very specific reframing, as well as very specific knowledge, skills, and resources.

The families of children with disabilities will be less susceptible to being overwhelmed by child needs when family stressors are acknowledged and potentially mediated. An array of resource and service options may be provided to families in their effort to meet their own and the individualized needs of their children with disabilities. The price of abuse and neglect is so high for both perpetrators and victims that its prevention is an emergency. Clearly it is apparent that we need to:

Recommendation 12: Design individualized family stressor protocols as needed in order to enhance the coping capacities of children with disabilities and their families.

***

Chapter Summary

The identification of the roles and relationships of the perpetrators of ANCD was the focus of this chapter. Aggregate data as well as data from the research in this area indicate that biological mothers acting alone are the most frequently cited perpetrators of CAN. Biological parents account for more than 80 % of CAN. The newspaper coverage on ANCD mirror these statistics and add that school professionals are implicated in almost 11 % of the stories of abuse and neglect in the lives of children with disabilities. We provided stories from the newspaper coverage to illustrate these data and conclude the chapter with a set of recommendations for researchers and practitioners.

References

Alriksson-Schmidt, A., Armour, B. S., & Thibadeau, J. K. (2010). Are adolescent girls with a physical disability at increased risk for sexual violence? *Journal of School Health, 80*(7), 361–367. doi:10.1111/j.1746-1561.2010.00514.x

Associated Press. (2006, December 23). Jury convicts 2 for keeping kids in cages. *Chicago Tribune.* Retrieved from http://search.proquest.com/chicagotribune/docview/420509362/D48463AE61E54D7APQ/1?accountid=11578

Barnum, A. (2005, July 14). Teen testifies about abuse in trial of foster parents. *Chicago Tribune*. Retrieved from http://articles.chicagotribune.com/2005-07-14/news/0507140261_1_youth-paddle-frank-barney

Barone, L., Bramante, A., Lionetti, F., & Pastore, M. (2014). Mothers who murdered their child: An attachment-based study on filicide. *Child Abuse & Neglect, 38*(9), 1468–1477. doi:10.1016/j.chiabu.2014.04.014

Bones, P. D. C. (2013). Perceptions of vulnerability: A target characteristics approach to disability, gender, and victimization. *Deviant Behavior, 34*(9), 727–750. doi:10.1080/01639625.2013.766511

Caldas, S. J., & Bensy, M. L. (2014). The sexual maltreatment of students with disabilities in American school settings. *Journal of Child Sexual Abuse, 23*(4), 345–366. doi:10.1080/10538712.2014.906530

Chicago Tribune. (2013, April 15). Authorities: Father smothered crying girl. *Chicago Tribune*. Retrieved from http://articles.chicagotribune.com/2013-04-15/news/chi-baby-dies-days-after-father-smothered-her-to-stop-her-crying-20130415_1_playpen-court-documents-records

Coorg, R., & Tournay, A. (2013). Filicide-suicide involving children with disabilities. *Journal of Child Neurology, 28*(6), 745–751. doi:10.1177/0883073812451777

Douglas, E. M. (2014). A comparison of child fatalities by physical abuse versus neglect: Child, family, service, and worker characteristics. *Journal of Social Service Research, 40*(3), 259–273. doi:10.1080/01488376.2014.893948

Douglas, E. M., & Mohn, B. L. (2014). Fatal and non-fatal child maltreatment in the US: An analysis of child, caregiver, and service utilization with the National Child Abuse and Neglect Data Set. *Child Abuse & Neglect, 38*(1), 42–51. doi:10.1016/j.chiabu.2013.10.022

Emerson, E., & Brigham, P. (2014). The developmental health of children of parents with intellectual disabilities: Cross sectional study. *Research in Developmental Disabilities, 35*, 917–921. doi:10.1016/j.ridd.2014.01.006

Fentiman, L. C. (2014). Are mothers hazardous to their children's health?: Law, culture, and the framing of risk. *Virginia Journal of Social Policy and the Law, 21*, 295–341. Retrieved from http://eds.a.ebscohost.com/eds/pdfviewer/pdfviewer?vid=4&sid=54b4bdbe-8c5d-4313-8a27-c81eeb97c249%40sessionmgr4005&hid=4202

Fergus, M. A., & Working, R. (2005, April 16). Adoptive mom guilty in boy's slaying; Convicted of involuntary manslaughter. *Chicago Tribune*. Retrieved from http://search.proquest.com/chicagotribune/docview/420276386/66B69AB0EB774CB0PQ/1?accountid=11578

Goldberg, A. P., Tobin, J., Daigneau, J., Griffith, R. T., Reinert, S. E., & Jenny, C. (2009). Bruising frequency and patterns in children with physical disabilities. *Pediatrics, 124*(2), 604–609. doi:10.1542/peds.2008-2900

Healy, V. O., Gutowski, C., & Walberg, M. (2013, June 23). Autism and the tragedy of Alex Spourdalakis. *Chicago Tribune*. Retrieved from http://articles.chicagotribune.com/2013-06-23/news/ct-met-autism-death-20130623_1_autism-society-severe-autism-mary-kay-betz

Khalifeh, H., Howard, L., Osborn, D., Moran, P., & Johnson, S. (2013). Violence against people with disability in England and Wales: Findings from a national cross-sectional survey. *Plus One, 8*(2), 1–9. doi:10.1371/journal.pone.0055952

Leeb, R. T., Bitsko, R. H., Merrick, M. T., & Armour, B. S. (2012). Does childhood disability increase risk for child abuse and neglect? *Journal of Mental Health Research in Intellectual Disabilities, 5*(1), 4–31. doi:10.1080/19315864.2011.608154

Long, J. & Starks, C. (2004, March 13). Mother of dead teen held on $1 million bail; officials try to piece together his life. *Chicago Tribune*. Retrieved from http://articles.chicagotribune.com/2004-03-13/news/0403130137_1_seamus-crystal-lake-north-middle-school

McDonald, J. L., Milne, S., Knight, J., & Webster, V. (2013). Developmental and behavioural characteristics of children enrolled in a child protection pre-school. *Journal of Paediatrics & Child Health, 49*(2), 142–146. doi:10.1111/jpc.12029

Moehler, E., Biringen, Z., & Poustka, L. (2007). Emotional availability in a sample of mothers with a history of abuse. *American Journal of Orthopsychiatry, 77*(4), 624–628. doi:10.1037/0002-9432.77.4.624

Rodriguez, C. M., & Tucker, M. C. (2015). Predicting maternal physical child abuse risk beyond distress and social support: Additive role of cognitive processes. *Journal of Child and Family Studies, 24*(6), 1780–1790. doi:10.1007/s10826-014-9981-9

Roe, S. (2011, March 29). More deaths at kids' facility: Equip for Equality investigation details pattern of neglect at Alden Village North, slated for shutdown. *Chicago Tribune.* Retrieved by http://search.proquest.com/chicagotribune/docview/858917512/8A411299340D4FD2PQ/1?accountid=11578

Roe, S., & Hopkins, J. S. (2011, January 11). Center is cited in 14th death. *Chicago Tribune.* Retrieved from http://articles.chicagotribune.com/2011-01-11/health/ct-met-disabled-alden-deaths-20110110_1_alden-village-north-alden-management-services-14-month-old-girl

Rozas, A., & Breslin, M. M. (2005, November 3). Aide charged in disabled patient's rape. *Chicago Tribune.* Retrieved from http://articles.chicagotribune.com/2005-11-03/news/0511030314_1_criminal-investigation-sexual-abuse-ed-fox

Sandberg, K. (2014). Statement by Kirsten Sandberg, Chairperson of the Committee on the Rights of the Child at the 69th session of the General Assembly. See more at: http://www.ohchr.org/EN/NewsEvents/Pages/DisplayNews.aspx?NewsID=15327&LangID=E#sthash.DR57tLfF.dpuf

Sidebotham, P., & Golding, J. (2001). Child maltreatment in the "Children of the Nineties": A longitudinal study of parental risk factors. *Child Abuse & Neglect, 25*(9), 1177–1200. doi:10.1016/S0145-2134(01)00261-7

Sinanan, A. N. (2011). The impact of child, family, and child protective services factors on reports of child sexual abuse recurrence. *Journal of Child Sexual Abuse, 20*(6), 657–676. doi:10.1080/10538712.2011.622354

Sobol, R. R. (2013, June 12). 2 charged in autistic boy's fatal stabbing. *Chicago Tribune.* Retrieved from http://articles.chicagotribune.com/2013-06-12/news/ct-met-autistic-dead-charges-0612-20130612_1_fatal-stabbing-river-grove-autism

Sobsey, D., Randall, W., & Parrila, R. K. (1997). Gender differences in abused children with and without disabilities. *Child Abuse & Neglect, 21*(8), 707–720.

Soylu, N., Alpaslan, A. H., Ayaz, M., Esenyel, S., & Oruc, M. (2013). Psychiatric disorders and characteristics of abuse in sexually abused children and adolescents with and without intellectual disabilities. *Research in Developmental Disabilities, 34*(12), 4334–4342.

Stalker, K., & McArthur, K. (2012). Child abuse, child protection and disabled children: A review of recent research. *Child Abuse Review, 21*(1), 24–40. doi:10.1002/car.1154

Starks, C., & Long, J. (2004, March 14). Sad tale of dead teen: None knew his plight. *Chicago Tribune.* Retrieved from http://articles.chicagotribune.com/2004-03-14/news/0403140388_1_united-cerebral-palsy-police-crystal-lake

Turriff, A., Levy, H. P., & Biesecker, B. (2015). Factors associated with adaptation to Klinefelter syndrome: The experience of adolescents and adults. *Patient Education and Counseling, 98*(1), 90–95. doi:10.1016/j.pec.2014.08.012

U.S. Department of Health and Human Services, Administration for Children and Families, Administration on Children, Youth and Families, Children's Bureau. (2013). *Child maltreatment 2012.* Retrieved from http://www.acf.hhs.gov/programs/cb/research-data-technology/statistics-research/child-maltreatment

Wells, M., & Mitchell, K. J. (2013). Patterns of internet use and risk of online victimization for youth with and without disabilities. *The Journal of Special Education, 20*(10), 1–10. doi:10.1177/0022466913479141

Wigham, S., Taylor, J. L., & Hatton, C. (2014). A prospective study of the relationship between adverse life events and trauma in adults with mild to moderate intellectual disabilities. *Journal of Intellectual Disability Research, 58*(12), 1131–1140.

World Health Organization (WHO). (2014). Child abuse and neglect by parents and other caregivers. Retrieved from http://www.who.int/violence_injury_prevention/violence/global_campaign/en/chap3.pdf?ua=1

Chapter 7
The Disabilities of Perpetrators Who Abuse and Neglect Children with Disabilities

> *The strength of a nation derives from the integrity of the home.* (Confucius, 551 BCE – 479 BCE)

Abstract Knowing perpetrators' disabilities has potential to inform child abuse and neglect (CAN) and abuse and neglect of children with disabilities (ANCD) intervention and prevention efforts in a variety of fields. This chapter focuses particularly on the disabilities of the perpetrators of ANCD. We examine the prevailing disabilities among the perpetrators as well as the unique challenges presented by "hidden" disabilities. We analyze the data in large databases as well as the literature on the disabilities of the people that are more prone to perpetrate ANCD. We focus on such questions as, what disabilities are more likely to be observed among the perpetrators of ANCD? We present the findings of a study on the newspaper coverage of the disabilities of the perpetrators of ANCD. We get behind the numbers and illustrate them with stories of real people who perpetrate ANCD. We conclude this chapter with a set of recommendations for researchers and practitioners.

Most people have difficulty thinking about the perpetrators of abuse and neglect of any kind. It is so much easier to label them as such and dismiss them to law enforcement personnel as quickly as possible. Why would anyone want to spend time thinking about people who hurt children with and without disabilities? Shall we notify the nearest law-enforcement officer and consider that our work is done? Sadly no! It is not that easy.

We cannot dismiss perpetrators as irrelevant in our herculean efforts to end the abuse and neglect of children with and without disabilities. Rather, we must get to know these people in order to prevent the abuse and neglect they effect on children's lives. We cannot dismiss perpetrators to law enforcement personnel without making every effort to get to know and understand them. This is essential in order to predict better their perspectives as well as the contexts that serve to sustain the occurrence of CAN and ANCD. Therefore, getting to know the perpetrators of abuse and neglect in the lives of children with and without disabilities is an essential step in the development of effective intervention and prevention programming.

© Springer International Publishing Switzerland 2016

E.P. Crowley, *Preventing Abuse and Neglect in the Lives of Children with Disabilities*, DOI 10.1007/978-3-319-30442-7_7

Exercise 7.1: Reflection
Do you believe that caregiver disability characteristics are relevant to the health and safety of children with disabilities? *Make at least three arguments to support your perspective.*

As we proceed with this chapter compelling questions emerge. Are adults and caregivers with disabilities disproportionately represented among the perpetrators of CAN and ANCD? Are parents, caregivers and other adults with learning disabilities, intellectual disabilities, physical and sensory disabilities, and psychiatric disorders more likely than nondisabled caregivers to abuse and neglect children with disabilities? Are adults with intellectual disabilities fit to be parents? Can we determine a point at which adults with disabilities are unable to provide appropriate care for children with and without disabilities? In short, what do we know about the relevance of having a disability and being more or less likely to perpetrate CAN or ANCD? Are there observable patterns of CAN and ANCD across alleged and confirmed adult caregivers with disabilities? The difficult questions go on. Here we focus on finding out as much as we can about the relevance of caregiver disability characteristics to the safety and protection of the children with disabilities in their care.

In this chapter we will focus on such questions as, do the perpetrators of CAN and ANCD have disabilities themselves? If so, what are they? Do children with disabilities become the human shields between their perpetrators and their lack of access to essential resources? Who educates and provides ongoing support to caregivers with special needs? First, we will examine data from the U.S. DHHS and other large databases that address this issue. We will then examine the research in this area and conclude the chapter with the findings from the study of the newspaper coverage and stories about the disabilities of perpetrators that were published in the *Chicago Tribune* from January 2004–December 2013.

The Disabilities of Perpetrators

The U.S. DHHS (2013) provides demographic data (Chaps. 3, 4 and 5) on the perpetrators of CAN and in Chap. 8 we will further examine the contexts in which CAN occurs. These demographic and contextual data are not disaggregated to focus specifically on the perpetrators of ANCD. Furthermore, these data provide no information about the disabilities of perpetrators. Perpetrators are not required to disclose their disabilities during the CAN investigation process and there is no requirement that the notification of perpetrators' disabilities is included in the state reports to NCANDS.

Perpetrators may have observable disabilities or they may have "hidden" disabilities across their lifespans. Physical disabilities such as paralysis, partial or complete amputation of limbs, limb deformity, and mobility impairments are all clearly observable. "Hidden" disabilities include learning disabilities, intellectual disabilities, emotional and psychological disorders, communication disorders or sensory impairments.

Learning disability (LD) and intellectual disability (ID) are examples of "hidden" disabilities that impact learners across the lifespan. LD is most clearly observable among children in school environments. Both LD and ID interrupt learning in childhood and in adulthood. LD is a neurological disorder that affects the brain's ability to receive, process, store, and respond to information. LD varies in how it impacts each individual child, adolescent and adult (Hallahan, Kauffman, & Pullen, 2015). Hallahan et al. describe ID as characterized by significant limitations in intellectual functioning and adaptive behavior that is expressed in deficits in conceptual, social, and adaptive functioning.

Individuals with both LD, ID and "hidden" disabilities may have difficulty with thinking, reasoning, understanding words, and with short-term and/or long-term memory loss. These individuals may have difficulty paying attention, solving problems, thinking abstractly, talking, and behaving. LD, ID, and emotional and psychological disorders challenge individuals' daily functioning in profoundly real ways, far beyond classroom environments and throughout their lifespans.

Discrimination between the characteristics of learning disabilities and intellectual disabilities offers unique challenges to researchers and practitioners. The most glaring difference between LD and ID is that individuals with learning disabilities have normal intelligence and those with ID do not.

Perpetrators with Intellectual Disabilities

Researchers have long been concerned about the health and welfare of children whose caregivers have intellectual disabilities (Brown & Schormans, 2003; Emerson & Brigham, 2014; Pestka & Wendt, 2014; Schormans & Brown, 2006; World Health Organization, 2014). The child development outcomes and the between-group differences for children whose caregivers do and do not have ID was the focus of a study by Emerson and Brigham (2014). The researchers generated data from 46,025 families. Adults with ID were the parents of children in 992 (2.16 %) of these families. Emerson and Brigham found significantly higher rates of poor outcomes across four measures of child health among the children of adult caregivers with ID.

Children with one or two parents with ID were more frequently exposed to environmental risks. Developmental delays and speech and language delays were also observed more frequently in the children of parents with ID. They were at an increased risk for exposure to poverty, poor housing, family isolation, violence, and abuse. They also failed to access appropriate medical intervention more frequently. Overall, parents with (ID) had more frequent parenting problems than parents without ID. Emerson and Brigham concluded that based on their observations "... it is likely that parenting difficulties may be an inevitable outcome of intellectual disability ..." (p. 921).

Collings and Llewellyn (2012) expressed concern about the possibility of unfair bias toward caregivers with ID. They reviewed research published from March 2010 to March 2011. They found mixed results in that some children of parents with ID fare well while others do not. They concluded that children grow and develop well when such variables as poverty, social isolation, high-risk pregnancies, birth complications, and troubled parental childhoods "are taken into account" (p. 80). In such circumstances, the social and academic characteristics of children whose parents have ID approach population norms. They acknowledged the data based findings that children of parents with ID will more likely experience social exclusion, bullying, and stigma. Collings and Llewellyn concluded by cautioning against the stereotype that the children of parents with intellectual disabilities should "be regarded as uniformly in need of protection from harm" (p. 81).

The role of intelligence cannot be separated from other confounding factors such as increased risk of abuse history, increased probability of family isolation and differences in detecting and reporting CAN. Azar, Stevenson, and Johnson (2012) examined the role of IQ in parenting risk. Azar and her colleagues were concerned that parents with ID were identified by IQ tests alone and were overrepresented in the child protective services (CPS). This overrepresentation gives the perception that there may be a positive correlation between low IQ and parenting ability; therefore mothers with ID might be perceived as having low parenting skills. Azar et al. investigated the utility of a Social Information Processing (SIP) model which included several domains such as schema (realistic expectations), executive functioning, knowledge structure, contextual factors, parent characteristics, and child characteristics.

Azar et al. examined the social information processing of 73 mothers with low IQs. Forty three (58.9 %) of these mothers had one and more than one contact with CPS and they formed the neglect group. The control group comprised 30 (41.1 %) mothers with low IQs and did not have CPS records. The neglect group had a lower mean IQ score (73.4) than the comparison group (83.5). The researchers administered questionnaires, wrote their observations and visited participants' homes during the course of the study.

Azar and her colleagues found that the mothers in the neglect group were younger, more frequently single, and poorer than the control group. They had fewer years of formal education and had more children than those in the control group. They also found that mothers with low IQs in the neglect group had higher scores in measures of unrealistic expectations, cognitive inflexibility, poorer problem solving skills and greater anticipation of negative outcomes. Mothers in the neglect group made "more negative misappraisals of child behavior in the form of hostile attributional biases compared with a demographically similar set of comparison mothers" (p. 120). These mothers interpreted child behaviors as specifically designed to annoy them more frequently than mothers in the control group. Azar et al. concluded that SIP factors appeared to be linked to neglectful parenting for a sample of mothers with low IQ. That is, mothers with more limited cognitive skills in the SIP domain areas were more likely to have low IQs and more likely to neglect their children.

Exercise 7.2: Reflection
Susan and her partner John are both 25 years old. Both of their IQ scores are in the 55–60 range. Susan is pregnant and her parents came to you for help. They are worried about Susan's and John's readiness for their parenting responsibilities. Imagine that you are in a unique professional position to guide them. *What guidance would you provide them? What will guide your own thinking?*

Perpetrators with Psychiatric Disorders

Traumatic experiences in childhood matter. Men and women who have childhood histories of abuse and neglect are at particular risk for psychiatric diagnoses in adulthood. Children who grow up in conflict, deprivation, fear, and overexposure to trauma need support not just during these events but for long after. Those who are denied the emotional and psychological support they need, often go on to live lives that remake the original trauma over and over again. They lack the skills to seek, accept and integrate the assistance they need. They go on to repeat, again and again, the cycle of trauma with which they are all too familiar.

Depression is a hidden disability which can be mild, moderate and severe as well as short-term and/or long-term. Capaldi (2014) conducted a longitudinal study of 125 pregnant women diagnosed with antenatal depression at 36 weeks of pregnancy. The women provided retrospective reports of their own experiences of abuse and neglect in their childhood. They each had a history of antisocial behavior, psychiatric problems, and depression. By age 11 years old their children had become the victims of CAN. During adolescence their children exhibited antisocial behavior. By age 16, their children were diagnosed with depression.

Capaldi found that maternal antenatal depression reliably sets women up for future psychopathology, to have families at-risk, and to abuse and neglect of their children. This finding and the findings of other researchers indicate that engaging mothers with depression in child abuse prevention programming is essential. They must learn how to access the resources that support them and their families. During pregnancy women and their partners are in contact with professionals in the health services and making it an appropriate time to participate in classes that would guide their understanding of and caring for their babies' healthy growth and development. They have an increased need to engage in parenting classes in order to learn how to avoid harsh discipline practices. Capaldi suggests screening for maltreatment among pregnant women. When abuse and neglect is indicated in their childhood experiences, they need to engage in focused development of self-awareness; the development of strong parenting skills; and in the development of a strong support system that will sustain them through their years of child caregiving.

Kaplan, Sunday, Labruna, Pelcovitz, and Salzinger (2009) examined the hypothesis that psychiatric disorders place parents at higher risk for physically abusing their adolescent children and that psychiatric disorders contribute to risk for being the parent of an abused adolescent. A total of 310 parents with psychiatric disorders were included in this study. Among them were 188 mothers (90 mothers in the abuse group and 98 in the comparison group) and 122 fathers (52 in the abuse group and 70 in the comparison group) were included in this study. Kaplan and her colleagues found that in all 142 (45.8 %) parents had physically abused their children and 168 (54.2 %) had not abused their children.

The parents who physically abused their adolescent children were younger and significantly less educated. They were more likely to either be divorced or separated than the comparison group. They had higher rates of psychiatric disorders than parents in the comparison group. Mothers and fathers in the abuse group showed significantly higher lifelong evidence of depression, anxiety, and/or dependence on alcohol and drugs. Fathers of physically abused adolescents had a greater lifetime incidence of conduct disorder (CD) and substance abuse/dependence than comparison fathers. Additionally, they found that mothers of abused adolescents had more unipolar depressive disorders than mothers in the comparison group. Kaplan et al. recommended mental health assessments and interventions for parents of adolescents who are physically abused. They observed that since parents' psychiatric disorders preceded their children's physical abuse, early recognition and treatment of parents' psychiatric disorders may contribute to the prevention of CAN and ANCD.

Who are the perpetrators of filicide? Neonaticide? Infanticide? Filicide is the murder of a child by a parent, neonaticide of the murder of a newborn by a parent and infanticide is the murder of a child by a parent in the first year of life. See also Chaps. 4 and 6 relative to the outcomes of ANCD and perpetrators' roles and relationships respectively.

Exercise 7.3: Reflection
Are you surprised, shocked, or perhaps speechless to hear that some parents, though a very small number, end the lives of their children with disabilities? *What might lead a parent to end the life of a child with a disability? List as many scenarios as you can.*

Filicide, neonaticide and infanticide occur all over the world. Coorg and Tournay (2013) conducted a study of filicide-suicide cases involving the deaths of 26 children with disabilities and the suicides or suicide attempts of 22 parent caregiver in the United States. They found that among those who perpetrated the deaths of their children with disabilities were 11 fathers (including one grandfather), 11 mothers. Five of the fathers and three of the mothers (38.1 %) who killed themselves and their children with disabilities had reported psychiatric disorders. Depression (3 cases), psychosis (3 cases), and bipolar disorder (3 cases) were the most common psychiatric conditions reported. Other psychiatric disorders included combinations of conditions for example, a father with paranoid delusions, obsessive compulsive disorder, psychosis and depression and a mother with "suspected bipolar versus psychosis (medicated)" (p. 748). No diagnosis was reported for 12 of the 21 (57.1 %) caregivers. Coorg and Tournay found that 87.5 % (7 out the 8) of the fathers with psychiatric conditions attempted and completed suicides and none of the mothers with psychiatric disorders who attempted actually completed suicide.

Barone, Bramante, Lionetti, and Pastore (2014) investigated variables that predict the engagement of mothers in filicide. They studied a group of 121 mothers; 61 were from a normal population, 37 were mothers with mental illness, and 23 of these mothers had committed filicide. The women were from 23 to 44 years old, and they came from low, medium, and high socioeconomic backgrounds. Barone and her colleagues found that 86.9 % (20) of the mothers in the filicide group experienced traumatic events whereas 75.0 % (28) and 44.3 % (27) of the mothers with mental illness and the normative group respectively experienced traumatic events. Traumatic events were described as the loss of a parent in childhood, the experience of frightening abusive experiences and the experience of extreme emotional threats.

Barone et al. found that mothers in the three groups differed in their emotional attachment to their children. Mothers in the filicide group scored highest in measures of helplessness and hostility toward their children. These researchers concluded that a combination of low socioeconomic status, a diagnosis of mental illness, traumatic events, unresolved experiences of traumatic events, and high hostility reliably predict filicide.

Exercise 7.4: Critical Thinking

Data indicate that caregivers with mental illness are at a higher risk of abusing and neglecting their children than are those who do not have mental illnesses. Data also indicate that they are at higher risk of being stigmatized due to societal stereotypes concerning mental illness and therefore they are at increased risk as perpetrators of CAN and ANCD. *Do you believe that mental illness and parenthood are compatible? Write at least three arguments to support your perspective.*

Child Perpetrators With and Without Disabilities

Do children themselves perpetrate CAN and ANCD? This area of study is complicated by theories of human development which promote the idea that it is quite normal for children to explore their physical, emotional, and sexual limits and boundaries (Banks, 2014; Bladon, Vizard, French, & Tranah, 2005; Firth et al., 2001; Martinello, 2015; Vizard, 2013). When does what initially may appear to be normal child curiosity become abusive and neglectful? When does play stop being play, and when does it become violent and abusive? When does resilience in the presence of deprivation stop? Where do normal life experiences end and abuse and neglect begin? When do children's interactions with their peers with disabilities stop being within socially acceptable boundaries? When do they become the perpetrators of abuse and neglect of their peers with and without disabilities?

In a recent study Allen, Tellez, Wevodau, Woods, and Percosky (2014) designed a study to examine the mental health status of 363 college students who had been sexually abused by child, teen, and adult perpetrators. Among the 363 participants,

144 (39.6 %) students acknowledged unwanted sexual contact prior to the age of 12. The participants reported that their perpetrators were child peers in 37 (25.7 %) cases, 39 (27.1 %) participants reported that their perpetrator was a teenager, and 48 (33.3 %) reported that their perpetrators were adults. Eleven (7.6 %) participants reported being abused by more than one perpetrator and 9 (7.6 %) failed to report the age of their perpetrators.

Allen et al. (2014) found that students with histories of sexual abuse scored higher in measures of anxiety, depression, and sexual problems. They found no differences among victims who were threatened with embarrassment or physical force. Victims who were abused by children were less likely to describe their experience as sexual abuse than those who were abused by teens and adults. Those who reported abuse by family members were more likely to indicate that their abuser was an adult. Allen et al. recommended continued efforts to understand child perpetrators. They also recommended the education of children using developmentally appropriate curriculum and materials that clarify the difference between physically, emotionally, and sexually appropriate and inappropriate behaviors among children.

Overall, data indicate that many of the perpetrators of CAN and ANCD are people with an assortment of disabilities themselves. Little attention has been given to this in large databases of U.S. DHHS and other international data bases. Independent researchers provide data on the disabilities of the perpetrators of CAN and ANCD. Research findings indicate that men, women, and children with observable and "hidden" disabilities perpetrate CAN and ANCD. They are more prone to doing so in contexts where they are exposed to poverty, social isolation, high-risk pregnancies, and previous exposure to trauma. We provide data from an analysis of the newspaper coverage in the next section.

Newspaper Findings

The disabilities of the perpetrators of ANCD were specified for 21 out of 78 (27.0 %) separate stories that were published in the *Chicago Tribune* from 2004 to 2013. Psychiatric disorders were associated with these individuals more frequently than any other disabilities (see Table 7.1). More than half of the stories described perpetrators with such psychiatric disorders as attention deficit disorder, antisocial personality disorder, obsessive paranoia, depression, paranoid sex addict,

Table 7.1 The disabilities of adult perpetrators (n = 21)

Type of disability	n[a]	%
Psychiatric disorders	11	52.4
Multiple disorders	9	42.8
Hearing impairment	1	4.7

[a]Only stories that included information about perpetrators' psychiatric disorders

Data from a study of the newspaper coverage in the *Chicago Tribune*

Table 7.2 The disabilities of child perpetrators (n = 8)

Type of disability	n	%
Emotional/Behavioral disorders	5	62.5
Intellectual disability	1	12.5
Learning disability	1	12.5
Unspecified disability[a]	1	12.5

[a]General reference to childhood disability such as disabled child, child with a handicap, child in special education

Data from a study of the newspaper coverage in the *Chicago Tribune*

posttraumatic stress disorder, and separation anxiety disorder. Almost half of these individuals had multiple disorders including such conditions as "anger, learning disorder, ADD and rage", "multiple sclerosis, psychosis, cognitive disorder, impulsivity and short-term memory issues" and "mental disorder and sexually violent person". These data reflected individuals with complex disabilities.

What are the characteristics of the remaining 57 out of 78 (73 %) perpetrators who ANCD and who were not reported to have had a disability themselves. What precipitates their ANCD? Do these individuals have undiagnosed disabilities? In Chap. 8 we will learn more about the perpetrators of ANCD and the contexts in which their ANCD occurs.

Children with disabilities were also among the perpetrators of ANCD described in stories in the *Chicago Tribune* (see Table 7.2). Disabilities were specified for 8 out of 13 (61.5 %) child perpetrators. Emotional and behavioral disorders were described most frequently among these children. These included such disorders as posttraumatic stress disorder, "emotional problems", ADHD, eating disorder, self-mutilation, and depression. Additional child perpetrator disabilities described included autism, Asperger's syndrome, and prenatal exposure to drugs.

Exercise 7.5: Critical Thinking

Are you surprised to observe that emotional and behavioral disorders among children with disabilities and psychiatric disorders among adult perpetrators are the disabilities most frequently associated with ANCD? *Write at least three reasons to support your observations. Then write at least three implications of these data for researchers and clinical personnel.*

The People Behind the Numbers

The following stories illustrate the findings of this study. These data confirm that mothers with disabilities abuse and neglect their children with disabilities. This is illustrated in a story on May 11, 2006 by Jeff Coen, *Chicago Tribune* staff reporter who described the death of a 9-year-old girl. ". . . Barwin Husan, who was deaf and blind . . . was tied to the radiator and left alone before she untied herself and plunged from a third-floor window of the family's apartment on the North Side." A neighbor discovered the child's body on the pavement nearly 2 h after the incident occurred.

Coen reported that "Investigators have said two cloth belts from bathrobes were knotted together and tied to a radiator, and they believe the child was bound there to keep her restrained." Coen added that "The girl's mother Balwa, 36, is charged with child endangerment and neglect... Barwin's stepfather, Shakir Alshahien, was [also] charged in the case and is awaiting trial."

Coen reported:

> ... the woman was imprisoned three times during Saddam Hussein's regime in her native Iraq, the first time when she was only 10 years old. Balwa was kept in a tiny cell for months, was forced to watch her father being beaten and was left with post-traumatic stress disorder...

Medical examinations showed that "Balwa's disorder 'left her out of touch with reality...'" She faced up to 5 years in prison and had been bailed out of the Cook County Jail. She was put on medication and regained custody of her other children. Her trial began in September of 2006.

Exercise 7.6: Reflection

What elements of this story disturb you most at this point? *Write at least five indicators that suggested this family needed help? Then, make a list of at least five ways this scenario might have been prevented?*

On September 7, 2006, Sadovi reported that: Sundas Blawa did not attend a scheduled court hearing. Her attorneys stated that "...she suffers from post-traumatic stress disorder and major depression... They submitted documents from psychiatrists saying that the woman had become mentally unhinged." On September 13, Sadovi reported that she is "... currently on trial in absentia for the 2002 death of her disabled daughter suffered from post-traumatic stress disorder and depression from being tortured by former Iraq President Saddam Hussein's soldiers, a torture expert testified Tuesday."

The case continued and Carlos Sadovi reported on September 14, 2006:

> A Cook County jury ruled Wednesday that an Iraqi woman whose disabled daughter fell to her death 4 years ago not guilty of criminal endangerment and neglect Wednesday.
>
> After more than six hours of deliberations, jurors said Sundas Balwa was not guilty by reason of insanity. Balwa, 37, was being tried in absentia for the death of 9-year-old Barwin Harsan in 2002. The child fell from a third-floor window in her family's apartment in the 2600 block of West Farragut Avenue after allegedly being tied to a radiator and left.
>
> Immediately after the verdict, Cook County Criminal Court Judge Clayton Crane issued a warrant for Balwa's arrest, requiring her to show up to court to determine what mental health services the woman required. The court could order her held in a state-run hospital.

This story continued. Sadovi's article "Iraqi mom faces psychiatric testing; woman acquitted in daughter's death" appeared in the *Chicago Tribune* on October 12, 2006. In this article he stated:

> An Iraqi woman who was acquitted last month of criminal endangerment for the 2002 death of her disabled daughter was ordered held by a Cook County judge Wednesday to undergo an inpatient psychiatric evaluation.
>
> Sundas Balwa, 37, was found not guilty by reason of insanity by a jury on Sept. 13 for the May 12, 2002, death of her 9-year-old daughter, Barwin Husan. The girl, who was deaf, blind and mentally disabled, fell out of a window in the family's North Side home when she was left alone.

> An emotional Balwa, 37, appeared before Cook County Criminal Court Judge Clayton Crane and tearfully pleaded not to be locked up in a psychiatric hospital.
>
> "I beg you, I cannot leave my children, I cannot stay away from my children. I will die if I am taken away from my children," Balwa said through an Arabic interpreter. "Just give me this chance, your honor. Do not leave me away from my children for one hour."

The final article in this story was written by Fitzsimmons and Heinzmann and published in the *Chicago Tribune* on November 23, 2006. The story titled, "Mother to reunite with family; woman released in daughter's death." Sundas Balwa was found not guilty by reason of insanity in the death of her disabled daughter. Fitzsimmons and Heinzmann reported that "An Iraqi woman, found not guilty by reason of insanity in the death of her disabled daughter, was released from a mental health facility Wednesday, in time to spend Thanksgiving with her husband and surviving children." Fitzsimmons and Heinzmann stated that "Doctors who evaluated her 'found that she has a supportive home to return to, and that there is no situation of abuse or extreme stress that would exacerbate her condition . . ..'"

Exercise 7.7: Reflection

Did you expect this outcome for this story? Do you believe that justice was done? *What are your thoughts and feelings as you read through the details of this story? What can we learn from this story about the intervention and prevention of abuse and neglect in the lives of children with disabilities?*

Males with disabilities in their 60s perpetrate ANCD. Greco (2006, June 7) reported a story about a man, 69-year-old Lawrence Lee Southwood, who was accused of repeatedly sexually molesting a 14-year-old girl with developmental disabilities. Police attempted to link Southwood to the death of a 3-year-old girl, but could not find one. Greco reported:

> George Lenard, his attorney, argued that a jailhouse confession Southwood made to police should be suppressed in that case. He told Judge Daniel Rozak that prosecutors tried to "pin" the Fox slaying on his client and are trying to do the same in the unrelated molestation.
>
> Lenard said that an investigator for the state's attorney's office effectively coerced the confession by not taking into account Southwood's mental and physical state during the December interview.
>
> Lenard said Southwood, who has an 8th grade education, was undernourished and psychologically confused when he agreed to waive his Miranda rights and talk to police. He also said Southwood has a hearing impairment that wasn't detected when police questioned him.

Southwood has a long history with the criminal justice system. In 1961 he pleaded guilty to rape, in 1967 he pleaded guilty to an attempted murder in the 1980s he pleaded guilty to sex acts with his daughter. In June 2007 he was accused of ". . . five counts of aggravated criminal sexual assault and abuse, he faces up to 97 years in prison. . .".

Exercise 7.8: Critical Thinking

Are you confident that Mr. Southwood's rights were protected by law enforcement personnel? Are his disabilities relevant? *Argue pro or con. Make at least three arguments to support your perspective.*

The details of an incident that occurred on February 1, 2012 in Calumet City first became known on October 19, 2012. Ryan Haggerty reaffirmed:

> The records of the investigation, obtained by the *Tribune* through a Freedom of Information Act request, give the most comprehensive summary yet of the events that led to Stephon's death.

The relationship between a child's disability and violence is captured by *Chicago Tribune* reporter Ryan Haggerty in 2012. Stephon Edward Watts' was 15 years old and diagnosed with Asperger's syndrome when he was 9 years old. He was 5 ft 7 in. (1.7 m) and he weighed 205 lb (93 kg). He was well known to the Calumet City police officers because they had been called to his home 10 times over a 2-year period before his death. On the morning of February 1, 2012 Stephon refused to go to school and his father called the police. Haggerty reported that:

> Extra officers were sent to the house in the 500 block of Forsythe Avenue because of Stephon's history of fighting with police, according to the investigation.
>
> Stephon's father met officers Robert Hynek, William Coffey and Jeff McBrayer when they arrived at the front door. He told them his son had left the house and that everything was under control, according to the investigation.
>
> All three officers had been at the house when Stephon locked himself in the bathroom, and they told his father they needed to check the house to make sure everyone was OK, according to the investigation. When they entered the house, Stephon's father told them his son was actually in the basement.
>
> Steven Watts told his son to come upstairs, but he refused. Stephon's father then led the three officers down the basement stairs.
>
> As they neared the bottom of the stairs, Stephon came around a corner holding a steak knife, ran past his father and charged the officers, who tried to go back up the stairs, according to the investigation. Stephon cut Hynek on the left forearm with the knife just before Hynek and Coffey fired one shot each, according to interviews with the officers included in the investigation.
>
> Autopsy reports and photos included in the state police investigation show Stephon was shot behind the right shoulder and below the right arm.

Stephon's parents and the police tell different stories about this incident. Haggerty stated that now they "...wish they hadn't called police the morning ... If they hadn't called police, they say, their son – who had autism – would still be alive." Stephon's parents insist that he used a butter knife when he approached and cut the arm of one of the police officers. The police insist that he used a steak knife "...to slash one of the officers." Haggerty stated that Stephon's parents "... are haunted by their son's death, replaying it in their minds while they're awake and having nightmares about it while they're asleep." His mother stated recently "'It's really hard,' she said ... struggling to speak through her tears. 'I can't understand that he's dead.'"

Exercise 7.9: Reflection
Are you surprised to read this story? *If so, why? What aspects of this story are most significant to you? Does this story cause you to reconsider how you think about perpetrators with disabilities? Write at least three suggestions of ways we can go about preventing abuse and neglect by perpetrators with disabilities.*

Perpetrators with and without disabilities wreak havoc on children's lives. What signs along the way do we miss? What might parents, teachers, and people who know these individuals do to prevent the violence they perpetrate? How might social service agencies more flexibly respond to the real and perceived needs of adults with disabilities? On October 7, 2009, *Chicago Tribune* reporter Matthew Walberg provided a close-up look at the violence people with disabilities perpetrate. He reported that James Degorski was convicted for the 1993 murders of seven workers from the Brown's Chicken restaurant in Palatine, Illinois. Walberg reported that the Cook County jury and members of the legal system had:

> ... one more decision to make: whether he should be sentenced to the death penalty. His accomplice, Juan Luna, was sentenced to life in prison in 2007.
>
> ... Degorski suffered from depression, post-traumatic stress disorder and other problems because of a horrifying childhood.
>
> Degorski's parents were both victims of abuse as children, and his father, a paranoid sex addict and alcoholic, walked naked around the house, spied on his children through peepholes in the walls and frequently beat Degorski and his four siblings, according to Smith.
>
> To escape, Degorski drank at age 10 and was abusing drugs and alcohol almost daily by age 18, Smith testified. Even now, Degorski is reluctant to discuss his childhood and sees alcohol and drugs as a proper escape from his past, he said.

Exercise 7.10: Critical Thinking

The references of this chapter contain the complete story written by Matthew Walberg on October 2009. *Following a careful analysis of this story, make a list of at least five ways which the violence perpetrated by Mr. Degorski might be interrupted? What are the implications of your list for the prevention of violence, abuse, and neglect perpetrated by people with disabilities?*

Are people with intellectual disabilities unfairly chastised for their behavior? Do they fully understand their actions? Members of the Hart family live with these questions every day. On April 8, 2009 Howard Witt, of the *Chicago Tribune* reported that:

> For more than six hours Tuesday, as a parade of witnesses testified about the severity of Aaron Hart's mental retardation and his inability to understand his legal rights, the 18-year-old defendant with an IQ of 47 sat silent and shackled in a chair, alternately fidgeting and making faces.
>
> ... His former special-education teacher testified that Hart functions below the level of a 1st grader.
>
> Last September, Hart confessed to police that he forced the boy to perform oral sex. The boy's stepmother had discovered them both behind a shed with their pants lowered. Hart's court-appointed attorney entered guilty pleas on his behalf to five related felony counts, a jury recommended multiple sentences and Clifford stacked the prison terms to run consecutively, for a total of 100 years.

The judge took only a few seconds to issue his decision. He stated, "Irregardless [sic] of whether he understood his Miranda rights, the evidence I have seen is overwhelming that he committed the offense ... The court finds that allegations of incompetence of counsel are unfounded." Witt reported that ineffective legal assistance, failure to present expert testimony about Hart's mental functioning, and Hart's own failure to understand the charges against him contributed to the outcome of this story.

Implications for Research and Practice

Children and adults with disabilities are among both perpetrators and victims of CAN and ANCD. Adults and children with disabilities who have been exposed to traumatic events themselves are at increased risk to perpetrate CAN and ANCD (Azar et al., 2012; Collings & Llewellyn, 2012; Emerson & Brigham, 2014). Do you expect that people with some disabilities are at increased risk of perpetrating CAN or ANCD? Are there predictable differences between male and female disability characteristics and their proneness to engage in specific types of abuse and neglect? To what extent are adults with disabilities aware of their own vulnerability as perpetrators of CAN and ANCD? What are the prevailing public perceptions of people with disabilities? In this section we will discuss the implications of perpetrators' disabilities for research and practice. We will focus on looming research questions in this area, the need for the development of focused programs that support people with disabilities and the need to build public awareness programs that focus on disability in childhood and adulthood.

Looming Research Questions

In this chapter we learned that caregivers with psychiatric disorders seem at increased risk of becoming potential perpetrators of CAN and ANCD (Capaldi, 2014; Kaplan et al., 2009). Perpetrators of filicide – that is, those who perpetrate the death of their children with and without disabilities, have higher rates of mental illness such as depression, anxiety disorders, and experience traumatic events early in their lives (Barone et al., 2014; Coorg & Tournay, 2013). Emerson and Brigham (2014) found that caregivers with intellectual disabilities are also particularly vulnerable as potential perpetrators of CAN and ANCD. Caregivers who perceive themselves as helpless and exhibit hostility are at increased risk to perpetrate CAN and ANCD. To what extent do people with disabilities perpetrate abuse and neglect in the lives of children with and without disabilities? The U.S. DHHS is in an ideal position to generate data on the disabilities of perpetrators. These data are not available at this time and we suggest that:

Recommendation 1: The U.S. DHHS generate data on the disabilities of the perpetrators of abuse and neglect in the lives of children with and without disabilities.

***

Kaplan et al. (2009) observed that existing research on the psychiatric illness of perpetuators of CAN and ANCD have been hampered by methodological limitations. These limitations include recruitment of families from service sites rather than directly from state agencies legally responsible for abuse documentation; recruitment of samples with multiple types of maltreatment and a wide range of ages; reliance on adults' retrospective reports of maltreatment, and on the use of nonstandardized diagnostic instruments. We observe the need to:

Recommendation 2: Focus on the generation of data from local, regional, and state level agencies that are legally responsible for the documentation of CAN and ANCD.

***

We need to know more about the risk factors associated with parenting children with disabilities, as well as, the risk factors associated with the parenting of adults with an assortment of disabilities (Azar et al., 2012). Is it possible that adults with some disabilities are more at-risk of engaging in CAN and ANCD than others? How do reciprocating child characteristics impact CAN and ANCD risk? Research, using longitudinal, population-based data would contribute greatly to our knowledge about the likely long-term outcomes for children and their parents with disabilities (Collings & Llewellyn, 2012). Finally, cases of filicide, neonaticide and infanticide are perhaps the most shocking and the worst possible outcomes for children who are exposed to abuse and neglect. Determining the risk factors that contribute to these behaviors is essential in order to intervene promptly, thus saving human lives. We observe the need to:

Recommendation 3: Develop research studies in order to understand the risk factors associated with parenting by adults with an assortment of disabilities. Focus particularly on adult disability and child characteristics relative to CAN or ANCD risk.

***

How can perpetrators with disabilities be reliably identified as being at-risk to perpetrate CAN and ANCD? Kaplan et al. suggest the use of screening protocols with those who are at particular risk of engaging in perpetrator behaviors. The data generated would reliably indicate those who are in need of learning how to negotiate the challenges of parenting and thereby increase awareness about their risk of perpetrating behaviors. Risk assessment checklists may focus on the assessment of a variety of parenting demands. The National Child Abuse Hotline (Childhelp®, 2015) recommends that caregivers:

- Begin today by being a positive parent or caretaker and help other family members, friends, and neighbors be positive parents too;
- Make children's lives a priority – regardless of disability;
- Show and tell your children that you love them every day;
- Let your children know you are happy to be with them;
- Give children the sense of security, belonging, and support;
- Catch your children being good and give them lots of praise;

Caregivers who communicate indicators that they are unable to engage in these behaviors or who do not believe in doing so might be at increased risk to engage in child perpetrator behaviors. We will predict and prevent CAN and ANCD more readily when:

Recommendation 4: Researchers examine caregiver attitudes and behaviors in order to predict the presence of perpetrator risk factors.

***

The U.S. DHHS indicate that biological mothers are the most frequent perpetrators of CAN and ANCD. Ethier, Couture, and Lacharité (2004) used the Child Abuse Potential Inventory (CAPI) to identify the characteristics of mothers who neglect their children. These included:

- limited education;
- having more than three children;
- living alone;
- lack of biological mother in their support system

Additionally, other critical characteristics included:

- mental health problems;
- childhood foster care placements; and
- past trauma

Neglect appears to be the most common form of ANCD amongst parents with intellectual disabilities (ID) (Azar et al., 2012; Brown & Schormans, 2003; Collings & Llewellyn, 2012; Emerson & Brigham, 2014; Pestka & Wendt, 2014; Schormans & Brown, 2006). These data indicate that the most common stressors in households headed by parents/caregivers of ID are exposure to poverty, poor housing, family isolation, frequent parenting problems, social exclusion, bullying, and stigmatization.

When we know more about the disability characteristics of perpetrators we will be in a better position to engage in the prevention of CAN and ANCD. Awareness of perpetrator disability characteristics and their attitudes toward children and children's behavior will guide decision making on resource provision and ongoing support. Kaplan et al. (2009) recommend mental health assessments and interventions for parents of adolescents who are physically abused. They observed that since parents' psychiatric disorders preceded their children's physical abuse, early recognition and treatment of parents' psychiatric disorders may contribute to the prevention of CAN and ANCD. These can most easily be conducted by school social workers and/or psychologists. Similarly, Boursnell (2014) recommends the use of risk assessment checklists for parents and caregivers with potential mental health problems.

We recommend:

Recommendation 5: Careful and systematic screenings to assess caregiver characteristics and evaluate their potential risk as perpetrators of the CAN and ANCD.

***

Focused Programs that Support People with Disabilities

The children of caregivers with intellectual disabilities, as well as those with a variety of other risk factors may approach age appropriate norms when provided appropriate supports and services (Collings & Llewellyn, 2012). These children are at increased risk for abuse and neglect by their caregivers. They are also at-risk for bullying and social isolation by their peers. Collings and Llewellyn advocate for providing appropriate supports and services to the children of adults with disabilities. We recommend that researchers and practitioners:

Recommendation 6: Evaluate and identify the specific supports and services needed by caregivers with disabilities and their children.

***

Exercise 7.11: Analysis
These recommendations require that professionals develop strong partnerships with families and caregivers of children with disabilities. What are some of the barriers you have found in your practice when trying to develop close relationships with adults and children with disabilities? *Identify at least five of these barriers. What infrastructure, supports and services may be put in place to enhance parent and professional partnerships?*

Adults with disabilities need a variety of supports and services. These include medical, social, emotional, and daily living supports. These supports and services are needed by adults with disabilities so that they can participate in society and engage in their communities, side-by-side with family, friends, and neighbors. Appropriate supports and services may include the provision of regular financial supports, medical and pharmaceutical check-ups, personal assistants who provide supports in daily living such as shopping, cleaning, laundry, and transportation; enrollment in dedicated recreational organizations that provide social and recreational supports to adults with disabilities such as Special Olympics and Best Buddies; and other social and emotional supports such that persons with disabilities can participate in their own family activities, church events, and maintain connections with a circle of friends who share their life experiences (Hallahan, Kauffman, & Pullen, 2015).

How can we ensure that the support needs of adults with disabilities in our communities are known and addressed in a systematic manner day-by-day? What infrastructure needs to be put in place so that adults with disabilities have what they need to live their lives without waiting for the next crisis? Awaiting crisis before the provision of needed supports is not an option. We have sufficient evidence to state that adults with disabilities need a variety of supports but we have yet to provide these supports systematically and predictably. We observe the need to:

Recommendation 7: Develop an infrastructure that ensures the provision of the resources and services adults with disabilities need in a systematic and predictable manner.

***

McConnell, Matthews, Llewellyn, Mildon, and Hindmarsh (2008) evaluated a national Australian program entitled *Healthy Start* that was designed to build capacity in the community service system to support parents with ID. The authors define capacity building as "the potential to act, including the will or commitment to act, and the knowledge, skills, and material resources needed to do so effectively" (p. 196). They define capacity building as an outcomes related practice involving three overall outcomes, including:

1. Proximal Outcomes

   (a)   Capacity
   (b)   Practice change

2. Intermediate Outcomes

   (a)   Family capacity/resources; and parent/child relationships

3. Distal Outcomes

   (a)   Child health and development

The authors posit that enhanced capacity will result in evidence-based practice that leads to improved parent and child outcomes. The strategies used to build capacity are spread across four different organizational levels. They include:

1. *Leadership and Managerial Support*

   (a)   State-based reference/advisory groups are formed;
   (b)   Develop local initiatives and provide support;
   (c)   Form learning hubs at the local level- a hub would include local practitioners;
   (d)   Local learning hub members *who* actively champion their agencies, their knowledge and the innovation disseminated through *Healthy Start;*

2. *Access to Knowledge and Innovation*

   (a)   Community asset mapping protocol;
   (b)   Dissemination of information through an information rich website;
   (c)   Online graduate course of study for learning hub;
   (d)   Parent education workshop training;

3. *Peer Networking (4 levels)*

   (a) The reference groups bring together the senior managers of government and non-government agencies in each state;

   (b) Program state leaders are brought together annually in face-to-face meetings to share experiences, exchange ideas, and promote innovation and change;

   (c) Bringing together of learning hub members online as students in the unit of study: reflect on the knowledge gained and application into evidence-based practice. Learning hub members also come together twice a year for face-to-face meetings at which innovative solutions and challenges are shared and resources distributed;

   (d) Bringing learning hub members together as practitioners in their local community from their different disciplines, sectors, and agencies;

4. *Adaptations to community contexts*

   (a) Learning hub members engage in community mapping to develop a local plan;

   (b) Local action plans are developed collaboratively by members of the learning hub members to integrate knowledge and innovation from research with local service strengths to address development needs. Examples of local action include the establishment of volunteer home-visiting services and parent–peer support groups, and the development of information/tip sheets and a training package for local health clinics, early childhood education, and social service providers; Thus, we recommend:

Recommendation 8: Coordination and commitment to the implementation of organized and systematic programs to support the parents of children with disabilities.

***

Exercise 7.12: Analysis
Read the article by McConnell et al. (2008). *Write six steps that need be taken in order to develop a program like this in your state, community, and/or local school.*

Perpetrators can also be children themselves. They perpetrate abuse and neglect in an assortment of ways. Bullying is perhaps the most common form of physical or emotional abuse that is seen in school settings by both children and adults. Bullying has been described as an immoral action because it humiliates and oppresses innocent victims (Gini, Pozzoli, Borghi, & Franzoni, 2008; Gini, Pozzoli, & Hauser, 2011). According to the U.S. Department of Justice, approximately 13 % of children ages 2–17 engage in physical bullying; 20 % engage in emotional bullying (Finkelhor, Turner, Ormrod, Hamby, & Kracke, 2009). These data indicate that approximately 6 % of children between the ages of 14–17 engage in internet harassment, or "cyberbullying."

While bullying may not be a "disability" in itself, it can manifest as part of the diagnosis of conduct disorder (American Psychiatric Association, 2013). Bullying may be considered a learned behavior; that is, learned from adult role models such as caregivers or other adults in the child's life. As professionals, it is important to determine where children are learning bullying behaviors and what can be done to address them. If it is determined that the child is learning these behaviors through the social modeling of an adult, or is learning through the pain of physical and emotional abuse, we must be willing to step in and help that child. We observe the need to:

Recommendation 9: Develop bullying awareness programs for both children and adults. Teach prosocial alternatives to bullying behaviors.

***

Exercise 7.13: Reflection
You notice that Johnny, an 8-year old child with ADHD is on your caseload and he exhibits bullying behaviors. For example, you noticed that he belittled a smaller boy by calling him a "sissy" and telling him he cannot do anything right. In your observation of Johnny's classroom you notice the teacher, Mr. Banks verbally humiliate Johnny in front of the class by asking him questions he does not know or yelling at him when he interrupts class. *Make a list of at least five ways that you can intervene to address both the child and the adult behaviors.*

CAN and the ANCD are predictable in a world where insufficient individualized support is provided to adults and children with disabilities. Such a world endangers children and adults with disabilities when punitive approaches are most assured. Law enforcement personnel become the only sure public responders. In such a world, children and adults with disabilities are disproportionately both victimized and punished. This cycle of abuse and neglect will continue until we build public knowledge about disability in childhood and in adulthood. We end this section with three recommendations that focus on the development of effective intervention and prevention programming. These are:

Recommendation 10: Build programs that promote public knowledge, awareness, and understanding of disability among children and their families.

***

Knowledge, awareness, and understanding of disability are the foundations of public embrace, respect, acceptance, and support of children with disabilities and their families. Children with disabilities will be best served in communities where their neighbors know and understand their physical, emotional, and intellectual characteristics and needs. Therefore we recommend that we:

Recommendation 11: Build programs that promote opportunities for public embrace, respect, acceptance, and support of children with disabilities and their families.

***

What can we do to sustain public and private programs that provide needed resources and services that meet the physical, emotional, and intellectual needs of children and caregivers with disabilities? These programs contribute richly to the prevention of CAN and ANCD. They provide members of their communities with essential resources and services. Such programs might be as simple as the provision of clothing and supplies to match seasonal changes, transportation to medical appointments or to recreation programs. Programs that make newspapers, magazines, books, school supplies, as well as, services, such as tutoring and job coaching that support intellectual growth and development, are essential ingredients of supportive communities. We recommend that we:

Recommendation 12: Reinforce supportive public and private programs that promote effective intervention and prevention of CAN and ANCD.

***

Chapter Summary

In this chapter we observed that people with an assortment of disabilities perpetrate abuse and neglect in the lives of children with disabilities. At this time the disabilities of perpetrators are not included in large national and international databases. We analyzed the research findings in this area and the newspaper coverage of the disabilities of the perpetrators of ANCD. We illustrated these findings with stories of disabilities among the perpetrators of ANCD. We concluded this chapter with a set of recommendations for researchers and practitioners. We provided exercises for reflection and critical thinking to support deeper reflection in this area.

Suggestions from Prevent Child Abuse Illinois

Begin today by being a positive parent or caretaker and help other family members, friends, and neighbors be positive parents too.
Make children a priority.
Show and tell your children that you love them every day.

Let your children know you are happy to be with them.

Give children the sense of security, belonging and support.

Catch your children being good and give them lots of praise.

Really listen to your children.

Give children your undivided attention when they are talking.

Be patient and remember that children move at a different pace when they tell a story about their day.

Spend time with your children.

Make some special time for each of your children.

Play with them, talk with them, and read with them.

Keep your promises.

Let your children help with household projects.

Tell your children about your own childhood.

Go to the zoo, museums and ball games as a family.

Make and fly a kite together.

Play outside, play a board game, do an art project or other creative activity.

Set a good example.

Use good manners.

Set clear, consistent limits.

Consider how your decisions will affect your children.

Open a savings account for college education.

Resolve conflicts quickly.

Take your children to your place of worship.

Allow yourself a time-out when needed. Taking care of yourself is as important as taking care of your family.

Reach out to other family members, friends and neighbors.

Talk to family, friends and neighbors about parenting.

Join a parent support group.

Get involved in something where you can socialize with other parents.

Seek help if you need it. If you feel out of control or like a bad parent, get help.

Isolation is often a contributing factor to child abuse. Lack of a support system and the feelings of being stressed and alone can intensify problems. Protecting children is everyone's responsibility. Need to talk to someone? Call: Childhelp® National Child Abuse Hotline 1-800-4-A-Child (1-800-422-4453) Prevent Child Abuse Illinois www.preventchildabuseillinois.org

References

Allen, B., Tellez, A., Wevodau, A., Woods, C. L., & Percosky, A. (2014). The impact of sexual abuse committed by a child on mental health in adulthood. *Journal of Interpersonal Violence, 29*(12), 2257–2272. doi:10.1177/0886260513517550

American Psychiatric Association. (2013). *Diagnostic and statistical manual of mental disorders* (5th ed.). Washington, DC: Author.

Azar, S. T., Stevenson, M. T., & Johnson, D. R. (2012). Intellectual disabilities and neglectful parenting: Preliminary findings on the role of cognition in parenting risk. *Journal of Mental Health Research in Intellectual Disabilities, 5*(2), 94–129. doi:10.1080/19315864.2011. 615460

Banks, N. (2014). Sexually harmful behavior in adolescents in a context of gender and intellectual disability: Implications for child psychologists. *Educational & Child Psychology, 31*(3), 9–21. http://eds.a.ebscohost.com/eds/pdfviewer/pdfviewer?sid=d62b5191-2161-4909-bc54-b4edbf8c8a6f%40sessionmgr4003&vid=8&hid=4208

Barone, L., Bramante, A., Lionetti, F., & Pastore, M. (2014). Mothers who murdered their child: An attachment-based study on filicide. *Child Abuse & Neglect, 38*(9), 1468–1477. doi:10.1016/j.chiabu.2014.04.014

Bladon, E. M., Vizard, E., French, L., & Tranah, T. (2005). Young sexual abusers: A descriptive study of a UK sample of children showing sexually harmful behaviours. *Journal of Forensic Psychiatry & Psychology, 16*(1), 109–126. doi:10.1080/14789940042000270265abc

Boursnell, M. (2014). Assessing the capacity of parents with mental illness: Parents with mental illness and risk. *International Social Work, 57*(2), 92–108. doi:10.1177/0020872812445197

Brown, I., & Schormans, A. F. (2003). Maltreatment and life stressors in single mothers who have children with developmental delay. *Journal on Developmental Disabilities, 10*(1), 61–66. Retrieved from http://www.oadd.org/publications/journal/issues/vol10no1/download/brown%26fudgeSchormans.pdf

Capaldi, D. M. (2014). Offspring of mothers who had antenatal depression and experienced maltreatment in childhood are more likely to experience child maltreatment themselves. *Evidence Based Nursing, 17*(2), 37–38. doi:10.1136/eb-2013-101378

Childhelp®. (2015). *National child abuse hotline. Prevent child abuse Illinois.* Retrieved from http://www.preventchildabuseillinois.org

Coen, J. (2006, May 11). Iraq torture to be defense in child's death. *Chicago Tribune.* Retrieved from http://articles.chicagotribune.com/2006-05-11/news/0605110259_1_radiator-iraq-torture

Collings, S., & Llewellyn, G. (2012). Children of parents with intellectual disability: Facing poor outcomes or faring okay? *Journal of Intellectual & Developmental Disability, 37*(1), 65–82. doi:10.3109/13668250.2011.648610

Coorg, R., & Tournay, A. (2013). Filicide-suicide involving children with disabilities. *Journal of Child Neurology, 28*(6), 745–751. doi:10.1177/0883073812451777

Emerson, E., & Brigham, P. (2014). The developmental health of children of parents with intellectual disabilities: Cross sectional study. *Research in Developmental Disabilities, 35*(4), 917–921. doi:10.1016/j.ridd.2014.01.006

Ethier, L. S., Couture, G., & Lacharité, C. (2004). Risk factors associated with the chronicity of high potential for child abuse and neglect. *Journal of Family Violence, 19*(1), 13–24. ISSN: 08857482.

Finkelhor, D., Turner, H., Ormrod, R., Hamby, S., & Kracke, K. (2009). *Children's exposure to violence: A comprehensive national survey.* Retrieved from http://www.ncjrs.gov/pdffiles1/ojjdp/227744.pdf

Firth, H., Balogh, R., Berney, T., Bretherton, K., Graham, S., & Whibley, S. (2001). Psychopathology of sexual abuse in young people with intellectual disability. *Journal of Intellectual Disability Research, 45*(3), 244–252. doi:10.1046/j.1365-2788.2001.00314.x

Fitzsimmons, E., & Heinzmann, D. (2006, November 23). Mother to reunite with family; woman released in daughter's death. *Chicago Tribune.* Retrieved from http://articles.chicagotribune.com/2006-11-23/news/0611230155_1_stress-disorder-and-depression-disabled-daughter-saddam-hussein

Gini, G., Pozzoli, T., Borghi, F., & Franzoni, L. (2008). The role of bystanders in students' perception of bullying and sense of safety. *Journal of School Psychology, 46*(6), 617–638. doi:10.1016/j.jsp.2008.02.001

Gini, G., Pozzoli, T., & Hauser, M. (2011). Bullies have enhanced moral competence to judge relative to victims, but lack moral compassion. *Personality and Individual Differences, 50*(5), 603–608. doi:10.1016/j.paid.2010.12.002

Greco, C. (2006, June 7). Sex assault suspect's DNA not linked to slain toddler – Cops find 'no link' between Wilmington girl, assault suspect. *Chicago Tribune*. Retrieved from http://search. proquest.com/chicagotribune/docview/420483341/738E54555FD04FD6PQ/1?accountid=11578

Haggerty, R. (2012, October 19). State police: Slain teen had steak knife. *Chicago Tribune*. Retrieved from http://articles.chicagotribune.com/2012-10-19/news/ct-met-calumet-city-police-shooting-20121019_1_steak-knife-extra-officers-butter-knife

Hallahan, D. P., Kauffman, J. M., & Pullen, P. C. (2015). *Exceptional learners: An introduction to special education* (13th ed.). Upper Saddle River, NJ: Pearson.

Kaplan, S. J., Sunday, S. R., Labruna, V., Pelcovitz, D., & Salzinger, S. (2009). Psychiatric disorders of parents of physically abused adolescents. *Journal of Family Violence, 24*(2), 273–281. doi:10.1007/s10896-009-9226-7

Martinello, E. (2015). Reviewing risks factors of individuals with intellectual disabilities as perpetrators of sexually abusive behaviors. *Sexuality and Disability, 33*(2), 269–278. doi:10.1007/s11195-014-9365-5

McConnell, D., Matthews, J., Llewellyn, G., Mildon, R., & Hindmarsh, G. (2008). "Healthy Start". A national strategy for parents with intellectual disabilities and their children. *Journal of Policy & Practice In Intellectual Disabilities, 5*(3), 194–202. doi:10.1111/j.1741-1130.2008.00173.x

Pestka, K., & Wendt, S. (2014). Belonging: Women living with intellectual disabilities and experiences of domestic violence. *Disability & Society, 29*(7), 1–15. doi:10.1080/09687599. 2014.902358

Sadovi, C. (2006, September 13). Iraqi mom ailing at time of child's death, court told; stress disorder linked to torture, expert says. *Chicago Tribune*. Retrieved from http://articles. chicagotribune.com/2006-09-13/news/0609130058_1_torture-kurdish-stress-disorder

Sadovi, C. (2006, September 14). Iraqi mom not guilty of neglect in daughter's death. *Chicago Tribune*. Retrieved from http://search.proquest.com/chicagotribune/docview/420479339/ 74303CC656A941BFPQ/3?accountid=11578

Sadovi, C. (2006, October 12). Iraqi mom faces psychiatric testing; woman acquitted in daughter's death. *Chicago Tribune*. Retrieved from http://articles.chicagotribune.com/2006-10-12/news/ 0610120036_1_crane-psychiatric-hospital-ordered

Schormans, A. F., & Brown, I. (2006). An investigation into the characteristics of the maltreatment of children with developmental delays and the alleged perpetrators of this maltreatment. *Journal of Developmental Disabilities, 12(2)*, 131–151. Retrieved from http://www.oadd.org/ publications/journal/issues/special/anniversary.pdf#page=145

U.S. Department of Health and Human Services, Administration for Children and Families, Administration on Children, Youth and Families, Children's Bureau. (2013). *Child maltreatment 2012*. Retrieved from http://www.acf.hhs.gov/programs/cb/research-data-technology/sta tistics-research/child-maltreatment

Vizard, E. (2013). The victims and juvenile perpetrators of child sexual abuse–assessment and intervention. *Journal of Child Psychology and Psychiatry, 54*(5), 503–515. doi:10.1111/jcpp. 12047

Walberg, M. (2009, October 7). Star witness tries to save Degorski. *Chicago Tribune*. Retrieved from http://articles.chicagotribune.com/2009-10-07/news/0910070147_1_juan-luna-james-degorski-death-penalty

Witt, H. (2009, April 8). IQ of 47 is no bar to a 100-year sentence. *Chicago Tribune*. Retrieved from http://articles.chicagotribune.com/2009-04-08/news/0904070638_1_molested-boy-judge-denies-new-trial-mental-retardation

World Health Organization. (2014). *Child abuse and neglect by parents and other caregivers*. Retrieved from http://www.who.int/violence_injury_prevention/violence/global_campaign/ en/chap3.pdf?ua=1

Part III
How Can We Predict and Thereby Prevent Abuse and Neglect in the Lives of Children with Disabilities?

Chapter 8
Understanding the Context of Abuse and Neglect in the Lives of Children with Disabilities

> *Safety and security don't just happen, they are the result of collective consensus and public investment. We owe our children, the most vulnerable citizens in our society, a life free of violence and fear.* (Nelson Mandela, President of South Africa, 1918–2013)

Abstract What contexts – backgrounds, environments, or situations characterize the settings that set the stage for the abuse and neglect of children with disabilities (ANCD)? If we anticipate the context variables that indicate the potential risk of abuse and neglect in the lives of children with disabilities, can we potentially anticipate and interrupt its occurrence. In this chapter, we will analyze the data from the large national database and take a brief look at our history. We will then analyze the data in the professional literature and conclude the chapter by analyzing the data from the newspaper coverage in the *Chicago Tribune*. We will illustrate the findings with excerpts from cases of ANCD which were published in this newspaper in the 10-year span between January, 2004 and December, 2013. We will provide exercises that promote reflection, analysis, and dialogue throughout the chapter. We will conclude this chapter with implications for research and practice.

Webster's New World Dictionary defines "context" as "the whole situation, background, or environment relevant to a particular event, personality, creation, etc." What contextual variables support the human growth and development of children with and without disabilities? Children have physical, emotional, and intellectual needs that must be met in order to promote their healthy growth and development. Children need food, shelter, clothing, and shoes to meet physical needs. They need warm emotional bonds and stimulating intellectual exchange to meet their emotional and intellectual needs.

Most children thrive even when the contexts of their lives only partly meet their needs, in one or more areas. However, to the extent that their physical, emotional, and intellectual needs are unmet, their healthy human growth and development is at-risk.

Children with disabilities need contexts that are designed to meet their unique and individualized growth and development needs. The physical, emotional, intellectual, and social needs of children with disabilities are such that if not met, further

© Springer International Publishing Switzerland 2016
E.P. Crowley, *Preventing Abuse and Neglect in the Lives of Children with Disabilities*, DOI 10.1007/978-3-319-30442-7_8

disability may follow. In more extreme cases, death may follow the unmet needs of some children with disabilities.

Exercise 8.1: Reflection
What contextual variables do you predict to be most relevant in the ANCD? *List as many variables as you can at the outset. Then write what you consider to be the top five most reliable contextual predictors of ANCD. Reexamine your list at the end of this chapter.*

Modern medical professionals can predict some disabilities in childhood prenatally. They can provide interested future caregivers with crucial information about the predictable unique needs of their children with disabilities. For example, the caregivers of children with Down syndrome and spina bifida may prepare to meet their unique needs of their babies by working with personnel in early intervention before their children are born.

More frequently, however, disability in childhood is unrecognized prenatally. In these cases it is revealed slowly as the child grows. Caregivers learn about the unique needs of their very young children with disabilities as they present unusual patterns in their growth and development. These caregivers can also learn about the contextual supports that are available and about those that are not available to meet their children's needs. Their physical, emotional, intellectual, and social needs are identified and addressed when early intervention personnel in the contexts in which they live are knowledgeable, resourceful, and supportive whenever possible.

Children are abused and neglected in contexts where their caregivers are oblivious to children's human growth and development needs. Recent studies reconfirm the disproportionate numbers of children with disabilities who are abused and neglected (Caldas & Bensy, 2014; Jones et al., 2012; Khalifeh, Howard, Osborn, Moran, & Johnson, 2013). Their special and individualized physical, emotional, and intellectual needs are addressed in contexts where caregivers have successfully acquired sufficient knowledge, skills, and resources to meet their own, as well as their children's unique and often unanticipated needs.

Children with disabilities all over the world are exposed to maltreatment in the form of neglect, physical abuse, emotional and psychological abuse, and sexual abuse. In this chapter we will analyze data in the national databases that address the contextual variables surrounding the maltreatment of children with and without disabilities. We will examine the data on situations, the backgrounds, and the relevant environmental characteristics associated with ANCD? We will then analyze the professional literature that addresses the contexts in which children with disabilities are abused and neglected. We will examine specific trends indicated in this literature and the particular contextual vulnerabilities to which children with disabilities are exposed. We will provide data about the contexts of ANCD based on the findings of the newspaper study described in Chap. 1. We will get behind the statistics and analyze the context of abuse and neglect in specific cases where children with disabilities have been abused and neglected. We will conclude this chapter with a set of recommendations for future research and professional practice.

Exercise 8.2: Reflection

Do you expect that some adults would find caregiving for children with disabilities particularly challenging? *List at least five circumstances in which you think that caring for a child with a disability would be more challenging than caregiving for a child without a disability?*

Context Variables Evident in the Large National Trends in the ANCD

What does the U.S. DHHS tell us about the contexts in which the abuse and neglect of children with and without disabilities occur? What do we know about how well children with disabilities fare in the context of their families, schools, communities, and in the world as a whole? Is disability relevant in the abuse and neglect of children? When does it matter that a child has a disability? What are the most relevant situational, background, and environmental effects around the lives of children with disabilities who have been abused and neglected? We will begin this section with an analysis of the statistics on caregiver risk factors that contribute to the development of abusive and neglectful contexts for children with and without disabilities. We will examine the statistics provided by U.S. DHHS on child fatality in the context of race and ethnicity.

Poverty and Public Assistance Risk

Did you list poverty among the risk factors that disposes for child abuse and neglect (CAN)? According to the U.S. DHHS (2015) children who live in families that are unable to provide sufficient financial resources to meet their basic needs are at greater risk for abuse and neglect. Furthermore, they are at greater risk for abuse and neglect when they live in families that participate in public assistance programs, including Temporary Assistance for Needy Families, Medicaid, Social Security Income, Special Supplemental Nutrition Program for Women, Infants, and Children (WIC). In 2013, 14.4 % of CAN victims and 8.8 % of nonvictims lived in homes that indicated financial problem caregiver risk factors. Furthermore, 29.9 % of victims and 23.4 % of nonvictims lived in homes with caregivers who received public assistance.

Domestic Violence Risk Factor

Did you list domestic violence among the top five predictors of CAN when you completed exercise 8.1 above? Though not disaggregated for childhood disability, the U.S. DHHS (2013) reports compelling data on domestic violence as a risk factor for CAN. Children with and without disabilities who live with caregivers who are at-risk for domestic violence will, more likely, be abused and neglected. In the United States the overall national average indicates that in 2012 28.5 % of children who were abused and neglected lived with caregivers who indicated domestic violence risk factors (see Table 8.1). At a National level and in 2012 only 8.6 % of children who lived with caregivers with domestic violence risk factors actually escaped involvement in domestic violence. These data indicate that children in the presence of caregivers with this factor are at least three times more likely to be abused and neglected.

The large numbers and percentages hide the gravity and clearly underestimate the problem here. In 2012 and in Texas alone, it would take 400 school buses to transport children who were documented victims of domestic violence. These numbers represent only the children who were brought to the attention of professionals and who were screened-in as victims of domestic violence. Predictably, at least 25.0–30.0 % of these children had disabilities.

Though the National numbers are astronomical, they too hide the gravity of this issue. In 2012 the U.S. DHHS reported that based on reports from 50 states and the District of Columbia, 3,165,572 children received a CPS response, which has increased from the preceding years since 2008 (see Table 8.2). During these years an average of 42 children per 1000 children were involved with services intended to protect children from abuse and neglect. These numbers estimate the extent of the problem and show only those cases in which the abuse and neglect was so apparent

Table 8.1 States where highest number of child victims of CAN who live with a caregiver with a domestic violence (DV) risk factor

State	Unique victims of CAN	% of Unique victims of CAN	Victims with DV risk	Nonvictims with DV	% victims with DV risk	% nonvictims with DV risk
Texas	62,551	9.0	23,954	27,342	38.3	14.5
Florida	53,341	13.3	22,465	11,133	42.1	4.6
Michigan	33,434	14.7	17,531	19,361	52.4	14.0
New York	68,375	16.0	14,587	6,556	21.3	4.4
Illinois	27,497	9.0	8,864	10,594	32.2	11.0
Georgia	18,752	7.5	6,814	6,419	36.3	7.0
	Average	*11.6*		*Average*	*37.1*	*9.2*
				National average	*28.5*	*8.6*

Data from the U.S. DHHS, *Child Maltreatment Report*, 2013

Table 8.2 Number of children who received a CPS response from 2008 to 2012

2008	2009	2010	2011	2012
3,034,305	3,003,142	2,987,485	3,049,871	3,165,572

CPS child protection service
Data from the U.S. DHHS, *Child Maltreatment Report*, 2013

that they were reported to CPS authorities. We may also conclude that at least 25.0–30.0 % of these children had disabilities and received a CPS response.

Alcohol Abuse Risk Factor

Did you list alcohol abuse as a risk factor for CAN? Children who live with caregivers who abuse alcohol have a higher chance of being abused and neglected. In the United States the national average indicates that 8.8 % of children who live with caregivers who abuse alcohol were abused and neglected and 4.9 % of these children escaped abuse and neglect (see Table 8.3). On average, in states where most children were abused and neglected by caregivers who had alcohol abuse risk factor 20.1 % were the victims of CAN and 9.6 % of them had caregivers with this factor but escaped abuse and neglect.

The percentages hide the gravity of the problem. For example, in Texas alone, 5726 children under the age of 18 were victims of CAN in 2012. These children lived with caregivers who indicated an alcohol abuse factor. To clarify the magnitude of these numbers – it would take 96 school buses with 60 children per bus to transport these children.

Drug Abuse Risk Factor

Children with and without disabilities are abused and neglected in the presence of caregivers who abuse drugs. Data from Texas, Ohio, Georgia, Oklahoma,

Table 8.3 States where highest number of child victims live with an alcohol abuse (AA) caregiver risk factor

State	Unique victims	Victims with AA	Nonvictims of CAN	Nonvictims with AA	% victims with AA	% nonvictims with AA
Texas	62,551	5,726	188,072	8,014	9.2	4.3
Michigan	33,434	2,747	*	*	8.2	*
New Mexico	5,882	2,305	16,017	3,749	39.2	23.4
Washington	6,546	1,984	37,184	3,916	30.3	10.5
Oklahoma	9,627	1,718	35,912	1,805	17.8	5.0
New Jersey	9,031	1,428	67,133	3,226	15.8	4.8
				Average	20.1	9.6
				National average	8.8	4.9

*Numbers not provided in the U.S. DHHS report, 2013
Data from the U.S. DHHS, *Child Maltreatment Report*, 2013

New Mexico, and Indiana indicate that children who live with caregivers who abuse drugs are more than twice as likely to be abused and neglected (see Table 8.4). At the National level these statistics hold as 20.0 % of children who live with a caregiver with a drug abuse risk factor are abused and neglected and 8.4 % of these children manage to escape CAN. These numbers too hide the gravity of this problem. Nationally 64,484 children or 1075 school buses with 60 children in each bus, were abused and neglected while living with caregivers with drug abuse risk factors. We may well expect that these statistics underestimate of the reality of CAN and that hidden among these children are 25–30 % with disabilities. Though underestimating and not disaggregating for childhood disability, these statistics indicate that when children live with caregivers with a drug abuse risk factor, they are at increased risk of abuse and neglect.

Children with and without disabilities are at increased risk for abuse and neglect when they live with caregivers with domestic violence, drug abuse, and alcohol abuse factors and domestic violence tops the list. They are at such risk that in 2012 1096 children who died as a result of abuse and neglect in the United States had caregivers with a risk for domestic violence as well as drug and alcohol risk factors (see Table 8.5). Combined child fatality resulting from abuse and neglect occurred among 1450 children who were living with caregivers with drug and alcohol abuse risk factors. These two factors were associated with 23.6 % of childhood fatalities resulting from abuse and neglect in 2012.

Table 8.4 States where highest numbers of child victims live with a drug abuse (DA) caregiver risk factor

State	Unique victims	Victims with DA	Nonvictims of CAN	Nonvictims with DA	% with DA	% Nonvictims with DA
Texas	62,551	18,254	188,072	24,594	29.2	13.1
Ohio	29,250	9,616	73,484	9,380	32.9	12.8
Georgia	18,752	3,855	91,571	4,416	20.6	4.8
Oklahoma	9,627	3,711	35,912	3,736	38.5	10.4
New Mexico	5,882	3,685	16,017	5,732	62.6	35.8
Indiana	20,223	3,683	72,252	2,044	18.2	2.8
				Average	*33.6*	*13.3*
				National average	*20.0*	*8.4*

Data from the U.S. DHHS, *Child Maltreatment Report*, 2013

Table 8.5 Child fatalities with caregiver domestic violence and drug and alcohol abuse factors

	States reporting	# of fatalities	% fatalities with caregiver risk
Domestic violence	31	1,096	20.1
Drug abuse	30	753	17.3
Alcohol abuse	27	697	6.3

Data from the U.S. DHHS, *Child Maltreatment Report*, 2013

Race and Ethnicity and Child Fatalities

What do we know about the racial, cultural, and ethnic backgrounds of children who die as a result of abuse and neglect? Are there patterns we need to be aware of? The U.S. DHHS (2013) statistics indicate that 1262 children were documented to have died as a result of trauma associated with abuse and neglect in 2012 (see Table 8.6).

The U.S. DHHS statistics are not disaggregated for disability, and it is safe to conclude that they underestimate the extent of the problem. Based on these data, we observe that children from African-American and Pacific Islander cultural backgrounds die at higher rates per 1000 children than those from any other cultural background. Furthermore, based on what we learned in Chap. 3, many of these children died following their exposure to neglect and physical abuse and that many of these children were under the age of 3 years old.

Research on the Context Variables Relevant in ANCD

Researchers observed the predictable relationship between childhood disability and abuse and neglect in recent history. Kempe, Silverman, Steele, Droegemueller, and Silver (1985) observed the contexts of abuse and neglect and made the connection with childhood disability as an outcome. Their historic paper, "The battered-child syndrome" was first published in 1962 and later republished in 1985. Kempe and his colleagues described the context in which they observed CAN and concluded that caregivers with and without psychiatric disorders, those with low intelligence, and from low socioeconomic backgrounds frequently abused and even traumatized their children. Additionally, they observed that:

Table 8.6 Child fatalities by race and ethnicity, 2012

Race	Child population	Number of child fatalities	% fatalities	Rate of fatalities per 1000 children
White	30,161,762	483	38.3	1.6
Hispanic	11,390,843	193	15.3	1.7
African-American	8,637,076	403	31.9	4.7
Two or more Races	1,995,195	48	3.8	2.4
Asian	1,972,578	11	0.9	0.6
American Indian or Alaskan Native	492,539	11	0.9	2.2
Pacific Islander	85,285	4	0.3	4.7
Unknown Race	*	109	8.6	*
Total	54,735,278	1,262	100.0	

*Data unknown
Data from the U.S. DHHS, *Child Maltreatment Report*, 2013

Alcoholism, sexual promiscuity, unstable marriages, and minor criminal activities are reportedly common amongst them. They are immature, impulsive, self-centered, hypersensitive, and quick to react with poorly controlled aggression. Data in some cases indicate that such attacking parents themselves had been subject to some degree of attack from their parents in their own childhood. . . . Not infrequently the beaten infant is a product of an unwanted pregnancy, a pregnancy which began before marriage, too soon after marriage, or at some other time felt to be extremely inconvenient . . . (Kempe et al., 1985, p. 145)

Kempe and his medical team made important strides in understanding the context of CAN and noted the connection with "death, . . . permanent brain injury . . . court action" (p. 142). Information about the context of disability remains uncovered and researchers today continue to unveil specific context variables in ANCD.

The examination of the contexts in which the ANCD occurs gives us some clues for intervention and prevention. Bones (2013) explains that perpetrators of abuse and neglect tend to prey on individuals who are vulnerable. Children with disabilities are especially vulnerable because they provide a motivated offender with an attractive target that often lacks guardianship (Bones, 2013; Hollis, Felson, & Welsh, 2013; Hollis-Peel, Reynald, van Bavel, Elffers, & Welsh, 2011; Spano & Bolland, 2013). Motivated offenders isolate the individuals they target for abuse and neglect.

Once an individual has been the target of physical abuse, sexual abuse, neglect or any combination thereof, that individual has an increased potential for continued exposure to abuse and neglect. Bones (2013) observed that abuse and neglect set the stage for further abuse and neglect, and that early victimization leads to repeated episodes of victimization. Often, individuals constitute both the repeated targets of and the perpetrators of abuse and neglect. Eventually, abuse and neglect becomes part of their lifestyles.

Data indicate unequivocally that disabilities as well as other risk factors play an important role in predicting higher potential for abuse and neglect. Researchers found that recipients of public assistance are at increased risk of abuse and neglect; isolation is correlated with disability and victimization; and disability enhances the potential vulnerability to ANCD (Bones, 2013; Miethe & Meier, 1994). Predictably, the contexts in which the ANCD happens are those that are overwhelmed by human needs, isolation, ignorance, and lack of appropriate resources.

Exercise 8.3: Reflection

What is the role of economic stability relative to the context variables of ANCD? Do you accept that a child with a disability who lives in the context of any level of economic advantage or disadvantage has an equal chance of being abused and neglected? *Argue the pro or con to this statement and list five convincing arguments to support your perspective.*

Attitudes Toward Disability as Contextual Variables

The attitudes of caregivers and professionals who work with children with disabilities are reflected in their words and in their actions. Their attitudes are the result of their search for meaning and determine their communication and behaviors. In the *World Report on Disability* (WHO, 2011) Dr. Margaret Chan, Director-General of the World Health Organization and Robert B. Zoellick, President of the World Bank Group stated that "Our driving vision is of an inclusive world in which we are all able to live a life of health, comfort, and dignity" (p. xi). Astrophysicist Professor Stephen W. Hawking states that "Disability need not be an obstacle to success" (p. ix, WHO). He has lived most of his life with a motor neuron disease and he reminds us that disability "has not prevented me from having a prominent career in astrophysics and a happy family life" (p. ix).

The attitudes we hold affirm and support the contextual fabric of our life experiences. What are the prevailing attitudes toward childhood disabilities at the local, national, and international levels? Hallahan, Kauffman, and Pullen (2015) reminded us that "We must not allow people's disabilities to keep us from recognizing their abilities or to become so much the focus of our concern that we overlook their capabilities" (p. 4). Inclusion of children with disabilities among their peers without disabilities is a concerted effort to build inclusive communities. Children with disabilities are children first. Inclusive language reflects this perspective when we make statements like, "My child has a disability and therefore ... " rather than "My disabled child ... " Children's disabilities may or may not be relevant depending on the context. Inclusive language is designed to focus on people first and disability only if it is relevant to the context of the conversation or experience. Special Olympics and Best Buddies are international programs that promote inclusive experiences for children and adults with disabilities.

The attitude of acceptance and inclusion of children with disabilities remains a dream in communities all over the world. Coorg and Tournay (2013) reminded us that even today children with disabilities are not always included and accepted in their own families. They conducted a study on filicide-suicide involving children with disabilities. They found that parents engaged in filicide due to their perceived altruism and concluded that death "releases their child from a real or imagined suffering" (p. 745). Other attitudes toward child disability are derived from religious explanations such as "God gave us a child with a disability because we are special people." Others conclude that "We have sinned so God punished us". Some people ignore children with disabilities and fail to count them in their families and communities. They remain hidden and their existence is denied.

Acceptance and inclusion of children with disabilities begins with the words we use to communicate. When people fail to use person first language they depersonalize children with disabilities and thereby increase their potential exposure to CAN. Children with disabilities are not regarded as real children in these circumstances. Rather, they are seen as enigmas. They become their disabilities. In this, they are rendered a new kind of vulnerability which exposes them to new threats of abuse and neglect.

Exercise 8.4: Reflection
What is the role of language in the communication of attitudes toward children with disabilities? *Examine the language you use when you talk about child disability. During the next week, listen to the words people around you use when they speak about children with disabilities? Characterize the extent to which the communication you hear fosters acceptance and inclusion of children with disabilities.*

Our attitudes determine our life experience and that of those around us. Children with disabilities and their peers without disabilities thrive when they, as well as their unique human characteristics, are accepted and valued. People who are interested in promoting inclusive and accepting attitudes toward children with disabilities will observe that a great deal of hard work remains for them.

In conclusion, our attitudes matter. When we communicate attitudes of acceptance and appreciation and inclusion we foster positive outcomes for children with disabilities and their caregivers. Attitudes that reflect rejection at any level will undermine the health and safe human growth and development experiences of children with and without disabilities.

What Else Do We Know About the Context of ANCD?

Disability and context variables contribute to the potential ANCD in a reciprocal dynamic, in that context affects disability and disability affects context. For decades, researchers have been studying the role of parents and caregivers with disabilities in the abuse and neglect of children (Azar, Stevenson, & Johnson, 2012; Herrenkohl, 2013; McGaw, Scully, & Pritchard, 2010). In what ways do the characteristics of children with disabilities challenge the parenting knowledge and skills of their parents and caregivers (Leeb, Bitsko, Merrick, & Armour, 2012). Parent and family characteristics as well as context characteristics such as poverty, marginal cultural, and familial ties all contribute to ANCD potential. Finally, when two or more disposing contextual variables are present the potential for ANCD increases (Stein, Leslie, & Nyamathi, 2002).

Contextual variables such as poverty, caregivers' childhood trauma experiences, disability, substance abuse, psychiatric disorders, stress, and isolation are repeatedly cited in the literature that describes the contexts where child maltreatment and disability converge (Bones, 2013; Coorg & Tournay, 2013; Hendricks, Lansford, Deater-Deckard, & Bornstein, 2014; Mueller-Johnson, Eisner, & Obsuth, 2014; Palusci & Vandervort, 2014; Sinanan, 2011; Tucker & Rodriguez, 2014; Yampolskaya, Greenbaum, & Berson, 2009). The significance of converging variables was reaffirmed in a recent study by Douglas and Mohn (2014). Males and females with converging histories of criminal behaviors, substance abuse, domestic violence, poor physical and behavioral health had an increased probability of perpetrating child abuse and associated child fatalities.

Sinanan (2011) identified contextual variables that correlate with the recurrence of child sexual abuse reports. Factors used in her analysis were divided into three categories: child characteristics (age, gender, ethnicity, disabilities, prior victimization, and relationship to the abuser), family factors (substance use, domestic violence, housing, and financial problems), and child protective services provided. Sinanan found that the prevalence of child disability, previous victimization, a caregiver with an abuse history, financial problems, and supportive services previously provided all increased the likelihood of child sexual abuse reports. White females between 6 and 11 years old, who had caregivers with a history of abuse were most vulnerable to child sexual abuse. Sinanan also found that children with disabilities are less likely to be believed or found "credible" when they attempt to self-report their own victimization.

Children's responses to their abuse and neglect are altered by the presence of a disability. The accuracy of the communication they provide may be compromised and perceived as either under or overinflating the actual situation, depending on the disability. They may not be able to respond to questions due to the influences of their disabilities. For example, a child with a communication disorder might not be able to tell the entire story of their abuse and neglect, whereas, a child with autism may be able to tell little to no part of the story of their abuse and neglect. Therefore, reported cases of abuse and neglect involving children with disabilities may be screened-out in error.

The ANCD is associated with contexts in which harsh and abusive parenting is observed. Hendricks, Lansford, Deater-Deckard, and Bornstein (2014) found that caregivers from 17 developing countries indicated that children with disabilities are disciplined more harshly than are their peers without disabilities. Hendricks et al. concluded that continued efforts are needed to develop policies and interventions, thereby working toward the United Nations' goals of ensuring that children with disabilities are protected from abuse, neglect, and violence.

Mueller-Johnson et al. (2014) extended the findings provided by Hendricks and colleagues. In their research Mueller-Johnson and her colleagues found, more specifically, that children with physical disabilities are sexually abused more frequently in contexts where harsh and abusive parenting is observed. They also found that boys and girls with physical disabilities are sexually abused more frequently in homes where they witness interparental violence, alcohol and drug use, violent delinquency, and engage in frequent internet use.

Substance abuse impairs human judgment and influences the discipline choices of caregivers (Bones, 2013). Caregivers' child-rearing styles become distorted and this has negative effects on the care and supervision they provide to their children with disabilities. The time and money parents spend seeking and using drugs or alcohol limit household resources. In addition, families affected by substance abuse often experience a number of other problems – including mental illness, domestic violence, poverty, and high levels of stress – which are also associated with CAN.

Drug use, social isolation, emotional neglect, and physical abuse are significant factors in predicting both future perpetrators and victims of abuse and neglect (Barone, Bramante, Lionetti & Pastore, 2014; Bones, 2013). Bones found that children with disabilities and their caregivers are at increased risk, as both perpetrators and victims, in contexts where poverty, isolation, drug use, and unemployment converge. Additionally, he found that "Early victimization leads to subsequent violations, creating a life full of pain for survivors of early abuse. ... having a disability increases the relative risk of sexual victimization by 123 % ..." (p. 742).

Barone et al. (2014) found that low socioeconomic levels, feelings of helplessness in caregiving, and the experience of past trauma lead mothers to engage in the abuse and neglect of their children. They observed the cyclical and intergenerational nature of abuse and neglect. The pain of abuse during childhood leads to the destructive cycle of ongoing abuse and neglect which eventually leads to subsequent generations of abuse and neglect. Bones (2013) found that females with disabilities who are isolated, use drugs, and engage in criminal offending behaviors are at high risk for sexual victimization. He found that females "who have used drugs in the past month are 93 % more likely to experience victimization than those who did not use drugs..." (p. 743).

Exercise 8.5: Reflection
What are your thoughts and feelings as you read about the contexts in which the abuse and neglect of children with disabilities occurs? *Are you angry? Are you sad? Are you propelled into action? What direction might your actions take? How might you contribute to the reduction of the ANCD?*

Looking for More Answers to Our Context Questions

Disability in childhood continues to challenge the boundaries of professional knowledge, and this contributes to the continued abuse and neglect of children with disabilities. Researchers and clinicians in the entire professional community have more to learn about disability in childhood. Professionals in such fields as psychiatry, psychology, counseling, special education, and other related disciplines continue to learn about autism, childhood schizophrenia, ADHD, learning disabilities, sensory and physical disabilities, and emotional and psychological disorders in childhood. We use words like "autism spectrum" in order to account for the variation that exists among children with autism. Would we benefit from adopting more specific terminology? Or, might we use the term "schizophrenia spectrum disorders" instead of using the term schizophrenia? Are there any possible benefits to the development of reliable and valid assessment instruments and procedures such that they identify accurately children with specific disabilities as early as possible? Is it possible that we waste valuable intervention time when we use such generalized diagnoses as developmental delay and other health impaired?

We may therefore question whether very young children might be better served with more specific diagnoses and focused intervention as early as possible.

Researchers continue to unveil findings about the importance of early intervention in the lives of young children with disabilities. These findings guide and direct the work of researchers, clinicians, and caregivers (Nahmias, Kase, & Mandell, 2014). Modern professionals in the areas of medicine, education, and law are deeply committed to early intervention programming for young children with disabilities. When children with disabilities have the familial, educational, social, medical, and financial supports they need, they are more likely to live healthy and happy lives that reflect their human potential.

What the Newspaper Tells Us?

The reasons given for the ANCD was provided in 75.2 % (85 out of 113) of the stories in the *Chicago Tribune* from 2004 to 2013) about children with disabilities who were abused and neglected (see Table 8.7). These reasons included lack of knowledge about how to care for the children and their disabilities. Among these stories was the account of a father who smothered his crying child (*Chicago Tribune*, April 15, 2013), caregivers who tied a child to a bed while engaging in errands and having lunch outside the home (Bowean, May 9, 2010), and lack of resources following childhood trauma (Hovitz, May 3, 2011).

The newspaper stories corroborated with the research findings, in that, stories about the ANCD provided clear evidence that perpetrators often have diagnosed disabilities and that they often live in the context of isolation, poverty, and high levels of stress. Additionally, congruent with research reports in this area, the ANCD occurred in the context of drug and alcohol abuse in 10.6 % of the newspaper stories.

The largest number of articles made no reference to a reason for the ANCD. These included newspaper stories which provided information about programs designed to address ANCD or which focused on either intervention or prevention. We present case examples that illustrate these findings in the next section of this chapter.

Table 8.7 Reasons for the abuse and neglect of children with disabilities (n = 113 articles)[a]

Context	# of stories	% of articles
No reason given	49	43.4
Lack of knowledge	30	26.5
Other (fear, lack of resources, discrimination)	18	16.0
Perpetrator had diagnosed disability	25	22.1
Perpetrator under the influence of drugs/alcohol	12	10.6

[a]n of specific cases exceeds 100 % due to some cases involved multiple reasons for ANCD
Data from a study of the newspaper coverage in the *Chicago Tribune*

Beyond the Numbers: Stories of Real Children Exhibit the Evidence – The Contribution of Disability to Context and Vice Versa

The neighbors in a Chicago suburb were surprised to find abuse and neglect of children in their quiet neighborhood. On May 9, 2010, Bowean broke the story of a 6-year-old boy, who remained unnamed in Park Forest, Illinois. He was "left alone for hours with his disabled 8-year-old cousin chained to a bed and covered in human waste, called police because he was scared, authorities said." Upon dialing 911 he "hung up when the operator answered . . . Operators thought it was a prank call, but when an officer conducted a wellness check . . . he discovered the children were living in squalor without running water." Both children are now in the custody of the Illinois Department of Children and Family Services (DCFS).

Following an investigation, "Renee Dennis, 35, and Paul Coleman, 38, were each charged with felony criminal neglect of a disabled person and endangering the life or health of a child . . .." Dennis and Coleman are the parents of the 6-year-old boy and Dennis is the aunt of the 8-year-old girl. These two children were left alone for a minimum of 6 h on May 1, 2010. Bowean stated that "When the officer arrived at the house, the girl was wearing a nylon harness attached to a bicycle chain that was padlocked to a crib in one of the bedrooms..." The 8-year-old girl "has cerebral palsy and is not able to speak. She was wearing a dirty diaper and appeared relieved when police arrived... They used a bolt cutter to free her, and both children were turned over to DCFS."

Since the couple's arrest their home has been declared uninhabitable and they have been told not to return. "The outside of the house is surrounded by construction debris, and an expired building permit is taped to the front window. Half of the house is covered in vinyl siding, but the other half is exposed." Bowean added that "The incident stunned the neighborhood in this quiet south suburb where residents don't normally see police cars, firetrucks and ambulances surrounding one house, said Stephen Anderson, who lives next door to the couple." The neighbors knew that the couple had a son but were unaware that they were also caring for a girl with cerebral palsy. One neighbor reported that "the case has become the talk of the block, especially since the couple isolated themselves from most of their neighbors."

Exercise 8.6: Reflection

Does this story surprise you? Why or why not? Read the entire story "Cops: Disabled child found chained to bed" (Bowean, May 9, 2010). *Note the contextual variables which contributed to the development of this story. How might the story of the abuse and neglect of these two children have been prevented in the first place? Who were the adults who failed to care for the wellbeing of these children?*

The dynamic interaction between context and disability is illustrated in the following excerpt from the article entitled, "Mother charged after boy's death:

Teen, 4 siblings lived in filth with 200-plus animals, officials say" by Gutowski, Sadovi, and Jaworski, *Chicago Tribune*, September 13, 2011:

> On Thursday, one of those children was found unresponsive in the yard wearing only a T-shirt and was later pronounced dead of natural causes related to bronchopneumonia.
>
> Authorities said the mentally disabled boy and his four siblings, ranging from 12 to 18, never went to school and were forced to live in filth among more than 200 animals – many of them dead. The home, officials said, was covered with feces and infested with spiders.
>
> Price, 49, was charged Monday with criminal neglect of a disabled child, a felony, as well as misdemeanors alleging child endangerment, animal hoarding and cruel treatment. Cook County Judge Pamela Leeming set a $100,000 bail.

This story continued to occupy the news for quite some time in 2011 and illustrated the complex dynamic of poverty, isolation from family members, an estranged ex-husband who is serving a 22 year prison term, and a single Mom.

The mother of the children provided no insight into what happened here other than to state 'I'm not some heartless monster,' Price told the reporter from the *Chicago Tribune*, that this was her first in-depth interview since one of her children died and she was charged with child neglect and animal hoarding. She stated,'My children were my absolute life. They were all loved and taken care of to the best of my ability' (Gutowski, October 3, 2011).

Exercise 8.7: Reflection

Lydia Price's neighbors thought that something was amiss inside her small brick bungalow on South Lombard Street, in Berwyn, Illinois. There lived Ms. Price, her elderly mother and her five children. One child had autism, and the other four had an assortment of disabilities. They were rarely seen and when they did go out, it was at odd hours of the night. Her neighbors contacted the police several times, but following a brief visit, these calls were dismissed as resulting from a trivial neighborhood dispute. *In this scenario, what variables contributed to the abuse and neglect of children with disabilities? Is it possible that this would happen in your neighborhood?*

Children with disabilities are more vulnerable to abuse and neglect in the context of drugs and poverty. On August 7, 2011 Vincent Bevins reported in the *Chicago Tribune* that in Rio de Janeiro, children are using drugs more frequently in the area known as "cracolandias" or crack lands, where children are living on the streets. Bevins reported that adults and hundreds of children, some with emotional and psychological disorders, were put into confined treatment against their will beginning in June 2011. Social worker Claudia de Castro, a social worker for the program stated:

> "The majority are desperate to leave, now. We've taken them from what they know, their lives, their friends," she said. "But we're trying to give them a better option. Here they get education and all kinds of medical and psychological treatment because we aren't just talking about drug addiction. Some have AIDS or other diseases, some have dementia or psychosis"

The program, led by social workers was attempting to deal with Brazil's problem of child homelessness and drug addiction. Usually, internment for treatment is illegal; however, city leaders in Rio de Janeiro found a way to work around the law in their city, saying "minors addicted to crack cocaine don't have the mental capacity to exercise the right to accept or deny treatment." Others disagree. Judge Siro Darlan said, "... children and adolescents are subjects, with rights, and they should be respected as citizens and not collected like human trash." The city attempts to find foster families once the children are fit to leave the center.

The stories go on. The contexts have common features. On August 12, 2011, Chicago Tribune reporter John Keilman began his story thus:

> Ask around this small rural town and people will tell you that something terrible was bound to happen at 50 Highland Court.
>
> That was the red brick apartment where Terry Payton, 16, lived with his mother, Kathie, in what his friends and neighbors describe as a den of dysfunction. They saw her drink heavily and scream at Terry for infractions. Sometimes she kept him isolated inside. Sometimes she locked him out.
>
> Investigators for the Illinois Department of Children and Family Services visited the home, as did police and mental health workers. But mother and son continued to live under the same roof even as their relationship grew more toxic.
>
> It reached an awful peak June 23. A quarrel allegedly escalated into violence, and when it was over, Kathie Payton was dead. Her son, an intelligent but socially awkward teen some say was as gentle as a lamb, was charged with her slaying.

On the nights before the incident, Kathie threw bottles and hit Terry across the face; she referenced killing Terry to his high school counselor. On the day of the incident, Kathie had cornered Terry, threatened to kill him, and reached for a knife. He quickly grabbed a knife and stabbed his mother in the chest. Some locals think DCFS should have removed him from the home long ago, and they see "Terry as a victim, not a criminal, a young man who was forced to strike back after a lifetime of unchecked abuse." Terry was confined to a juvenile detention center until his court case played out and was given psychiatric testing before the case. No update is provided in the *Chicago Tribune* on the Terry Payton's case as of October 1, 2014.

On April 14, 2010, *Chicago Tribune* reporter John Kass told the story of a woman who did not know how to care for her child with disabilities. Torry Hansen adopted a 7-year-old boy from an orphanage in Russia and:

> ... A few months later, she decided she couldn't handle him anymore.
>
> So the other day, she pinned a note to his shirt that read as if written by a lawyer. She put him on a United Airlines jet, by himself, and sent him back to Moscow alone.
>
> "This child is mentally unstable," Hansen wrote. "He is violent and has severe psychopathic issues/behaviors. I was lied to and misled by the Russian Orphanage workers and director regarding his mental stability and other issues. ... After giving my best to this child, I'm sorry to say, for the safety of my family, friends and myself, I no longer wish to parent this child."
>
> "Sincerely, Torry Hansen."

Ms. Hansen faced the criticism of observers at home and abroad. Russian Foreign Minister, Sergey Lavrov weighed in and according to John Kass he was quoted as saying that the abandonment of Artyem was "the last straw." He added, "...We have taken the decision to suggest a freeze on any adoptions to American families until Russia and the U.S. sign an international agreement. . ." Kass continued that at home Ms. Hansen's critics stated ". . . Her best was only a few months? What about parents – adoptive and biological – who give their lifetime? Naturally, Americans and Russians were horrified. You have a child, you don't return it to the Child Store."

Exercise 8.8: Reflection
Let us revisit your list of the contextual variables you predict to be relevant in the ANCD. *How did your list match with the content of this chapter? Do you have contextual variables on your list which were not discussed in this chapter? Were there relevant contextual variables introduced to you in this chapter which you had not predicted? What contextual variables most surprise you? Which of these variables disturb you most of all?*

Implications for Research and Practice

We began this chapter with an understanding of "context" as the whole situation, background, and environment into which a child with a disability in born. To what extent does the context meet the physical, emotional, intellectual, and social needs of a child with a disability? The first step in determining the answer to this question will come from a careful analysis of the child's needs and of the strengths and challenges in the context around the life of the child. In addition to understanding the child's unique needs, imperative questions include, does the child have adequate food and shelter? Does the child have responsible caregivers? Are the child's educational and social needs met? Are the child's unique needs as indicated by his/her disability met? The questions posed here are imperative to the work of researchers and practitioners in this area.

Exercise 8.9: Analysis
What do you think is the most significant contextual variable professionals need to address in order to prevent ANCD? If you were to write the top six aspects of a context that need to be addressed in order to protect children with disabilities from abuse and neglect, what would you write? *Now prioritize the top three contextual variables that need to be addressed.*

Indeed context matters. The top six contextual variables will differ depending on who makes the list. The unique needs of each child and family, and the context in which they live will determine priorities. These variables will differ across each community, city, region, and country. This assumes that our work will be highly contextualized. Yet, common variables may be recognized. In the next section we will address the need to ameliorate poverty, engage in self-advocacy, enhance human capacity, and address the unique needs of children with disabilities.

Ameliorating Poverty

How many of us know can imagine a life lived in poverty? How do children and adults fare when, on a daily basis, they encounter a scarcity of food, shelter, and clothing? Child and adults who live in poverty are marginalized and have limited access to public and private institutions. When children with disabilities are born into poverty they are at an increased risk for abuse and neglect (McConnell, Savage, & Breitkreuz, 2014). It threatens, undermines, and often robs the possibility for safe and appropriate housing, appropriate food, and nourishment. It isolates children with disabilities from appropriate emotional interactions, educational programming, and social exchanges. Poverty increases the risk of added disabilities, ill health, and increased childhood vulnerability in every form (Abdullah et al., 2014; Gennetian, Kessler, & Sanbonmatsu, 2014; McConnell et al., 2014).

The very survival of children with disabilities who live in poverty is at stake. Those who do manage to survive impoverished circumstances will more likely experience increased adversity in the areas of physical, emotional, academic, and social development. When poverty remains unaddressed, a culture of poverty grows deeper and wider. These declines widen further and further and drill deeper and deeper. Children with disabilities who live in poverty grow to adulthood with needs that are so severe that they drain every modicum of their own internal human resources. As adults, rather than contributing members of their communities, they are at-risk to be overwhelmed by their own needs and thereby wind up in custodial care. Everyone loses in these circumstances.

Sheehy-Skeffington and Haushofer (2014) examined the behavioral effects of poverty. A careful consideration of the implications for their findings leads to the following recommendations for researchers and practitioners:

Recommendation 1: Design local infrastructures so that scarcity of essential resources is ameliorated and local capacity and resources become accessible.

***

Children with disabilities who live in poverty are uniquely vulnerable. They have unique medical, emotional, and educational needs. If these needs go unmet, children with disabilities are at-risk for further ill health, emotional instability, and intellectual deprivation. It is therefore essential that we have an infrastructure in place to identify the needs of children with disabilities and:

Recommendation 2: Develop supportive, proactive, and targeted programming that addresses the unique needs of children with disabilities and their families who live in poverty.

***

The development of reliable and stable infrastructures that give consistent access to essential life-giving resources to children and families who are deprived of them remains a creative challenge in every community. We live in a world that is technologically connected more than ever before but somehow we have not managed, as yet, to provide the most vulnerable children and their families with the basic essentials that meet their most basic human needs. How might we use our technological ingenuity to:

Recommendation 3: Address resource scarcity and establish, in contracts, the ongoing availability, actual distribution, and provision of such basic human essentials as safe housing, sufficient food, and clothing for the most vulnerable children and their families.

***

Exercise 8.10: Reflection
Consider your own community. In what ways are the material needs of children with disabilities and their families being addressed? What is missing? What might you do to address these needs? Make a list of activities you might engage in so these children and their families have access to the shelter, food, and clothing they need. Consider community activities such as serving on a committee that addresses local housing needs, supporting local food and clothing drives. *List the programs, services or activities you could engage in. Select one with which you could be involved and make a least a one- year commitment to participate in it.*

Engaging in Self-Advocacy

When children with disabilities are born into families that do not understand their own needs or the needs of their children with disabilities, they are at increased risk of abuse and neglect. Poor self-advocacy skills lead to deprivation in every imaginable area. When children with disabilities are born to parents who do not advocate for their own or their children's needs we can only expect that these needs will grow greater and greater. Poor self-advocacy skills among children and their families with disabilities will lead to denied rights, unaddressed human needs, and ever-growing reduction of human capacity. Furthermore, poor self-advocacy skills lead to lethargy, hopelessness, learned helplessness, and eventual despair. Without self-advocacy skills resentments become frustration and frustration becomes either seething anger or explosive aggression.

Exercise 8.11: Analysis
When did you last engage in self-advocacy? Describe what you did and how it worked out for you. Imagine your experience had you not engaged in self-advocacy. *Make a list of at least three ways that children with disabilities and*

their families might have particular difficulty engaging in self-advocacy. What helped or hindered you in your own experiences with self-advocacy? What did you need to have in place before you could self-advocate?

Sheehy-Skeffington and Haushofer (2014) consider that some people in adverse circumstances may be prone to disengagement in self-advocacy. Is it possible that some families do not recognize the subtle ways that childhood disability influences the healthy growth and development of their children? Is it possible that families do not engage in self-advocacy because they do not accept their children and their disabilities? Researchers, policymakers and practitioners engage in essential work when they encourage the engagement of children with disabilities and families in self-advocacy. Therefore we must:

Recommendation 4: Provide families in need with essential support services for their children with disabilities. These supports services include access to agencies, professional personnel, and ongoing services that address the unique needs of families of children with disabilities.

***

How might we teach families and caregivers how to self-advocate? Focused training might be essential to teach parents of children with disabilities about the needs of their children and their legal rights to have these needs met. We recommend:

Recommendation 5: Putting in place incentives to encourage self-advocacy. These include campaigns that show the long- and short-term benefits of services as well as the long- and short-term costs of denial of access to legitimate rights and services.

Families and caregivers need to know that consistent and long-term commitment to their own and their children's special needs is essential. This long-term commitment is essential in order to maximize the potential of their children with disabilities. Failure to make this commitment diminishes the possibility of long-term positive outcomes. We recommend that we:

Recommendation 6: Put in place child- and family-centered processes for monitoring the progress of children with disabilities as well as the processes and procedures for filing legitimate grievances when denied access to essential resources.

***

Exercise 8.12: Reflection
Which of the above recommendations fits best with your own knowledge and skills? Consider engaging in a local effort to encourage children with disabilities to engage in self-advocacy. *How do your see yourself making a contribution to such an effort? Describe what you can do tomorrow or in the near future.*

Enhancing Capacity

Disability in childhood poses new life challenges for children with disabilities themselves, as well as for their immediate and for their extended family members, neighbors, and friends. When a child is born with a disability or when a disability emerges after one, two, three, or more years, expectations are altered; dreams are shifted or they vanish in the stress of the daily routine. Indeed, under these circumstances, instead of going to Paris, we go to Holland (Kingsley, 1987). Childhood disability causes relationships shifts within families. Is the child with a disability the firstborn? Is the child male or female? How severe is the disability? What is the family's understanding of the basis for the disability? The answers to these and other related questions will determine essential capacity enhancing activities.

Exercise 8.13: Analysis
Do you know a family with a child with a disability? In what ways did the arrival of this child change the dynamics as well as the day-to-day life of this family? What enhanced the capacity of this family? Were there ways that the capacity of this family met or did not meet the challenges of parenting a child with a disability? *Support your response with at least three observations.*

Child-by-child differences, disability manifestation differences, and contextual differences render capacity enhancement a case-by-case effort. Some families and caregivers seem to slip seamlessly into their roles as mothers, fathers, brothers, and sisters of children with disabilities. We have much to learn from these families. Variables such as child characteristics, age of onset of the disability, disability characteristics, the behavioral manifestations and demands of the disability all contribute to the capacity of the family and the overall capacity of the context to embrace the child and his or her unique physical, emotional, medical, educational or other needs.

How can we build and enhance the capacity of families to embrace their children with disabilities? What needs to be put in place in order to ensure that children with disabilities will get the care, education and treatment they need? What can we do to enhance the capacities of families and communities in order to provide appropriately for children with disabilities? Based on the work of Sheehy-Skeffington and Haushofer (2014) we recommend:

Recommendation 7: Develop and support ongoing and targeted educational and service programs for children with disabilities and for their families. Such services and educational programs must be sufficiently flexible, such that, they address the unique and individualized needs of children with disabilities and their families.

***

Can we imagine a day when children with disabilities grow up in families that meet their needs reliably? This level of consistency and support is necessary in order to establish a solid foundation for the child's life in the community. Programs like Goodwill, Special Olympics, and the Salvation Army are enduring sources of support for many children with disabilities and their families. These programs are models for new and creative programs that meet the remaining unmet needs of children with disabilities and their families. We must find new ways to:

Recommendation 8: Ensure that needed capacity enhancing programs are reliably funded, staffed, and offer certainty and security to children with disabilities and their families.

***

Disability in childhood is here to stay. We might as well embrace it and accept it. We might as well stretch our imaginations and consider that living with a disability is no different from living with any other unique feature such as our cultural heritage, our genetic make-up, and our unique attributes. We will be wise to:

Recommendation 9: Develop and support programming that focuses on the present and the future. A present and future orientation inspires hope, commitment, and the belief that children and families will fare well as future days unfold. Future oriented programs might include child and/or parent educational programs, financial planning, savings programs, and job shadowing, among others.

***

Exercise 8.14: Reflection
How might you be involved in enhancing the capacity of families of children with disabilities? Consider at least five ways that you could be involved in family capacity enhancement. *Which of these activities best matches your own knowledge, skills, interest and lifestyle? Are you willing to make a commitment to be engaged in this activity for at least one year? Why or why not?*

Addressing Unique Needs

Data indicate that the families of children who are exposed to abuse and neglect have unique needs. Poverty, domestic violence, alcohol abuse, drug, and substance abuse in general are more prevalent in families where children are abused and neglected. Data indicate also that children are abused and neglected more often in families with diverse cultural backgrounds. The data on the characteristics of the perpetrators and the families of children with disabilities are not disaggregated from the data on their nondisabled peers at this time.

Disability in childhood offers its own unique challenges in that it manifests itself uniquely across children. Families respond uniquely to disability manifestation. No two children are the same; no two children even with the same disability are the same. We may think that just because we know one child with autism, we know what autism looks like in childhood. Or, we may think that just because we know one child with Down syndrome, we know how Down syndrome will manifest itself in the next child we will meet. Just as autism and Down syndrome are uniquely manifested across children, so is blindness, deafness, physical disability, ADHD, learning disability, intellectual disability, cerebral palsy, depression, anxiety and more. The hard work here involves engaging in getting to know the unique needs of each child and family.

Painstakingly challenging work is required in order to get to know and understand the unique needs of children with disabilities and their families. This careful work is also essential in order to meet the needs of each individual child and those of each individual family of which they are a part.

Exercise 8.15: Reflection

Consider two children you know who have the same disability. The children might have any imaginable disability. For example, the two children might have intellectual disabilities. Speak to the parents of these children to find out what these two children have in common. *Record your interview and following an analysis of these data, what do the children have in common and what is unique to each one? State at least three characteristics they share and three that are unique to each one.*

Children with disabilities are at an increased risk when they have parents who do not know how to meet their own needs or the needs of their children. In addition to domestic violence, poverty, alcohol abuse, drug abuse, race, and ethnicity factors, attitudes toward disability, and poor educational outcomes contribute to caregiver abuse and neglect. What sets up families to engage in domestic violence? Why do people abuse alcohol? Why do people engage in behaviors that, rather than reduce the impact of childhood disability, instead increase and exaggerate its impact to the point that the lives of children with disabilities are further destabilized and at increased risk?

Based on the work of Sheehy-Skeffington and Haushofer (2014) we make the following recommendation:

Recommendation 10: Provide children with disabilities and their families with adequate time, individual counseling, and group support programs, among others, in order to develop their understanding of childhood disability manifestation, and mitigate the stress induced by disability.

***

We often forget that each one of us and each one of our children is one step away from a disability. The next accident might be the one that impairs our physical, emotional, sensory, or cognitive functioning. How might we develop our awareness that children with disabilities and their families are much more like us than unlike us? How might we get beyond our superficial sympathies and accept children with disabilities, their families, and their caregivers as the unique and fascinating people that that are? Thereby we:

Recommendation 11: Encourage and support the ongoing development of processes and programs that are designed to promote understanding, social acceptance, and emotional support for children with disabilities and their families.

***

Parents and caregivers of children with disabilities have unique needs for flexibility in their work and social lives. How can we accept and honor these needs? Parents and caregivers need increased flexibility so that they can provide for their children with disabilities. Is it possible to provide them with flexible work schedules and flexible support systems that make it possible for them to fulful their roles as parents and caregivers of the children with special needs? What infrastructure needs to be put in place in order to:

Recommendation 12: Provide flexible work schedules, reliable and regular child- care assistance, and paid leave to the parents and families of children with disabilities.

***

Proactive programming would require that, from the outset, every possible effort would be made to educate families and caregivers about resources that are available. Parents and caregivers of children with disabilities will be in the best position to provide for their children when they understand and accept their own needs as well as the needs of their children.

In conclusion, children with disabilities fare best in homes where the effects of poverty are ameliorated and were their caregivers and the children themselves have learned how to advocate for themselves. They fair best in homes and contexts that have the capacity to meet their physical, emotional, and intellectual needs. Finally, children with disabilities and their families will be poised to respond to the challenges of everyday life when their own unique needs as well as those of their children are met.

Chapter Summary

In this chapter we uncovered the context in which child maltreatment occurs. We found that children with disabilities are more vulnerable in situations where abuse and neglect disposing variables converge. Child disability itself increases vulnerability to abuse and neglect. Domestic violence and adult caregivers' abuse of drugs and alcohol increase the potential for abuse and neglect. Poverty, attitudes toward disability, and history of caregiver maltreatment also increase child vulnerability to abuse and neglect. Lack of a clear professional understanding of intervention and prevention of disability both contribute to the development of contexts that promote ANCD. We find evidence of these findings in newspaper coverage all over the world daily. This coverage takes us beyond the numbers and permits us to get a deeper understanding of how abuse and neglect plays out in the lives of children with disabilities locally, at the state, national, and international levels. We concluded this chapter with specific implications for research and practice.

References

Abdullah, M. A., Basharat, Z., Lodhi, O., Wazir, M. H. K., Khan, H. T., Sattar, N. Y., & Zahid, A. (2014). A qualitative exploration of Pakistan's street children, as a consequence of the poverty-disease cycle. *Infectious Diseases of Poverty, 3*(1), 1–8. http://www.idpjournal.com/content/3/1/11

Azar, S. T., Stevenson, M. T., & Johnson, D. R. (2012). Intellectual disabilities and neglectful parenting: Preliminary findings on the role of cognition in parenting risk. *Journal of Mental Health Research in Intellectual Disabilities, 5*(2), 94–129. doi:10.1080/19315864.2011.615460

Barone, L., Bramante, A., Lionetti, F., & Pastore, M. (2014). Mothers who murdered their child: An attachment-based study on filicide. *Child Abuse & Neglect, 38*(9), 1468–1477. doi:10.1016/j.chiabu.2014.04.014

Bevins, V. (2011, August 07). Rio's newest drug treatment effort sparks controversy. *Chicago Tribune*. Retrieved from http://search.proquest.com/docview/881404179?accountid=11578

Bones, P. D. C. (2013). Perceptions of vulnerability: A target characteristics approach to disability, gender, and victimization. *Deviant Behavior, 34*(9), 727–750. doi:10.1080/01639625.2013.766511

Bowean, L. (2010, May 09). Cops: Disabled child found chained to bed. *Chicago Tribune*. Retrieved from http://search.proquest.com/docview/251761409?accountid=11578

Caldas, S. J., & Bensy, M. L. (2014). The sexual maltreatment of students with disabilities in American school settings. *Journal of Child Sexual Abuse, 23*(4), 345–366. doi:10.1080/10538712.2014.906530

Chicago Tribune. (2013, April 15). Authorities: Father smothered crying girl. *Chicago Tribune*. Retrieved from http://articles.chicagotribune.com/2013-04-15/news/chi-baby-dies-days-after-father-smothered-her-to-stop-her-crying-20130415_1_playpen-court-documents-records

Coorg, R., & Tournay, A. (2013). Filicide-suicide involving children with disabilities. *Journal of Child Neurology, 28*, 745–751. doi:10.1177/0883073812451777

Douglas, E. M., & Mohn, B. L. (2014). Fatal and non-fatal child maltreatment in the US: An analysis of child, caregiver, and service utilization with the National Child Abuse and Neglect Data Set. *Child Abuse & Neglect, 38*(1), 42–51. doi:10.1016/j.chiabu.2013.10.022

Gennetian, L. K., Kessler, R., & Sanbonmatsu, L. (2014). Moving to more affluent neighborhoods improves health and happiness over the long-term among the poor. *Policy research brief*, MacArthur Foundation. http://www.macfound.org/media/files/HHM_Research_Brief-Moving_to_More_Affluent_Neighborhoods.pdf

Gutowski, C. (2011, October 03). 'I'm not some heartless monster'. *Chicago Tribune*. Retrieved from http://search.proquest.com/docview/895851071?accountid=11578

Gutowski, C., Sadovi, C., & Jaworski, J. (2011, September 13). Mother charged after boy's death. *Chicago Tribune*. Retrieved from http://articles.chicagotribune.com/2011-09-13/news/ct-met-berwyn-hoarding-charges-0913-2-20110913_1_animal-hoarding-animal-hoarding-exotic-animals

Hallahan, D. P., Kauffman, J. M., & Pullen, P. C. (2015). *Exceptional learners: An introduction to special education* (13th ed.). Upper Saddle River, NJ: Pearson.

Hendricks, C., Lansford, J. E., Deater-Deckard, K., & Bornstein, M. H. (2014). Associations between child disabilities and caregiver discipline and violence in low-and middle-income countries. *Child Development, 85*(2), 513–531. doi:10.1111/cdev.12132

Herrenkohl, T. I. (2013). Person-environment interactions and the shaping of resilience. *Trauma Violence Abuse, 14*(3), 191–194. doi:10.1177/1524838013491035

Hollis, M. E., Felson, M., & Welsh, B. C. (2013). The capable guardian in routine activities theory: A theoretical and conceptual reappraisal. *Crime Prevention & Community Safety, 15*(1), 65–79. doi:10.1057/cpcs.2012.14

Hollis-Peel, M. E., Reynald, D. M., van Bavel, M., Elffers, H., & Welsh, B. C. (2011). Guardianship for crime prevention: A critical review of the literature. *Crime, Law and Social Change, 56*(1), 53–70. doi:10.1007/s10611-011-9309-2

Hovitz, H. (2011, May 3). Putting bin laden and pain behind me. *Chicago Tribune*. Retrieved from http://articles.chicagotribune.com/2011-05-03/opinion/ct-oped-0502-recovery-20110503_1_panic-attacks-bin-childhood

Jones, L., Bellis, M. A., Wood, S., Hughes, K., McCoy, E., Eckley, L., ... Officer, A. (2012). Prevalence and risk of violence against children with disabilities: A systematic review and meta-analysis of observational studies. *Lancet, 380*(9845), 899–907. doi:10.1016/S0140-6736(12)60692-8

Kass, J. (2010, April 14). Adopting Russian children isn't a trip to kids R us. *Chicago Tribune*. Retrieved from http://articles.chicagotribune.com/2010-04-14/news/ct-met-kass-0414-20100413_1_adoptive-parents-russian-orphanage-russian-child

Keilman, J. (2011, August 12). Small town comes to the defense of teen accused of killing his mom. *Chicago Tribune*. Retrieved from http://articles.chicagotribune.com/2011-08-12/news/chi-the-surprise-while-reporting-this-murder-in-paris-ill-20110812_1_kathie-notebook-down state-town

Kempe, C. H., Silverman, F. N., Steele, B. F., Droegemueller, W., & Silver, H. K. (1985). The battered child syndrome. *Child Abuse and Neglect, 9*(2), 143–154.

Khalifeh, H., Howard, L. M., Osborn, D., Moran, P., & Johnson, S. (2013). Violence against people with disability in England and Wales: Findings from a national cross-sectional survey. *PloS One, 8*(2), 1–9. doi:10.1371/journal.pone.0055952

Kingsley, E. P. (1987). *Welcome to Holland*. http://www.our-kids.org/Archives/Holland.html

Leeb, R. T., Bitsko, R. H., Merrick, M. T., & Armour, B. S. (2012). Does childhood disability increase risk for child abuse and neglect? *Journal of Mental Health Research in Intellectual Disabilities, 5*(1), 4–31. doi:10.1080/19315864.2011.608154

McConnell, D., Savage, A., & Breitkreuz, R. (2014). Resilience in families raising children with disabilities and behavior problems. *Research in Developmental Disabilities, 35*(4), 833–848. doi:10.1016/j.ridd.2014.01.015

McGaw, S., Scully, T., & Pritchard, C. (2010). Predicting the unpredictable? Identifying high-risk versus low-risk parents with intellectual disabilities. *Child Abuse & Neglect, 34*(9), 699–710. doi:10.1016/j.chiabu.2010.02.006

Miethe, T. D., & Meier, R. F. (1994). *Crime and its social context: Toward an integrated theory of offenders, victims, and situations.* Albany, NY: SUNY Press.

Mueller-Johnson, K., Eisner, M. P., & Obsuth, I. (2014). Sexual victimization of youth with a physical disability: An examination of prevalence rates, and risk and protective factors. *Journal of Interpersonal Violence, 29*(17), 3180–3206. doi:10.1177/0886260514534529

Nahmias, A. S., Kase, C., & Mandell, D. S. (2014). Comparing cognitive outcomes among children with autism spectrum disorders receiving community-based early intervention in one of three placements. *Autism, 18*(3), 311–320. doi:10.1177/1362361312467865

Palusci, V. J., & Vandervort, F. E. (2014). Universal reporting laws and child maltreatmentreport rates in large U.S. counties. *Children and Youth Services Review, 38*, 20–28. http://dx.doi.org/10.1016/j.childyouth.2013.12.010

Sheehy-Skeffington, J., & Haushofer, J. (2014). The behavioural economics of poverty. In D. P. Bhawuk, S. C. Carr, A. E. Gloss, & L. F. Thompson, (Eds.), *Barriers to and opportunities for poverty reduction* (pp. 96–112). Retrieved from http://www.undp.org/content/dam/undp/library/Poverty%20Reduction/Private%20Sector/undp-psd-Barriers%20and%20Prospects%20for%20Poverty%20Reduction%202014.pdf#page=65

Sinanan, A. N. (2011). The impact of child, family, and child protective services factors on reports of child sexual abuse recurrence. *Journal of Child Sexual Abuse, 20*(6), 657–676. doi:10.1080/10538712.2011.622354

Spano, R., & Bolland, J. (2013). Disentangling the effects of violent victimization, violent behavior, and gun carrying for minority inner-city youth living in extreme poverty. *Crime & Delinquency, 59*(2), 191–213. doi:10.1177/0011128710372196

Stein, J. A., Leslie, M. B., & Nyamathi, A. (2002). Relative contributions of parent substance use and childhood maltreatment to chronic homelessness, depression, and substance abuse problems among homeless women: Mediating roles of self-esteem and abuse in adulthood. *Child Abuse & Neglect, 26*(10), 1011–1027.

Tucker, M. C., & Rodriguez, C. M. (2014). Family dysfunction and social isolation as moderators between stress and child physical abuse risk. *Journal of Family Violence, 29*(2), 175–186. doi:10.1007/s10896-013-9567-0

U.S. Department of Health and Human Services, Administration for Children and Families, Administration on Children, Youth and Families, Children's Bureau. (2013). *Child maltreatment 2012.* Retrieved from http://www.acf.hhs.gov/programs/cb/research-data-technology/statistics-research/child-maltreatment

U.S. Department of Health and Human Services, Administration for Children and Families, Administration on Children, Youth and Families, Children's Bureau. (2015). *Child maltreatment 2013.* Retrieved from http://www.acf.hhs.gov/programs/cb/research-data-technology/statistics-research/child-maltreatment

World Health Organization. (2011). *World report on disability.* Geneva, Switzerland: WHO Press. Retrieved from http://whqlibdoc.who.int/publications/2011/9789240685215_eng.pdf?ua=1

Yampolskaya, S., Greenbaum, P. E., & Berson, I. R. (2009). Profiles of child maltreatment perpetrators and risk for fatal assault: A latent class analysis. *Journal of Family Violence, 24*, 337–348. doi:10.1007/s10896-009-9233-8

Helpful Resources for Further Study

Karr-Morse, R., & Wiley, M. S. (2011). *Ghosts from the nursery: Tracing the roots of violence.* New York, NY: The Atlantic Monthly Press.

National Council on Child Abuse and Family Violence. *Parental substance abuse a major factor in child abuse and neglect.* Retrieved from http://www.nccafv.org/parentalsubstanceabuse.htm

Parental substance abuse. Retrieved from http://www.childwelfare.gov/can/factors/parentcaregiver/substance.cfm

Chapter 9
Our Professional Failures at Predicting and Preventing Abuse and Neglect in the Lives of Children with Disabilities

... this extension is unavailable, goodbye! (State of Illinois Child Service Agency)

Abstract The focus of this chapter is on our professional failures to protect the lives of children with disabilities from abuse and neglect. Specifically, we will describe the maltreatment of children by professionals. These professionals include doctors, lawyers, educators, and related professionals. We will analyze the data provided by the U.S. DHHS on the professional perpetuators of child abuse and neglect (CAN) and abuse and neglect of children with disabilities (ANCD). We will present an analysis of the newspaper coverage over a 10-year span and provide examples of professionals who abuse and neglect children with disabilities. We will address the unique challenges inherent in this area of research and practice. We will conclude this chapter by making recommendations for future researchers and practitioners in this area.

Do you expect that professional personnel, such as educators, doctors, hospital staff, as well as staff in group homes and residential facilities, are perpetrators of abuse and neglect in the lives of children with and without disabilities? If not perpetrators themselves, are you surprised to learn that some professionals stand by, observe CAN and ANCD and fail to report the abuse and neglect of children with disabilities? Who suspects that professional personnel, into whose care we entrust children, including those with disabilities, are indeed potential perpetrators of abuse and neglect? After all, we expect that their personal commitment, as well as their professional expertise, and their ongoing professional development will protect them from any possible allegations of CAN and ANCD.

Exercise 9.1: Reflection
Does the title of this chapter surprise you? Have you considered that professionals might be perpetrators of abuse and neglect in the lives of children with disabilities? How do you feel when you think about medical, legal, educational, and related professionals who perpetrate CAN and ANCD?

Data across disciplines indicate our professional failures to protect children with and without disabilities from abuse and neglect in the legal system (Cederborg, Danielsson, La Rooy, & Lamb, 2009; Cederborg & Gumpert, 2010;

© Springer International Publishing Switzerland 2016
E.P. Crowley, *Preventing Abuse and Neglect in the Lives of Children with Disabilities*, DOI 10.1007/978-3-319-30442-7_9

213

Cederborg & Lamb, 2006; Ford, 2011); in educational environments (Bryant, 2009; Goldman, 2010; Gore & Janssen, 2007; Hogelin, 2013; Kenny, 2004); and in hospitals and other health care service environments (Cooke & Standen, 2002; Mallén, 2011; Sanghera, 2007; Schols, Ruiter, & Öry, 2013). Kenny and McEachern (2002) found that even though professionals are mandated reporters of abuse and neglect of children with and without disabilities in the United States, 40 % of them failed to report the abuse and neglect of children they observed at some point in their careers. They also found that 6 % of professionals consistently fail to report their observations of CAN and ANCD. Furthermore, in their review of recent research, Stalker and McArthur (2012) and Cooke and Standen (2002) provided evidence that professionals contribute to the continuation of abuse and neglect of children with disabilities in the United States and worldwide.

In this chapter we will examine the database on professionals as perpetrators of CAN and ANCD. We will analyze the research on professionals relative to their roles in the ANCD specifically. We will examine stories published in the *Chicago Tribune* that illustrate the prevailing evidence of the ANCD by professionals. We will observe trends in these data and propose essential considerations for a research agenda and for improved professional practice in this area.

National and State Level Data

The database of the U.S. DHHS (2013) confirms that professionals are included among the identified perpetrators of abuse and neglect children from birth to 18 years old. Though perhaps vastly underestimated, these data indicate that combined, professionals perpetrate 0.6 % of all CAN. More specifically, day care providers perpetrate 0.4 % of the abuse and neglect of children, 0.1 % is perpetrated by other professionals and 0.1 % is perpetrated by staff in group homes.

Methodological issues plague these data. For example, in 2012, only 28 out of 50 states and the District of Columbia reported abuse and neglect by professionals, 36 out of 50 states and the District of Columbia reported abuse and neglect by group home and residential facility staff and 38 out of 50 states and the District of Columbia reported abuse and neglect by day care staff. Furthermore, data from the U.S. DHHS are not disaggregated thus; we do not know specifically, the extent to which professionals perpetrate abuse and neglect in the lives of children with disabilities. Cleary, these data provide an incomplete picture of the extent to which professionals perpetrate abuse and neglect in the lives of children with disabilities.

Scott Reeder (2007), an investigative reporter with the *Small Newspaper Group Springfield Bureau,* found that in the 10 years between 1997 and 2007 the teaching certificates of 124 teachers were suspended or revoked in Illinois. Reeder observed that the costs associated with dismissing educators, so burdens educational institutions, that their dismissal is discouraged. For example, what school district has more than $200,000.00 to spend on attorney fees? Reeder found that "Over a 5-year period school districts that retained attorneys and attempted to fire a tenured teacher spent an average $219,000 per case in legal fees alone." Reeder also observed that no investigators of educators' misconduct are employed by the Illinois State Board of Education.

Reeder reported that from 1999 to 2007, the DCFS received 3,871, at times superficial, complaints against educators. However, in 323 cases, credible evidence of abuse by teachers was found. Based solely on the DCFS findings, the Illinois State Board of Education did not once suspend or revote a teacher's teaching certificate. Reeder also observed that the licenses of physicians and lawyers were 43 and 25 times respectively, more likely to be suspended than were educators. Furthermore, Reeder concluded that teachers hired before 2004 were not required to undergo State-mandated national criminal background checks.

In 2012, the U. S. DHHS data indicated that 58.7 % of all reports of CAN were made by professional personnel including child daycare providers, education personnel, foster care providers, legal and law enforcement, as well as medical and social service personnel. Even though educational professionals spend substantial time with children daily, they were the report sources for only 16.6 % of the abuse and neglect allegations made by professionals.

Exercise 9.2: Critical Thinking

What information in this chapter surprises you most up to this point? *What did or did not surprise you? Do you have new questions that you want to explore further?*

Research on Professionals Who Abuse and Neglect Children with Disabilities

Kenny (2004), using the Educators and Child Abuse Questionnaire (ECAQ), conducted a study on educators' knowledge of the signs and symptoms of CAN, reporting procedures and their knowledge of the legal aspects of CAN. Kenny found that 25 % of educators had made at least one report of child abuse. Only 34 % reported that they received professional preparation about CAN and of these and only 23 % considered this preparation adequate. Seventy six percent of these educators believed that the administrators with whom they work would not support them if they were to make a report of child abuse. Among these educators, 56 % believed they could be sued by the family if the allegations they made were unfounded. Only 13 % reported they had knowledge of their school's reporting procedures. Finally, Kenny found that two out of three educators reported having received no professional preparation on CAN in their preservice professional preparation.

As mandated reporters, teachers have three main responsibilities relative to CAN detection, treatment, and prevention. Data indicate that they lack knowledge of CAN as well as knowledge of their reporting obligations and the mandated legal processes involved (Walsh, Rassafiani, Mathews, Farrell, & Butler, 2010). They are often misinformed or are trained in ways that do not reflect formal legal policy. This lack of training and knowledge may, in turn, affect educators' roles and their compliance as mandated reporters.

Similarly, in a study conducted in England, Cooke and Standen (2002) found that social workers and members of social service departments considered that they lacked the professional preparation necessary to work with children with disabilities who have been abused and neglected. They observed that the disabilities children have often go unreported in the context of abuse and neglect. Social workers and child protection agency staff often lack knowledge of child disability characteristics, as well as of their potential as human beings. This renders their estimates as mere approximations of the extent to which the ANCD occurs. The professional preservice and in-service preparation of social workers and child protection agency staff for increased awareness of the abuse and neglect of children with disabilities remains a critical need (Child Welfare Information Child Welfare Information Gateway, 2012; Cooke & Standen, 2002; Farrell, 2014a, 2014b; Orelove, Hollahan, & Myles, 2000).

In the world of law and law enforcement, much work remains to be done. To the amazement of many readers, there is legal support for the corporal punishment of children by adults, including professionals, in many countries all over the world (Farrell, 2015). In the United States corporal punishment is legal in 19 States and it is common practice in Alabama, Arkansas, and Mississippi (Farrell, 2014a, 2014b).

There is growing support for universal reporting laws in the United States (Palusci & Vandervort, 2014). Universal reporting laws would extend mandated reporting laws to all adults. Palusci and Vandervort conducted a study of the effects of universal reporting laws on CAN report rates in the United States. They found that states with universal laws had higher rates of reported and confirmed cases of CAN. Additionally, under mandated reporting conditions psychological maltreatment and neglect were more frequently reported. Under conditions when adults were not mandated reporters of CAN, physical and sexual abuse were more frequently reported. Based on Palusci and Vandervort's findings, we may well conclude that when mandated reporters report child neglect, they are actually preventing more serious forms of CAN.

Cederborg and Lamb (2006) investigated the response of the Swedish legal system in cases which involved evidence that children with disabilities were the victims of CAN. Cederborg and Lamb contacted prosecutors and asked them to send as much information as possible about all the cases they had processed within the previous 5 years in which children with disabilities were purportedly victimized. Of 69 cases, 39 (56.5 %) were brought to court. Thirty one (45.0 %) of these cases led to prosecution, and seven of those decisions were then reversed. The children involved in these cases averaged from age 11 years-8 months to 12 years-7 months. Sexual abuse of children was observed in 33 (85.0 %) of the 39 cases and the data indicated that children with developmental disabilities, autism, psychiatric disorders and deafness were among those who were identified. Physical abuse was indicated in 5 (13 %) of the 39 cases. Multiple factors, such as misinformation, determined the legal system's role and appropriateness in handling these cases and multiple findings indicated the inappropriateness of many of the courts' procedures.

In 22 (56.4 %) out of 39 of these cases, the judges argued that credible accounts should have the same, clear characteristics that previous decisions had sought by alleged victims who did not have disabilities (Cederborg & Lamb, 2006). Basically, it is conceivable that a child who is deaf who sits in silence in a courtroom is nonverbally communicating consent, agreement or even culpability. Cederborg and Lamb found that expert guidance was provided for the people involved in only 18 (46.0 %) out of these 39 cases. Largely unrequested, and thereby, unavailable to the members of the court, this expert knowledge would have helped to increase the courts' understanding of how to proceed with the investigation and adjudication of these cases. Incomplete psychological and medical assessments also created problems for members of the court in being well-versed in factors associated with understanding disability characteristics, capabilities, and limitations as well as miscommunication between the court staff regarding sources of expert information. Overall, based on the findings of this study, we may conclude that even when children with disabilities do get their day in court, we cannot assume that justice will prevail.

Children and adolescents with disabilities are abused and neglected in hospitals and among medical teams in social service settings and educational settings (Benbenishty et al., 2014; Brachear & Rohde, 2010; Caldas & Bensy, 2014; Hoffman, 2014; Sanghera, 2007). Abusive practices in hospitals are often subtle and can include inappropriate assessments of pain for children with disabilities, over-medicating, administering unexplained and unconsented procedures, failing to honor the child's privacy and dignity, assuming that those with more severe disabilities do not need to be consulted, rough and hurtful handling, and removing food when the assigned eating time has passed.

Mallen (2011) found that medical and social service personnel are reluctant to report the ANCD. A major obstacle to their reporting of CAN is their own perceived closeness to the parents and their consideration or belief that such reporting is merely a last resort. They employ other remedies such as house calls or conversations with caregivers and through these methods they maintain their closeness to families of children with disabilities. Furthermore, Mallen found that medical and social service personnel find explanations for the bruises and other injuries they observe and their observations become blurred by their alignment with caregivers. Mallen found that only clear cases of abuse and neglect are reported by medical and social service personnel.

Caldas and Bensy (2014) investigated sexual abuse of students with disabilities in schools in the United States. The researchers generated data on the sexual abuse to which children with disabilities between 14 and 17 years were exposed. The children came from diverse backgrounds and from 41 States. Males accounted for 53.4 % of the students and females accounted for 46.6 %. The students had an assortment of disabilities including autism (25.8 %), intellectual disability (14.8 %), and multiple disabilities (14.5 %). Caldas and Bensy found that 78.2 % of these children were "very upset" by their experiences of sexual abuse and 37.7 % of "the victims were doing poorly and failing in school" (p. 356). Comments, jokes, and gestures (68.5 %) and being "touched, pinched and rubbed" (62.3 %) represented the most frequent types of the sexual abuse to which these children were exposed in school settings. They were also exposed to other such severe types of sexual abuse as "pulled off or down clothing" (41.0 %), "forced intercourse" (30.1 %), and "forced kissing" (14.2 %). Caldas and Bensy found that in 35.0 % of the cases the abuse they experienced was reported as having occurred "more than 10 times" and in 75.6 % of the cases the sexual abuse of the child occurred more than once.

Exercise 9.3: Critical Thinking
If you were a child with a disability or if your child had a disability, what country in the world would you most like to live? Are there safe havens for children with disabilities in any part of the world? Do you support the development of safe havens?

Findings and Cases from the Newspaper Study

An analysis of the newspaper coverage in the *Chicago Tribune* from January, 2004 to December, 2013 indicated that professionals are among the active and passive perpetrators of ANCD. They were involved in stories which described physical, sexual, and emotional abuse and in stories that indicated their failure to protect children and adolescents with disabilities from abuse and neglect. Overall, professionals were implicated directly in 18.6 % (21 of the 113 stories) of the stories about ANCD. This is a conservative estimate because it does not include the 6.1 % of the stories which involved perpetrators unknown to the children with disabilities. These stories conceivably included professionals who were unknown to the children. School professionals were involved in 13.7 % of these stories. General education teachers, teacher assistants, administrators, and other school staff were the focus of 10.5 % of these stories and 3.2 % of these stories involved special education teachers and their assistants. Priests and ministers were implicated in 4.2 % of the stories about the ANCD. These findings are illustrated in the following stories about the ANCD and by professionals into whose care children with disabilities were committed.

The Legal System

On September 8, 2013, *Chicago Tribune* reporters, Dizikes and Lighty described an extraordinary saga of what appears to be a comedy of errors, implicating the ineptitude of the court system and its capacity to deliver justice to Cristina Zvunca following a tragic accident. In 2002, Cristina Zvunca, then a 7 year child, was diagnosed with post-traumatic stress disorder after a fatal accident during which she witnessed the death of her mother when a Greyhound bus driver ran over her in a parking lot. Recurring nightmares continued for Cristina during which she watched other family members die. Dizikes and Lighty observed that "Cristina's odyssey through the courts involves allegations of unethical behavior and conflicts of interest. It involves questions about William Maddux, one of Cook County's most powerful judges, and his relationship with a lawyer in the case" (Dizikes & Lighty, September 8, 2013a, 2013b).

Many years have passed and Cristina is now an adult. This case alleges the culpability of a Greyhound bus driver who did not respond to her mother's knock on the bus door when she feared the bus was leaving. While unresolved, this case "spawned 13 other lawsuits, more than 25 appeals and a series of questionable decisions by Cook County judges" (Dizikes & Lighty, September 8, 2013a, 2013b). This case was valued at $8 million or more and it resulted in a settlement that was later thrown out by the court system. A judge pronounced this case as "'one of the most unholy messes' he'd ever seen" (Dizikes & Lighty, 2013b). According to Dizikes and Lighty, on December 29 (2013b) this case was back in Cook County court system with little reason to believe that it will be resolved any time soon.

Exercise 9.4: Critical Thinking
Are you surprised to read that the incident involving the death of a 31 year old mother perpetrated by a Greyhound bus driver remains unresolved? The woman's daughter Cristina, at 19 years old stated, "This case destroyed my life...in 12 years we did not receive justice" (Dizikes & Lighty, September 8, 2013a, 2013b). *What contributing variables do you observe in this scenario? Are your disappointed? What may be done to avoid such injustice?*

Abusive and neglectful decision-making by personnel in the legal system is further illustrated in the case of a 7-year-old African-American boy who was arrested in 1998. The child was accused of murdering 11-year-old Ryan Harris. The case resurfaced in 2005. At the time of his arrest, the boy "had a disability that prevented him from processing communication properly" (Washburn, 2005). The family of the 7-year old received a $2 million settlement from the city of Chicago for his wrongful arrest. Though the charges were dismissed, a month after his detainment, the wrongfully accused boy is now diagnosed with post-traumatic stress disorder. The lawyer for the boy and his family agreed to the settlement "because the child needed treatment, [and] he needed to conclude this episode in his life" (Washburn, 2005). The child was severely traumatized by the event, but he received treatment while attending a school for children with special needs.

Washburn stated that a spokesman from the state's attorney's office, John Gorman, said at the time of the arrest, "there was no felony review for juvenile cases, so we did not approve the charges. Since then, we have instituted felony review for murder cases involving juveniles."

Our Professional Failure in Educational Settings

On November 13, 2012 Jackson and Marx reported that "Sometimes, Yajaira Rivera would storm out of school in frustration during the middle of the day."

At other times, Yajaira was either asked to leave school or she simply chose to stay at home in hope of avoiding both the day's trouble and school failure. Since second grade she missed 213 school days which amounts to far more than the 180 days which constitutes a school year.

Meeting the academic and social demands of school was a constant struggle for Yajaira. Though she was diagnosed with learning and emotional disabilities, a school social worker described her as "motivated to learn." Without careful intervention, conflicts with both teachers and students are highly predictable for students with learning and emotional disabilities. *Chicago Tribune* reporters, Jackson and Marx indicate that:

> Attendance data provided by Chicago Public Schools show that students like Yajaira who are diagnosed with a learning or emotional disability – and there are thousands of them in grades K-8 – miss far more school days on average than children without a disability.

Yajaira's mother, Maria Figueroa, told the *Chicago Tribune* reporters that she reached "an agreement with the principal at Nobel: When Yajaira is upset, I will not send her to school." Clearly illegal, the school principal, Manuel Adrianzen denied that he made this agreement. Regardless, this information fits with prevailing patterns:

> Consider the 17,000 students in grades K-8 whose "primary diagnosis" in CPS' database is a learning disability – a disorder generally affecting the ability to use or understand language. On average, each of these students racked up two weeks of truancy and excused absences in the 2010–2011 school year – about 20 percent more than those with no disability.
>
> Also frequently gone from school were the 1500 elementary students with an emotional disorder as their primary diagnosis – children whose behavior or feelings impede their learning and ability to get along with others.
>
> On average, K-8 students with an emotional disorder missed about four weeks of school because of truancy and other absences, the Tribune's analysis found. They also accrued 10 times as many suspension days as children without a disability. (Jackson & Marx, November 13, 2012)

Jackson and Marx add ". . . While not commenting specifically on Yajaira's case, Harvard University education professor Thomas Hehir said that excessive suspensions and informal exclusions from school are a nationwide problem for youths with disabilities." Yajaira's discipline records indicate that she "was suspended for 2 days for refusing to take off her hoodie in a classroom, then cursing. Days later she got another 2-day suspension for swearing at a teacher before walking out of class." Another day "a Nobel official called police after Yajaira threw a plastic spider at a girl and threatened to "beat" and "kill" her." Absences and suspensions became routine for Yajaira as indicated on her school record:

> By the end of November 2011 she already had "22 school absences, due to out-of-school suspensions, and her mother's attempts to keep her out of school so Yajaira will not engage in inappropriate behaviors," according to an evaluation from that month. . .
>
> "The general education teacher finds it 'impossible' to teach when she is in the class," the school report said. "Sometimes she will sit quietly and not work, those are the times when teaching can occur.". . .

> The school social worker's report from that month stated that the principal was "verbalizing intent to remove Yajaira from his school." (Jackson & Marx, November 13, 2012)

The school personnel conducted a new education evaluation and diagnosed Yajaira with an added disability – an emotional disorder. Her new education plan required her to be placed in a specialized setting that involved her removal from general education classes. Eventually Yajaira attended eighth grade in a therapeutic day school in which 90 students with learning and behavioral problems were enrolled. Jackson and Marx conclude their story thus:

> As the school year began, Yajaira displayed a new knapsack, proudly unpacking pristine notebooks with Tinker Bell covers and a quiver of markers, highlighters and colored pencils.
>
> "I am going to a new school. I don't have the bad friends that I had. I can control my temper," Yajaira said.
>
> Yajaira's first interim report card, issued at the end of October, showed she got A's and B's with only one C, in physical education. She had missed five school days at Near North – two of them after a second brother, age 15, was locked up while facing attempted murder charges in juvenile court.
>
> On a recent afternoon, Yajaira carefully completed an enrollment application to five Chicago high schools, noting that she wanted to focus on health sciences, a step toward her dream of becoming a veterinarian.
>
> "I'm doing a good job in school," she said. "I need to keep it up." (Jackson & Marx, November 13, 2012)

Our systematic and collective professional failures as educators dispose children like Yajaira to live lives that often grossly undermine their potential. Far from receiving the special education that is their hard won right in the United States, they are often pushed to the sidelines and deprived of both the education they need and the future they deserve. This is not the failure of children like Yajaira, rather it is an all-systems failure and we all lose out in the process.

Our Professional Failures Among Medical Personnel

The first sentence of an article by Megan Twohey in the *Chicago Tribune* on July 29, 2010 read as follows: "A 17-year-old girl reported to Berwyn police in 2003 that her doctor, Ricardo Arze, had pulled off her clothes and sexually assaulted her in his exam room, state records show." For years following, reports like this remained unattended while Dr. Arze claimed that he was treating depression in women and girls. Even after 21 patients reported sexual assault, Twohey reported that "Cook County state's attorney's office said it lacked enough evidence to prosecute Arze." Though the women made the reports to the police, they stated that "law enforcement officials brushed them aside." After years of complaints, information provided by an undercover investigator was used in a case against Dr. Arze (Twohey, 2010a, 2010b, July 30). Following his eventual day in court, Dr. Arze said that:

... he was treating more than 6000 patients at Arze Doctors Center at the time of his arrest
and that his practice had a "great emphasis on mental health" – including treatment for
depression and other mood disorders.

According to Twohey "After Arze's arrest made news, the charges against him
multiplied – in court and with the state, painting a picture of a chronic sex abuser
who allegedly preyed on vulnerable patients suffering from depression." Eventually
Arze was charged with sexual assault and battery of patients and the state
suspended his license to practice medicine.

This case not only showed blatant sexual abuse of women and girls by a trusted
professional who, as a physician, had pledged to do no harm, it also revealed:

... a disconnect between the criminal justice system and the state agency in charge of
policing doctors. The Illinois Department of Financial and Professional Regulation and its
medical disciplinary board did not learn of the 2003 and 2005 allegations against Arze until
2007, said Sue Hofer, the department's spokeswoman. State law does not require the
department and police to share such complaints, she said.

In Illinois, the state Medical Practice Act is interpreted to mean that Arze cannot
permanently lose his license to practice medicine "unless a doctor has been twice
convicted of felonies involving controlled substances or public aid offenses"
(Twohey, 2010a, 2010b).

The needs of children with disabilities often defy the imaginations of many
members of the medical profession. For years, Mary Gabel appealed for help from
medical professionals and found none. Her son, Chris Marciano was in the care of a
psychiatrist since age 8 when he was diagnosed with anxiety and depression. At age
24 he was diagnosed with paranoid schizophrenia. During his life he bounced
between emergency rooms, jails and the streets. Gable cared for her troubled
child for so long that she was drained financially and emotionally. She navigated
the barriers of the mental health care system which, according to her, was broken.
The American Academy of Child and Adolescent Psychiatry indicates ". . . Of the
15 million U.S. youths with bipolar disorder, schizophrenia and other mental
illnesses, less than half will get medical attention. . . in Illinois, which slashed
more than $100 million in mental health services from 2009 to 2011. . ." (Rubin
& Haggerty, 2013).

Chris and his parents were constantly engaged in conflict. They divorced when
the boy was 10. He attended St. Christina Catholic School until his behavior
became so challenging that he was asked to leave. His mother enrolled him in
Mount Greenwood Elementary school where he began the 7th grade and qualified
to receive special education services. His problem behaviors increased throughout
high school and so did his hospital visits and diagnoses. He was diagnosed with
bipolar, conduct, and narcissistic personality disorder later, and he was abusing
drugs. At 15 years old, he had a re-evaluation by Dr. Alan Ravitz, a child and
adolescent psychiatrist who concluded:

'The only appropriate . . . placement for him given his severe mental illness and his
significantly dangerous behaviors is a 24-hour residential facility,' Ravitz concluded.
'Any educational intervention less intensive will result in a continuing downward spiral

and the likelihood that Chris will act out in some type of dangerous fashion, endangering his life or those of the people around him.' (Rubin & Haggerty, 2013, May 6)

The cost of this around-the-clock placement ran $10,000 per month. His mother's application for an Individual Care Grant was denied despite his need. His application was among the 92.5 % that were rejected 2012. It took Chris Marciano hurting his mother to have him sent to a home for youth with emotional and behavioral disorders, where he made progress. A court ordered that he no longer needed to stay at the residential placement. Upon his return home, he resumed his use of drugs, engaged in burglary, sexually abused a 3-year old child, and he was arrested on several occasions, and imprisoned. He was convicted of aggravated criminal sexual abuse, and he spent 3 years in Dixon Correctional Center where he made no progress.

Chris Marciano's life may have been very different had he been provided effective treatment at a young age. Currently, he lives at the Chicago Read Mental Health Center, the only long-term, state-operated psychiatric facility in the city. Today, Rubin and Haggerty state that "Taxpayers are covering the cost of his care at roughly $250,000 per year." His mother indicates that he is safe and has made progress.

The professional ignorance of both law enforcement and medical personnel is illustrated in a story of a wrongfully accused mother of four children. Weber (2008, March 20) reported:

It was lunchtime at Loma Linda Academy when the social workers arrived, escorted by a deputy sheriff.

They were there to collect the Udvardi children. Amid dozens of students eating sandwiches and chips, school officials found 6-year-old Esther, then Abram, 11, and Sam, 14. They got the eldest, Matthew, 16, just as he arrived at his American Literature class.

The children were hustled one by one to a white van in the parking lot, then whisked away even before their father, the school's band teacher, knew what was happening.

Their mother "Leslie had been deemed a danger to her children." A doctor-in-training at the local hospital evaluated her daughter Esther and entered in her medical record "suspected Munchausen by proxy syndrome." This condition involves a caregiver – usually a mother – who fabricates real or apparent symptoms of an illness in her children in order to gain attention.

This family engaged in a long trail of experiences in medical and legal circles. Eventually a judge concluded:

The evidence ... "does not support a finding that these are severely damaged children, let alone a finding that their parents caused it."

At home, there was a tearful, almost giddy reunion.

The only acknowledgment from the hospital came from its attorney. At the end of a three-page letter defending the hospital, E. Nathan Schilt wrote: "I am deeply sorry for the ordeal you and your family have undergone."

Hospital and social-service officials, including Sheridan-Matney, declined to discuss any aspect of the case with the Los Angeles Times.

A geneticist at University of California, Irvine, Medical Center, recommended by Francomano, is keeping watch over the children's health. All of them have been diagnosed with "EDS-plus." By March 2007, based on new tests, the children had been diagnosed with Chiari as well, Leslie said. How their health will be affected in the long term remains unknown.

Our Professional Failures in Residential Treatment Centers

Despite the data in the investigative report by the *Chicago Tribune* that uncovered a 10-year pattern of abuse and neglect of such a magnitude of harmful and neglectful care, Alden Village North remained open on appeal (Chicago Tribune, 2012, January, 3). Alden Village is designated as a residential treatment center for children and adults with developmental disabilities. Roe and Hopkins (2011a, 2011b, January 11) illustrate the neglectful care of children with disabilities at this facility in the following excerpt:

> … Alden has been under fire since October, when a Tribune investigation revealed a high number of deaths at the home and the worst safety record in Illinois for facilities of its kind. The girl's death [14-month-old child] brings to 14 the number of children and young adults who have died at the home since 2000 in cases that resulted in state citations.
>
> The Illinois Department of Public Health finished investigating the girl's death last week, an agency spokeswoman said. About 90 people live at the North Side facility, most of them children and young adults with profound cognitive impairment.
>
> "We care for a very fragile patient population who suffer from very serious medical conditions," Alden Management Services, which oversees the facility, said in a statement Monday. "Our residents are like family to us and we grieve whenever one of them passes. We continually evaluate the care that we provide to all of our patients to see if there are areas for improvement."
>
> State inspection records show that the girl, whose identity was not disclosed, suffered from heart ailments and a seizure disorder. On the morning of July 3, test results showed she had "heavy growth" of MRSA, or methicillin-resistant Staphylococcus aureus, a kind of staph bacterium that is resistant to some antibiotics. Yet her doctor was not notified until the evening of July 5.
>
> The girl arrived at a hospital with a temperature of 105.4 degrees and a pulse of 180. She died the next day of septic shock, a drop in blood pressure brought on by infection.
>
> While investigating the girl's death, state inspectors learned that another Alden Village North resident, a 14-year-old boy with profound mental disabilities, was also sent to the hospital in July after a lengthy delay.
>
> Records show that after the boy began breathing rapidly, Alden staff paged his doctor six times over 19 hours before the physician responded. In citing the facility, regulators concluded the home should have contacted its medical director instead of waiting for the doctor to respond.
>
> The teenager died two months later, but records do not state whether the delayed trip to the hospital was a factor.

Roe (2011, March 4) provided more details on the neglect of children with disabilities at Alden Village. For example, a 9-year-old boy with profound disabilities who grew mortally ill at this facility, while no one called a doctor. Not his case manager. Not his day nurse, nor his night nurse. As the third day dawned, a nurse finally called for help. But it was too late. When the child died he became the most recent fatality following the pattern of harmful and neglectful care provided by the staff at Alden Village North.

The *Chicago Tribune* reporters Roe and Hopkins (2011a, 2011b, June 1) indicated that new rules for nursing homes would preclude the rampant abuse and neglect to which children with disabilities were exposed at Alden Village. During the last 10 years, the State of Illinois issued at least 13 citations of neglect or failure to investigate the deaths of its residents with disabilities at Alden Village.

On June 30, 2012, Patrick Quinn, Governor of Illinois signed a law requiring sweeping reforms designed to protect thousands of children and adults with disabilities who live in residential centers. Following citations of neglect, the new law will impose stiffer fines, fewer roadblocks to shuttering facilities, stricter rules on the use of medicines and increased requirements to report deaths.

Exercise 9.5: Reflection

Are you surprised to read stories about children with disabilities who are abused and neglected by designated personnel in residential treatment centers and in organizations designed to care for them? *Make at least five observations about why children with disabilities might be abused and neglected by personnel in such placements and in such organizations. Make a list of as many suggestions as you can on how to increase appropriate care to children with disabilities by designated personnel.*

The failure of organizations such as the Department of Children and Family Services (DCFS), designed to provide appropriate care to children with and without disabilities, is once again illustrated in the Chicago Tribune on June 8, 2013, "DCFS failed 23-lb teen girl: 'No excuse' for taking 4 months to report her, agency says." Reporter Christy Gutowski described the dismay of medical staff upon their observation of this child:

> When teenager Darlene Armstrong arrived at the emergency room curled on a stretcher, she weighed a skeletal 23 pounds.
>   In serious condition, the 16-year-old had cerebral palsy and couldn't walk or talk, but the stunned medical staff also focused on her shriveled 3-foot-10-inch frame, her sunken cheeks and protruding ribs.

Gutowski went on to describe the severe, long-standing neglect and starvation, as well as the unacceptable medical neglect of this child. The staff at DCFS was alerted about the neglect of this child on November 17, 2011 but it was not until March 14, 2012 that during a home visit they actually heard the cries of this child and immediately dialed 911.

A series of errors were made by the staff at DCFS. Kendal Marlowe, a spokesperson for DCFS acknowledged these errors and attributed them to high caseloads and inadequate staffing. Upon closer examination, Darlene Armstrong was diagnosed with fetal alcohol syndrome at birth and it was clear even in 1996 that her mother neglected her. In 2000 she removed Darlene from her special education classes and she could not recall when she last attended a medical appointment or even had been outside her home.

Gutowski reported that the DCFS violates federal guidelines when they assign caseworkers more than 12 new cases per month. Furthermore, their caseloads may

Table 9.1 Alleged and indicated victims of CAN in Illinois over 30 years (DCFS, 2014)

Victims	1981	1990	2000	2010	2013
Alleged victims	51,674	103,420	103,577	109,185	108,613
Indicated victims	20,977	38,209	32,712	28,855	30,038
% alleged victims	71.1	73.0	76.0	79.1	78.3
% indicated Victims	28.9 (−42.2 %)	27.0 (−46 %)	24.0 (−52 %)	20.9 (−58.2 %)	21.7 (−56.6 %)

Data from Illinois DCFS

not exceed 15 cases for more than 3 months. DCFS caseworkers must close their cases within 2 months; no caseworker is expected to work on more than 24 cases at any one time. Darlene's investigator had a caseload above the assigned limit. The DCFS agency reports indicate that "Darlene's investigator had ... more than 30 cases pending when given the hotline call about Darlene. She was assigned about 60 additional cases in the months that case languished, the reports show" (Gutowski, 2012).

At this time the DCFS in Illinois is understaffed and underfunded (DCFS, 2014). While the number of staff employed in this agency was reduced by 33 % since 2000, the demand for their investigative services has increased. For example, both the alleged and indicated statistics on CAN have been increasing since these statistics have been available in 1981 (see Table 9.1). Furthermore, proportionately fewer actual victims were identified in both 2010 and 2013. Overall, these data indicate a reversing trend. Although there are more than double the alleged victims of CAN from 1981 to 2013, there is a 7.3 % decrease in indicated victims of CAN over this period of time.

Exercise 9.6: Critical Thinking The *alleged* and the *indicated* child victims of abuse and neglect in Illinois from 1981 to 2013 have both increased. Specifically, there is a 47.6 % increase in *alleged* child victims in that 32 year span. However, during the same 32 years, the number of *indicated* victims has disproportionately dropped. In 1981, 40.6 % of *alleged* child victims of abuse and neglect were designated as *indicated* victims that year. In 2013, 27.7 % of these children were designated as *indicated* victims of abuse and neglect. *In your analysis, is this good news or bad news? What facts can you use to support your argument either pro or con?*

Getting to Know the People Behind the Numbers

Children with and without disabilities who are abused and neglected get stuck in crowded shelters for months, far longer than the permitted waiting period. The Illinois DCFS is required by a 1991 consent decree to place children who are abused and neglected in safe alternative homes which need to be found for these children within 30 days. Gutowski (2013) reported that this 30-day limit has been broken in many shelters, forcing infants, children, and teens to remain in overcrowded shelters:

> After being beaten with a pan and left in the dark for hours bound to a pole, the 11-year- old girl escaped from their abusive home through a basement window and walked barefoot six blocks to the La Grange police station one summer night in 2011. . . .
> The girl's mother had been deported, and a woman who was caring for her and a sister was arrested for the beating. (Gutowski, January 8, 2013)

Far from a haven from the physical abuse to which she was exposed, Gutowski adds, "Police reports, provide data and confidential documents that show that the shelter, Aunt Martha's Children's Reception Center, has been plagued by overcrowding and problems with runaways that require hundreds of police visits a year". Though designed to serve 50 children, newborns to 21 years old, "An e-mail from Martha's on Oct. 11 said the shelter had 62 children, including 14 babies and toddlers."

While Aunt Martha's claims to be a safe place with therapeutic programs, Fred Pennix, an investigator and union leader stated, "I try to avoid bringing them there, but sometimes you have no choice. I've seen kids wait for weeks for a caseworker to get assigned. Meanwhile, the kid just sits there."

The complaints raised about Aunt Martha's Center included:

> On Oct. 8, two 6-year-old boys were moved to another floor reserved for older males because the 16 beds on the floor where they normally stay with infants and toddlers were filled. . .
> More than two dozen shelter teens were arrested since 2010 on misdemeanor and felony charges, according to police and court records. That does not include juvenile arrests, which are not public record.
> Police used a Taser on a teenage boy Aug. 30 after they said he became violent in the shelter when questioned about a robbery. (Gutowski, January 8, 2013)

Over the course of 3 years, the police came to Aunt Martha's Children's Center 2,063 times due to complaints about runaways, fights, drugs, theft, and vandalism. Incidents at the Center involved teens with gang ties, children with emotional and behavioral disorders, bipolar disorder and mild mental retardation.

Additional professional failures occur because an emergency shelter becomes a placement. Richard Calica, DCFS Director argued that an emergency shelter is ". . . supposed to be emergency intervention, not placement. Ideally a child would get out of the shelter within 48 hours." DCFS data shows that Illinois failed to achieve the 30-day standard for 13 % of children in the past 4 years, a total of 417 children. In a 3-month period through November 2013, 24 % of children stayed longer than 30 days. Six teens stayed at the shelter for more than 100 days. Experts state that "Overburdened shelters put children at further risk and are a symptom of larger systemic issues, such as a shortage of placement options and delays in finding permanent outcomes for children." Other DCFS problems include "clogged child abuse hotline, high worker caseloads, delayed day care inspections, staffing short-ages and deep cuts to family services programs."

Exercise 9.7: Reflection

How do you feel when you read that the staff at Aunt Martha's did not live up to their own self-proclaimed mission? What approach would you take with the staff at places like Aunt Martha's? Would you close them down immediately? Would you investigate the abuse and neglect with the intent to reorganize and refocus the services? What other thoughts do you have about the failure of trusted organizations to live up to their own missions?

More Failures of Trusted Organizations

Our trusted organizations fail when reports of CAN are ignored or when their investigations are thwarted. The *Chicago Tribune*, February 4, 2013 reported that Cardinal Roger M. Mahoney and other church officials prevented investigations concerning the sexual abuse of hundreds of children. They protected priests in the Roman Catholic Church who were alleged perpetrators of CAN. Since 2002 widespread corruption among church officials is well documented.

The documentary "Mea Maxima Culpa" exposes the first known case of a priest accused of molesting children with disabilities. The priest, Father Lawrence Murphy, worked at Milwaukee's Saint John's School for the Deaf. The priest raped and abused more than 200 students during the 24 years he worked at the school. The author states that "the fact that these children were deaf makes physical some of the issues of silence that allowed this abuse to occur in so many other places to so many other children" (Sanchez, February 4, 2013). Four former pupils of the school gave signed testimonials years after the abuse, and several students did everything they could to have Murphy arrested. Haphazard investigations of Murphy were conducted and no concrete evidence of abuse was found. The men were told that "the statute of limitations had run out." Eventually, Murphy was removed from St. John's due to "health reasons." Therapists provided by the church stated that Murphy had made detailed confessions of his abuse of children, yet he remained free and a priest until he died in 1998.

Including Murphy's, every sex abuse case went to the office of then-Cardinal Joseph Ratzinger, and now Pope Benedict XVI. Year after year, known pedophiles were allowed to be free and remain priests, even in parishes where they had access to children. Only after victims of Murphy's and other victims filed a civil suit against the Vatican was the church forced to release documents; this made it clear that many officials knew about the abuses and did not take action. The author states that ". . . no member of the hierarchy of the Catholic Church is innocent in this almost unbelievably ubiquitous wave of abuse. . ."

Psychiatric disorders in children still confound the medical profession. Dr. Stuart Kaplan, expert in child and adolescent psychiatry brought this to the attention of readers of the *Chicago Tribune* on June 29, 2011. He reported:

> I have been a child psychiatrist for nearly five decades and have seen diagnostic fads come and go. But I have never witnessed anything like the tidal wave of unwarranted enthusiasm

for the diagnosis of bipolar disorder in children that now engulfs the public and the profession. Before 1995, bipolar disorder, once known as manic-depressive illness, was rarely diagnosed in children; today nearly one-third of all children and adolescents discharged from child psychiatric hospitals are diagnosed with the disorder and medicated accordingly. The rise of outpatient office visits for children and adolescents with bipolar disorder increased 40-fold from 20,000 in 1994–1995 to 800,000 in 2002–2003. A Harvard child-psychiatry group led by Dr. Joseph Biederman, a prominent supporter of the diagnosis, recently insisted, "Juvenile bipolar disorder is a serious illness that is estimated to affect approximately 1 percent to 4 percent of children."

I believe, to the contrary, that there is no scientific evidence to support the belief that bipolar disorder surfaces in childhood. In fact, the opposite seems to be the case: The evidence against the existence of pediatric bipolar disorder is so strong that it's difficult to imagine how it has gained the endorsement of anyone in the scientific community. And the effect of this trendy thinking can have devastating consequences. Such children are regularly prescribed medications that are not effective in kids and have unwelcome side effects.

Exercise 9.8: Reflection

Read the story of Rebecca Riley by Dr. Stuart Kaplan cited in the referenced that follow this chapter. *Do you expect that when most parents bring their children with emotional and behavioral disorders to see a medical professional they expect expert medical care? How do you feel when doctors refer to medication as "the common cocktail"? What contribution is Dr. Stuart Kaplan making toward the prevention of our professional failures?*

In summary, children with disabilities are abused and neglected by professionals across disciplines and by staff in organizations designated to the care and welfare of children with disabilities. How can this stop? In the following section we outline a set of recommendations for researchers and practitioners. These recommendations focus on three overarching themes that include: (a) fostering respect and regard for the human dignity of children with and without disabilities and that of their families; (b) encouraging the development of personal professional competence as well as that of peer professionals whenever this is possible; and (c) fostering collaborative professional relationships.

Implications for Research and Practice: Being Your Best Professional Self!

The acknowledgement that professionals and designated related service providers perpetrate abuse and neglect in the lives of children with and without disabilities is an important first step. Data from the U.S. DHHS (2013), from research studies in a variety of disciplines, as well as from an analysis of the *Chicago Tribune* newspaper coverage all confirm that professionals as well as related service providers in a variety of fields are implicated as perpetrators of abuse and neglect in the lives of children with disabilities. The Council for Exceptional Children (CEC) outlines a set of principles that guide ethical professional conduct. We make the following recommendations based on these guidelines.

Professionals perpetrate abuse and neglect in the lives of children with disabilities either actively or passively. Active perpetrators hurt children with disabilities physically, sexually and/or emotionally. Passive perpetrators of abuse and neglect are those who know that abuse and neglect is happening and do nothing. They engage in benign forms of CAN such as ignoring children's needs or failing to report evidence of observed abuse and neglect. Practitioners in the areas of education, law, medicine and related service professionals respect the rights of children with disabilities well when they:

Recommendation 1: Practice professionalism by engaging the highest ethical standards of conduct, and embrace the policies, laws, rules and regulations of professional practice; and, when necessary, advocate for the improvement of professional laws, regulations and policies.

***

Data indicate that even though professionals and related service providers are mandated reporters, they frequently ignore their professional responsibility when it comes to reporting CAN. Why? Are they afraid to embrace this responsibility? Are there any trends in these data that might help us understand the characteristics of children who are more or less prone to being supported by the existing laws of mandated reporting? For example, are professionals and related service providers more prone to report the abuse and neglect of children with or without disabilities? What supports need to be put in place in order to ensure that when a child with a disability is abused and neglected professionals and related service providers:

Recommendation 2: Engage as eager whistle-blowers upon the observation of any practice that harms children with disabilities, their families and their communities.

***

As professionals we must examine our own attitudes, behaviors and biases relative to disability in children in childhood. When we uncover and acknowledge our own internal dispositions we can then get to work on educating ourselves and our institutions about the dignified care and protection of children with disabilities from deadly abuse and neglect. We may wonder whether researchers and practitioners might develop interventions that will lessen, if not end, the participation of professionals and related service providers in the abuse and neglect in the lives of children with disabilities who are so frequently the most vulnerable children. What variables serve as protective factors for those who might be prone to perpetuate abuse and neglect in the lives of children with disabilities? What layer of professional knowledge, support or service might be missing? At the outset professionals and designated staff with responsibilities for children with disabilities will increase their potential to enhance the lives of the children in their care when they regard the human dignity of each child with a disability and:

Recommendation 3: Respect the human dignity, culture and linguistic background of each child with a disability.

***

Professionals in the fields of education, medicine, law, and related areas and organizations entrusted with the care and welfare of children with disabilities must be aware that they comprise only part of a community of care. They must foster relationships with significant others in the lives of the children they serve. They will do well to:

Recommendation 4: Develop and foster positive relationships with children with disabilities and their families based on mutual respect and welcome their active participation.

***

Researchers and practitioners in a variety of related disciplines have unique roles to play in the provision of needed as well as innovative medical, educational and legal services. They provide unique services through designated organizations such as state and national government agencies, DCFS, and residential programs. Professionals and practitioners fulfil their responsibilities in their designated roles when they acknowledge, get to know and collaborate to meet the individualized needs of children with disabilities and their families. Thereby they:

Recommendation 5: Provide appropriate support and care for children with disabilities and their families in their efforts to achieve the best possible quality of life for themselves and their children.

***

Educators, medical personnel, law enforcement personnel and in related professional areas are in unique positions to enhance the lives of children with disabilities. In their work they have the opportunity to make a difference such that the lives of the children in their care will be lived to their fullest potential. Professionals will be wise to engage in collaborative program planning and implementation in order to focus on the realization of the children's potential and thereby:

Recommendation 6: Promote meaningful participation of children with disabilities in their homes, schools, and communities in every part of the world.

***

Researchers and practitioners innovate our understanding of abuse and neglect in the lives of children with disabilities when they use ongoing reliable and valid observation methods. Professionals in varied disciplines need to become more knowledgeable about disability in children's lives and about effective methods of observing and reporting their ongoing observations. They protect children with disabilities from abuse and enhance their own professionalism when they:

Recommendation 7: Use data based observation methods and engage in decision- making to inform their professional practice.

***

The ongoing development of one's own professional competence is the challenge of every professional person. Professionalism requires the willingness as essential and often very difficult questions. There is no place for professionals to ignore real issues. Professionalism requires relentless engagement with the frontiers of our knowledge. Professionals engage in professional development through continuing education, attendance at seminars and engagement with colleagues in professional communities and:

Recommendation 8: Maintain a high level of professional competence and integrity when exercising ethical judgment that dignifies the lives of children with disabilities, their families, and their communities.

***

Professional organizations play a critical role in the continued professional development of preservice and in-service professionals. These organizations provide professionals with opportunities to participate in a professional community, get to know one another and engage in collaborative work that would otherwise be impossible. Memberships in professional organizations provide professionals with ongoing support and protection in their efforts to maintain their professionalism. We observe that professionals are obliged to:

Recommendation 9: Participate in organizations, service projects, as well as in the development and dissemination of professional knowledge and skills.

***

The unique needs of children with disabilities will at times puzzle even the most experienced professional. New disability manifestations continue to challenge the established knowledge base. Conversely, in our modern era new knowledge is generated in every professional arena at a speed that defines our capacity to keep abreast of professional developments. When professionals become aware of innovative data-based developments that enhance the lives of children with disabilities they have a professional obligation to share and use that knowledge. Collaboration and coordination of information across professionals in their unique roles, as well as among and between organizations will serve to protect children with disabilities from abuse and neglect. Such collaboration and coordination will serve to protect personnel and institutions from allegations of abuse and neglect, as well as, stop when necessary the abuse and neglect that may be occurring. When professionals in legal, educational, medical and related fields work together, children with disabilities will more likely be protected from abuse and neglect by professionals and have a higher chance of living lives that honor their human dignity. Thus, we recommend that professionals:

Recommendation 10: Practice professional collegiality and innovative professional collaboration across a variety of disciplines in the provision of resources and services to children with disabilities and their families.

***

Professional practice that focuses on protecting the lives of children with disabilities from abuse and neglect requires new professional awareness. It requires the implementation of protocols that acknowledge the reality that abuse and neglect is disproportionately present in the lives of children with disabilities. What existing protocols, such as, individualized education plans and hospital admission procedures, might provide a professional with an opportunity to check "yes" or "no" relative to the suspected presence of abuse and neglect? We observe the need for professionals to:

Recommendation 11: Advocate for conditions and resources that will protect the lives of children with disabilities from abuse and neglect.

***

Abuse and neglect in the lives of children with disabilities is manifested differentially across professionals. For example, doctors and medical staff have unique obligations to protect the privacy and the dignity of children with disabilities. The medical community has a unique obligation to acknowledge pain and seek information before initiating medical procedures that are intrusive and even potentially painful. Furthermore, they have unique obligations to find ways to communicate directly with the children with disabilities in their care.

Kenny (2004) recommends that school personnel need to educate themselves thoroughly in order to protect the lives of children with disabilities from abuse and neglect. Additionally, they need to provide their staff with appropriate education and training about detecting, preventing, and reporting CAN. Schools and school districts must have clearly written policies regarding the detection and reporting of CAN. School personnel must implement these policies and procedures on an ongoing and daily basis. In addition, training for educators should be more extensive. This professional development must be directed to preservice professionals as well as to in-service professionals. Professionals in every discipline will be well served to spend time reflecting on their roles relative to intervention and prevention of the abuse and neglect of all children, with a particular focus on the unique vulnerability children with disabilities have to abuse and neglect.

Law and law enforcement personnel are obligated professionally to protect the rights of all children, including those with disabilities. They must be aware of and respect children with disabilities who have unique physical, intellectual, emotional, and communication needs. When they do not understand the behavior or communication of children with disabilities, they have an obligation to involve professionals who can provide them with the information they need. We observe the need to:

Recommendation 12: Engage in the ongoing improvement of educational, medical and legal policies, procedures, resources and services for children with disabilities.

***

Exercise 9.9: Reflection
Upon reflection on these 12 recommendations, what are your observations? What is missing? What would you add? What would you delete? Is there one recommendation that stands out to you as particularly important? Among these recommendations, are there three or more of them that seem of particular relevance in your own professional life?

Chapter Summary

This chapter focused on our continued professional failures to protect the lives of children with disabilities from abuse and neglect. Professionals and trusted service providers in every discipline contribute to these professional failures. We analyzed the data available on our personal professional and organizational failures and provided stories of people and organizations implicated in the perpetuation of abuse and neglect in the lives of children with disabilities. We concluded this chapter by providing recommendations for future researchers and practitioners.

References

Benbenishty, R., Jedwab, M., Chen, W., Glasser, S., Slutzky, H., Siegal, G., ... & Lerner-Geva, L. (2014). Predicting the decisions of hospital based child protection teams to report to child protective services, police and community welfare services. *Child Abuse & Neglect, 38*(1), 11–24. doi:10.1016/j.chiabu.2013.06.011

Brachear, M. A., & Rohde, M. (2010, March 28). Priest's victims have questions, but few answers. *Chicago Tribune*. Retrieved from http://articles.chicagotribune.com/2010-03-28/news/ct-met-priest-abuse-victim-20100328_1_dorm-room-milwaukee-lawsuit

Bryant, J. K. (2009). School counselors and child abuse reporting: A national survey. *Professional School Counseling, 12*(5), 333. doi:10.5330/PSC.n.2010-12.333

Caldas, S. J., & Bensy, M. L. (2014). The sexual maltreatment of students with disabilities in American school settings. *Journal of Child Sexual Abuse, 23*(4), 345–366. doi:10.1080/10538712.2014.906530

Cederborg, A. C., Danielsson, H., La Rooy, D., & Lamb, M. E. (2009). Repetition of contaminating question types when children and youths with intellectual disabilities are interviewed. *Journal of Intellectual Disability Research, 53*(5), 440–449. doi:10.1111/j.1365-2788.2009.01160.x

Cederborg, A. C., & Gumpert, C. H. (2010). The challenge of assessing credibility when children with intellectual disabilities are alleged victims of abuse. *Scandinavian Journal of Disability Research, 12*(2), 125–140. doi:10.1080/15017410902909134

Cederborg, A. C., & Lamb, M. E. (2006). How does the legal system respond when children with learning difficulties are victimized? *Child Abuse & Neglect, 30*(5), 537–547.

Chicago Tribune. (2012, January 3). Deadly neglect. *Chicago Tribune,* 7. http://www.chicagotribune.com/news/watchdog/chi-watchdog-alden-deadly-neglect-storygallery,0,6966836.storygallery

Child Welfare Information Gateway. (2012). *The risk and prevention of maltreatment of children with disabilities.* Washington, DC: U.S. Department of Health and Human Services, Children's Bureau. https://www.childwelfare.gov/pubs/prevenres/focus/focus.pdf

Cooke, P., & Standen, P. J. (2002). Abuse and disabled children: Hidden needs . . .? *Child Abuse Review, 11*(1), 1–18. doi:10.1002/car.710

Department of Children and Family Services. (2014, January). *Child abuse neglect statistics.* http://www.state.il.us/dcfs/docs/canstat.pdf

Dizikes, C., & Lighty, T. (2013a, September 8). Justice for Cristina: A fatal bus accident leaves a 7-year-old girl motherless – And at the mercy of the Cook County court system. *Chicago Tribune,* 1. http://articles.chicagotribune.com/2013-09-08/news/ct-met-cook-county-justice-20130908_1_cook-county-circuit-court-romania-mother

Dizikes, C., & Lighty, T. (2013b, December 29). Daughter of bus victim faces more legal twists and turns 19-year-old's decadelong journey through Cook County court system seems far from an end, *Chicago Tribune,* 1. http://articles.chicagotribune.com/2013-12-29/news/ct-cristina-zvunca-update-met-20131229_1_death-case-new-judge-bus-victim

Farrell, C. (2014a). Corporal punishment in US schools. *World Corporal Punishment Research.* Retrieved from http://www.corpun.com/counuss.htm

Farrell, C. (2014b). Laws, rules and procedural details for the administration of corporal punishment. *World Corporal Punishment Research.* Retrieved from http://www.corpun.com/rules.htm

Farrell, C. (2015). *World corporal punishment research.* www.corpun.com

Ford, A. (2011). State child emotional abuse laws: Their failure to protect children with gender identity disorder. *Family Court Review, 49*(3), 642–656. doi:10.1111/j.1744-1617.2011.01399.x

Goldman, J. G. (2010). Australian undergraduate primary school student-teachers' responses to child sexual abuse and its mandatory reporting. *Pastoral Care In Education, 28*(4), 283–294. doi:10.1080/02643944.2010.530679

Gore, M. G., & Janssen, K. G. (2007). What educators need to know about abused children with disabilities. *Preventing School Failure, 52*(1), 49–55.

Gutowski, C. (2012, June 8). DCFS failed 23-pound teen girl: 'No excuse' for taking 4 months to locate her, agency says. *Chicago Tribune,* 1.1. http://articles.chicagotribune.com/2012-06-08/news/ct-met-dcfs-starved-girl-20120606_1_dcfs-data-kendall-marlowe-neglect

Gutowski, C. (2013, January 8). Kids get stuck in crowded shelter. *Chicago Tribune.* Retrieved from http://articles.chicagotribune.com/2013-01-08/news/ct-met-child-abuse-shelters-20130108_1_emergency-shelter-dcfs-aunt-martha

Hoffman, L. C. (2014). Hospital medical futility policy & the severely disabled child: Is disability a death sentence? *Hamline Law Review, 36*(2), 12. Retrieved from http://digitalcommons.hamline.edu/hlr/vol36/iss2/12

Hogelin, J. M. (2013). To prevent and to protect: The reporting of child abuse by educators. *Brigham Young University Education & Law Journal,* (2013), 225.

Jackson, D., & Marx, G. (2012, November 13). A challenge unmet: Students with emotional or learning disabilities are entitled to an education, but in Chicago they often miss weeks of school, more than other children. *Chicago Tribune*. http://articles.chicagotribune.com/2012-11-13/news/ct-met-truancy-yajaira-20121113_1_school-social-worker-disability-more-school-days/3

Kaplan, S. L. (2011, June 29). Mommy, daddy, am I really bipolar? *Chicago Tribune*. Retrieved from http://articles.chicagotribune.com/2011-06-29/opinion/ct-oped-0629-bipolar-20110629_1_bipolar-disorder-psychiatrist-diagnosis

Kenny, M. C. (2004). Teachers' attitudes toward and knowledge of child maltreatment. *Child Abuse & Neglect, 28*(12), 1311–1319. doi:10.1016/j.chiabu.2004.06.010

Kenny, M. C., & McEachern, A. G. (2002). Reporting suspected child abuse: A pilot comparison of middle and high school counselors and principals. *Journal of Child Sexual Abuse, 11*(2), 59–75. doi:10.1300/J070v11n02_04 http://dx.doi.org/10.1300/J070v11n02_04

Mallén, A. (2011). 'It's like piecing together small pieces of a puzzle': Difficulties in reporting abuse and neglect of disabled children to the social services. *Journal of Scandinavian Studies in Criminology & Crime Prevention, 12*(1), 45–62. doi:10.1080/14043858.2011.561622

Orelove, F. P., Hollahan, D. J., & Myles, K. T. (2000). Maltreatment of children with disabilities: Training needs for a collaborative response. *Child Abuse & Neglect, 24*(185–194), 2000. http://dx.doi.org/10.1016/S0145-2134(99)00134-9

Palusci, V. J., & Vandervort, F. E. (2014). Universal reporting laws and child maltreatment report rates in large U.S. counties. *Children and Youth Services Review, 38*, 20–28. http://dx.doi.org/10.1016/j.childyouth.2013.12.010

Reeder, S. (2007). Teachers get fired, but don't leave classroom. *Small Newspaper Group*. http://hiddenviolations.com/stories/?prcss=display&id=358596

Roe, S. (2011, March 4). Nursing home targeted: State acts to close site with history of neglect, death. *Chicago Tribune*. Retrieved from http://search.proquest.com/docview/854907861/B0301175CC27410DPQ/1?accountid=11578

Roe, S., & Hopkins, J. S. (2011a, January 11). Center is cited in 14th death: Nursing facility sent girl to hospital after 2-day wait, state says. *Chicago Tribune*. Retrieved from http://search.proquest.com/docview/830400992/60AA8C76C114320PQ/1?accountid=11578

Roe, S., & Hopkins, J. S. (2011b, June 1). Nursing home rules passed: Deaths of disabled patients will need to be reported to state. *Chicago Tribune*. Retrieved from http://search.proquest.com/docview/869392897/2C8D6B61CF554A55PQ/1?accountid=11578

Rubin, B. M., & Haggerty, R. (2013, May 6). 'A slow, gradual spiral downward'. *Chicago Tribune*. Retrieved from http://articles.chicagotribune.com/2013-05-06/health/ct-met-search-for-treatment-20130506_1_health-system-school-shootings-mother

Sanchez, M. (2013, February 4). Chilling view of church sex abuse. *Chicago Tribune*. Retrieved from http://articles.chicagotribune.com/2013-07-04/opinion/sns-201307041200--tms--msanchezctnms-a20130704-20130704_1_sexual-abuse-archdiocese-priests

Sanghera, P. (2007). Abuse of children with disabilities in hospital: Issues and implications. *Pediatric Nursing 19*(6), 29–32. Retrieved from http://europepmc.org/abstract/MED/17694891

Schols, M. A., Ruiter, C., & Öry, F. G. (2013). How do public child healthcare professionals and primary school teachers identify and handle child abuse cases? A qualitative study. *BMC Public Health, 13*(1), 1–16. doi:10.1186/1471-2458-13-807

Stalker, K., & McArthur, K. (2012). Child abuse, child protection and disabled children: A review of recent research. *Child Abuse Review, 21*(1), 24–40. doi:10.1002/car.1154

Twohey, M. (2010a, July 29). Dr. Ricardo Arze and sex abuse cases shows disconnect between law enforcement, state regulators of doctors. *Chicago Tribune*, p. 1. http://articles.chicagotribune.com/2010-07-29/health/ct-met-doctor-sex-charges-20100729_1_berwyn-police-ricardo-arze-policing-doctors

Twohey, M. (2010b, July 30). Sex-abuse claims filed; doctor still practiced: Police were slow to act, say some of physician's alleged victims. *Chicago Tribune* p. 1. http://search.proquest.com/chicagotribune/docview/734327161/fulltext/CDB158583D2F438FPQ/2?accountid=11578

U.S. Department of Health and Human Services, Administration for Children and Families, Administration on Children, Youth and Families, Children's Bureau. (2013). *Child maltreatment 2012*. Retrieved from http://www.acf.hhs.gov/programs/cb/research-data-technology/statistics-research/child-maltreatment

Walsh, K., Rassafiani, M., Mathews, B., Farrell, A., & Butler, D. (2010). Teachers' attitudes toward reporting child sexual abuse: Problems with existing research leading to new scale development. *Journal of Child Sexual Abuse, 19*(3), 310–336. doi:10.1080/10538711003781392

Washburn, G. (2005, January 11). Aldermen slam cops in Ryan Harris case; City settlement of suit advances. *Chicago Tribune*. Retrieved from http://articles.chicagotribune.com/2005-01-11/news/0501110325_1_ryan-harris-case-ald-million-settlement

Weber, T. (2008, March 20). Kids' illnesses spark battle with state. *Chicago Tribune*. Retrieved from http://search.proquest.com/docview/420676664?accountid=11578

Chapter 10
Preventing Abuse and Neglect in the Lives of Children with Disabilities

Happy children are the hope of a nation. (Nano Nagle, Irish Activist, 1718–1784)

Abstract The abuse and neglect of children with and without disabilities is a choice. Our efforts to stop child abuse and neglect (CAN) and the abuse and neglect of children with disabilities (ANCD) need to take on a new urgency and bring about immediate positive and sustained change. To this end we will discuss the high price of ignorance, the existing barriers to prevention, and how we can engage in our roles as professionals in order to stop CAN and ANCD. This includes concrete and multidisciplinary strategies to prevent ANCD. Aspects of these strategies may be used by family members, friends, neighbors, teachers, social workers, lawyers, medical professionals and all who have unique roles in the care and protection of children with and without disabilities. The ability to use prevention strategies in order to promote healthy outcomes for children is paramount in our efforts to end this horrendous societal ill. We conclude this chapter with a set of recommendations for researchers and practitioners.

The physical, emotional, medical, and educational needs of children with disabilities often stress the parents, caregivers, and other people in their lives. As stress levels increase, the inappropriate conduct of children and adults increases. Self-control and rational decision making may decrease while depression and anxiety levels increase.

Biological parents are the most frequent perpetrators of CAN (see Chap. 6). The challenges of parenting are increased when the necessary resources to meet childrens' needs are unavailable (see Chap. 8). We can predict increased probability of CAN and ANCD if we stop long enough to try to figure out why it occurs on a case-by-case basis. Too often the abuse an neglect of children with and without disabilities is predictable.

© Springer International Publishing Switzerland 2016
E.P. Crowley, *Preventing Abuse and Neglect in the Lives of Children with Disabilities*, DOI 10.1007/978-3-319-30442-7_10

Beginning with Our Attitudes

The realization that children with disabilities are abused and neglected is so disturbing that many people want to turn away from it, or trivialize the frequency of its occurrence. Turning away and refusing to think and talk about this topic serves only to perpetuate it. This is surely one of the best ways to prevent the work of prevention (Kauffman, 1999).

The abuse and neglect of children with and without disabilities is so prevalent that countless dedicated people, in a variety of fields, all over the world, work hard every day to prevent it (Collin-Vézina, Daigneault, & Hébert, 2013; Dunn & Burcaw, 2013; Johnson, 2012; Mepham, 2010). How can we increase the awareness of the general public that children with disabilities are at greater risk for abuse and neglect than their peers without disabilities?

In the Preface to the *World Report on Disability* (WHO, 2011) Dr. Margaret Chan, Director-General of the World Health Organization and Robert B. Zoellick, President of the World Bank Group stated "Our driving vision is of an inclusive world in which we are all able to live a life of health, comfort, and dignity" (p. xi). The WHO is focused on enhancing the health and quality of life of individuals with disabilities. The objectives of the *Better Health of Persons with Disabilities* program, 2014–2021 include:

1. Address barriers and improve access to health care services and programs.
2. Strengthen and extend habilitation and rehabilitation services including community based rehabilitation and assistive technology.
3. Support the collection of appropriate and internationally comparable data on disability and promote multi-disciplinary research on disability (WHO, 2014).

Prevention and intervention go hand-in-hand. The procedures, practices, and programs designed to prevent CAN involve indirect and direct intervention. In this chapter, we focus on the impediments to prevention and intervention programming. Then we discuss a three tiered and interdisciplinary approach to the prevention of the abuse and neglect of children with disabilities (ANCD). Here we will focus on primary, secondary, and tertiary prevention across the disciplines of education, law, and medicine.

Impediments to Prevention of Abuse and Neglect Programming

Child abuse and neglect prevention is a broad endeavor that encompasses multiple aspects of human life, and it is not the work of any single professional endeavor. In Chap. 1 we outlined particular challenges relative to the definitions of abuse, neglect, and disability. Here we focus on how particular impediments, such as ignorance of disability, lack of consensus on important topics, such as medical care and child behavior management, and cost of prevention, serve to block efforts to prevent the abuse and neglect of children with and without disabilities. We will conclude this section with a discussion of how the lack of a specific disciplinary focus contributes to the continuation of CAN and ANCD.

Ignorance of Disability

Beginning prenatally, parents-to-be, those they look to for support, those who provide them with medical care, and generally supportive environments all contribute to the future health and welfare of children. In the following reflection, examine the quality of the support Rona and Mara provide to Susan?

Exercise 10.1: Reflection
Three friends Susan, Rona, and Mara met in a local restaurant for a glass of wine or two and shared stories about their experiences while raising their children. Susan is pregnant with her first child and just found out that her child has been diagnosed prenatally with spina bifida. None of the women had ever heard of this diagnosis and they congratulated Susan while stating that she must be very happy, as a baby is a baby first and foremost. They celebrated that soon Susan will be a Mom. They raised their wine glasses and toasted happily, "To The New Mom." *Is this a credible scenario? What do you think of the responses of Susan's friends? Do you consider that they might be putting this baby at- risk for further disability? Defend your perspective with at least three observations.*

Ignorance of disability in childhood is an impediment to the prevention of CAN and ANCD. Ignorance of the abundant threats perpetrated by nature and nurture compromises the potential health and wellbeing of children. Too many children are exposed to people and environments that fail to promote their health, safety, and welfare.

In the scenario above Susan, Rona, and Mara, not only seem unconcerned about Susan's use of alcohol, they also lack knowledge about spina bifida. Even more serious, they appear to lack the curiosity needed to learn about this disability and about the resources that are available for Susan and her family at this time. In the absence of knowledge and skills, Susan and her baby are at increased risk.

Lack of Consensus

Lack of professional consensus impedes prevention of ANCD. A striking example of this is despite the strong predictive relationship between the use of alcohol by women who are pregnant and its potential harm to an unborn child, some professionals advocate for the moderate use of alcohol during pregnancy. On September 10, 2013, an article by Lisa Black published in the *Chicago Tribune* titled, "A glass of wine a day OK with baby on the way?: U. of C. economist's new book Oks moderate drinking while pregnant, but others adamantly oppose her advice" (p. 1). The author of this newspaper article challenges the nonchalance with which Emily Oster (2013) wrote, *Expecting better: Why the conventional pregnancy wisdom is wrong – and what you really need to know*. Lisa Black describes the outrage provoked by this book while doctors, patients, as well as families of children with a host of fetal alcohol spectrum disorders (FASD) decry the publication of this work.

For decades, scientific evidence indicates that the consumption of alcohol during pregnancy has potential to cause a host of possible birth defects but Oster trivializes doctors' concerns. She is not alone among those who recommend the use of alcohol during pregnancy. Abel, a professor of obstetrics, gynecology, and psychology at Wayne State University in Detroit, updated a book he wrote in 1984 and published *Fetal alcohol abuse syndrome* in 1998. In this book he encouraged debunking myths about alcohol use by pregnant mothers and expressed support for the intake of light or moderate amounts of alcohol during pregnancy.

Clearly we do not have consensus on the consequences of using alcohol during pregnancy (Abel, 1998; Carpenter, Blackburn, & Egerton, 2014; Chasnoff, 1998, 2010; Chasnoff et al., 2005; Oster, 2013). Based on the scientific evidence that relates the use alcohol during pregnancy with a host of childhood disorders, Chasnoff (1998) concluded that the use of alcohol and other drugs during pregnancy may be "Silent violence …" (p. 145). Chasnoff, a pediatrician and member of the National Association for Families and Addiction Research and Education, is a specialist in the disorders of infants who have been exposed to drugs, including alcohol prenatally, and cautions that the prevention of induced disability is a moral obligation. How much alcohol is too much? How much drug use is acceptable? Members of communities, one-by-one all over the world, must recognize that, generally speaking, alcohol, and drugs are toxins for women who are pregnant.

Corporal Punishment

Debates still rage about how to manage children's behavior. We discussed corporal punishment in Chap. 9, and here we add that this practice remains a behavior management option for parents, caregivers, and teachers in the United States and across the world. In the United States, 31 States have banned hitting children but this practice remains protected by law in the following 19 states: Alabama, Arizona, Arkansas, Colorado, Florida, Georgia, Idaho, Indiana, Kansas, Kentucky, Louisiana, Mississippi, Missouri, North Carolina, Oklahoma, South Carolina, Tennessee, Texas, and Wyoming (World Corporal Punishment Research, 2014). Corporal punishment is most widespread in Alabama, Arkansas, and Mississippi. Is it is ever acceptable to hit a child? Does hitting children invite more prevalent abuse of children with disabilities who have a reduced or little or no ability to avoid engaging in challenging behaviors? If a parent considers that striking a child is acceptable conduct under certain circumstances, are they more likely to strike a child with a disability under circumstances that any objective person would consider inappropriate?

Exercise 10.2: Critical Thinking
In fourth grade, Ramon, small in stature for his age and diagnosed with mild cerebral palsy was the target of teasing by his peers. Following PE, he could not find his pants. Marcus, a peer stayed behind to help him find his pants and returned to class late for the third time in a row. His teacher talked with Marcus about his tardiness after PE already and this time she decided to refer him to the principal's office to receive corporal punishment. She thought that this would finally teach him that she does mean what she says. *In your opinion is there a difference between the terms corporal punishment, spanking, and hitting? If so, define each one and provide three arguments which either support or refute their place in the management of children's behavior.*

Some parents and professionals staunchly continue to defend the necessity to use corporal punishment in the management of children's behavior despite the evidence that hitting children is harmful, ineffective, and often perpetrates life-long emotional, intellectual, and physical disabilities (Chavis et al., 2013; Gershoff, 2013; Kempe, Silverman, Steele, Droegemueller, & Silver, 1985). The National Child Protection Training Center (NCPTC) is working to end all forms of child abuse and neglect in the next three generations. NCPTC promotes the care and welfare of children through education, training, advocacy, and through the justice system.

The Fine Line Between Perpetrator and Victim

When caregivers lack the knowledge and resources they need to work with children with disabilities they put their children and themselves at-risk. Persistent impediments to child abuse prevention include staff and resource shortages, as well as denial, reluctance or unwillingness to embrace the real needs of children with disabilities. Children and their caregivers are put at risk for further perpetrating abuse and neglect when they lack the knowledge and skills essential to their roles and relationships. The roles of perpetrators of harm and victims of maltreatment are fluid; caregivers as well as children with disabilities may move flexibly from one role to another. Consider the following scenario that is based on a true story that occurred in a large metropolitan area in the Midwest:

Exercise 10.3: Critical Thinking A 14 year old boy with an intellectual disability loved to swim in the local public swimming pool. While he was playing with a group of young children one sunny afternoon, he held a small five year old boy for so long and so tightly under water that the child drowned. Despite the efforts of a quick and highly efficient crisis team, all attempts to revive the child failed. *What* *happened here? Who is the perpetrator? Who is the victim? Who is abused? Who is neglected? How could this be avoided?*

When parents, caregivers, and professionals understand and accept the real needs of children with disabilities, they are in the best position to maximize their own potential and that of their children with disabilities. All too often, errors are made that either under or overestimate the true capacity of children with disabilities. For example, caregivers and professionals who vehemently advocate for the inclusion of children with severe emotional, intellectual or sensory disabilities in the mainstream of life without the supports they need to meet their needs, run the risk of child neglect. They also run the risk of denying children the development of the knowledge and skills they really need in order to participate authentically in society.

Do some teachers really recommend the placement of children with severe intellectual disabilities in high school physics classes for social reasons? Might this be construed as educational neglect? A teacher who lacks an understanding of the needs of children with disabilities fails to use their individualized education plans to guide educational decision making and thereby denies children the opportunity to learn appropriate knowledge and skills that addresses their real and individualized needs. When it is time for them to graduate from high school, such children are often unprepared for independent and meaningful participation in the world around them.

On the contrary, caregivers and professionals create impediments for children with disabilities when they assume that just because the child has a disability, they need to be cared for, catered to, pleased and protected at every turn. In these circumstances, children with disabilities are denied the development of their true potential. They rapidly become 18 or 21 years old and often remain unaware of their own capacities to make choices, and navigate through their daily lives safely, productively, and as independently as they can be. They are relegated to a life of dependence and helplessness and to a level of vulnerability that puts them at serious risk of abuse and neglect.

Cost – Are We "Willing to Pay the Piper"?

Corso, Ingels and Roldos (2013) found that we are reluctant to pay the price of preventing child abuse and neglect in the United States. In their study, they found that comparatively, the people of Ecuador are more willing to spend money on the prevention of child abuse and neglect than are people in the United States. We might wonder why? Is it because they do not really understand the extent of child abuse and neglect that exists? Is it because the people of the United States do not know the overall general and aversive effects of abuse and neglect in their own lives? Is it because that they are unaware that these effects spill over into every dimension of human endeavor now and for generations to come?

Everybody Business Becomes Nobody's Business!

The prevention of abuse and neglect of children with and without disabilities is not housed under the auspices of any one discipline, nor by any one particular professional group or effort. The amorphous nature of abuse and neglect prevention is both a strength and a weakness. In essence, we are all obliged to prevent CAN, yet, no single one of us is so obliged, nor is any one professional pursuit solely responsible for CAN prevention. Thus, it is everyone's business and quickly becomes no one's business. In the context of tight budgets and scarce personnel, the prevention of CAN and ANCD runs the risk of being ignored. These circumstances exacerbate the needs of children with and without disabilities and put many more of them at increased risk for abuse and neglect, as well as for additional disabilities.

Preventing the Abuse and Neglect of Children with Disabilities – Discourse on Global Strategy

Again and again research findings suggest that children with disabilities are at increased risk of abuse and neglect in their own homes, schools, residential centers, and hospitals (Bones, 2013; Bowman, Scotti, & Morris, 2010; De Bellis, Spratt, & Hooper, 2011; Sanghera, 2007; Stalker & McArthur, 2012). Researchers continue to extend this area of research while addressing crucial definitions, characteristics, reporting, and other research methodological issues (Leeb, Bitsko, Merrick, & Armour, 2012) while others focus on prevention (Child Welfare Information Gateway, 2013; Johnson, 2012).

The Child Welfare Information Gateway (2013) provides guidelines on prevention of CAN, though these guidelines do not differentiate between the prevention of abuse and neglect of children with and without disabilities. They provide a framework for prevention activities. This framework needs to be extended in order to address the unique challenges of children with disabilities and the caregivers who care for them. Johnson (2012) focuses on the unique protection needs of children with disabilities. He encourages the acknowledgement of disability as a risk factor by pinpointing potential vulnerability to abuse and neglect. Johnson addresses the need for the implementation of policies and procedures that are designed to protect children with disabilities from abuse and neglect.

An undisputable need exists to prevent the ANCD. A multi-tiered approach to prevention organizes the knowledge in this area and focuses on effective practices to address primary, secondary, and tertiary levels of abuse and neglect prevention (Skarbek, Hahn, & Parrish, 2009). In the following sections, we will provide a discussion of the prevention of abuse and neglect of children with disabilities at each of these levels and across the disciplines of education, law, and medicine.

What is Primary Level Prevention?

Primary level prevention engages broad approaches involving both child (Kenny, Bennett, Dougery, & Steele, 2013) and context variables (Herrenkohl, 2013; Scheuermann & Hall, 2012) in order to promote the individual and collective health and welfare as well as safety and success of children with disabilities. This pre-supposes the development of individual and collective awareness of the unique safety and protection needs of all children, and particularly those with disabilities. Prevention at this level focuses on the promotion of the healthy development of children with a focused consideration for their success by addressing their medical, emotional, social, and academic needs on an hour-by hour and day-by-day basis. This level of prevention begins with awareness and moves forward to the eventual implementation of larger contextual processes and procedures that ensure the safety and wellbeing of all children.

Newspaper coverage provides an opportunity for broad based consciousness-raising, and it has potential to educate its audiences about the prevention of the ANCD. Over a 10 year span, we found 113 unduplicated newspaper articles that focused on the ANCD were published in the *Chicago Tribune*. Criminal cases topped the list of these article types (see Table 10.1). More than half of them provided direct information or engaged a reader in a personal story which involved the ANCD. The fields of education, law, and related disciplines are all involved in the prevention of the abuse and neglect of children with disabilities at the primary level.

Education and Related Fields

We engage in primary prevention of ANCD when we embrace generally accepted prosocial cultural knowledge that serves us well as human beings and across cultures. Children are safer and more protected when their caregivers employ accepted, prosocial, and shared cultural knowledge that is handed down from generation to generation. Children are protected when practices and procedures derived from scientific research are in place. Primary level prevention requires the search for knowledge, engagement, and collaboration with needed personnel,

Table 10.1 Type of stories that focus on child disability and abuse and neglect

Type of story (n = 113)[a]	# of Stories	%
Criminal case	78	69.0
Informational	47	41.6
Personal	10	8.8

Data from a study of the newspaper coverage in the *Chicago Tribune*

[a]Percentages can be over 100 % due to duplicate story type designations

programs and supportive resources in the midst of unfamiliar and uncharted life experiences such as preparing for the birth of a child with a disability.

An essential first step in prevention of abuse and neglect is learning about the interplay between abuse, neglect, and disability. We discussed the reciprocal relationship between disability, abuse, and neglect in Chap. 1. Clearly abuse and neglect often bring about disability and disability often increases the vulnerability of children with disabilities to abuse and neglect. Educators in prevention programs will be wise to focus on the egregious short- and long-term effects of abuse and neglect of children at the local, state, regional, national, and international levels (Fang, Brown, Florence, & Mercy, 2012). Educational programs at the primary prevention level promote awareness that poverty, social, political and cultural isolation and instability are especially devastating to children and families who, once subjected, will likely become the repeated targets of abuse and neglect (Bones, 2013).

Based on the data from the U.S. DHHS (2013) and corroborated with studies in the field as well as with the data from the study on the newspaper coverage, fostering prosocial behavior in children might well be a centerpiece in abuse and neglect prevention. In an article in the *Chicago Tribune*, Bonnie (2010, October 6) explained:

> In 2004, Illinois became the first state in the nation to require all school districts to teach social and emotional skills as part of their curriculum and daily school life. That means students are expected to meet certain benchmarks, such as recognizing and managing feelings, building empathy and making responsible decisions.
>
> The social homework: Focus on teaching students interpersonal skills can lead to better behavior, higher grades.

How well do we know that in the process of managing a child's behavior, both the child and the caregiver are at-risk? What belief systems does the caregiver have about behavior management? How well does the caregiver understand the child's behavior? What attributions does the caregiver associate with the child's behavior? Children with disabilities exhibit behaviors that characterize their specific disabilities and require caregivers to have unique behavior management skills. For example, how often do caregivers know that children with autism have particular difficulty responding to changes of any kind and that children with attention deficit disorders are often disorganized and unpredictable? Additionally, though children with disabilities may have some characteristics in common, no two children with the same disability will exhibit exactly the same disability characteristics. Therefore it is imperative that parents, caregivers, and teachers get to know their children and their disabilities one-by-one.

Children with emotional and behavioral disorders (EBD) are the most frequently abused and neglected group (U.S. DHHS, 2013). This finding has implications for educational programming. The behavior of children with EBD is challenging by definition, and the behavior of these children can challenge even the most knowledgeable and experienced professionals (Walker & Gresham, 2014). The care and management of children who exhibit challenging behaviors is an essential topic in abuse and neglect prevention programming. Through such programming, from the outset parents and professionals who mismanage the behavior of children with EBD perpetrate disability and set children on course for acquiring additional disabilities.

Primary level educational programming may be provided in hospitals, schools, libraries, and online. Through these programs the life-long care, health, and well-being of children is promoted. Memberships and involvement in local, state, national, and international organizations also provide support and information to parents, caregivers, teachers, prevention specialists, and others with the support and information they need in order to foster their own development as well as the prosocial development of the children in their care. Primary level prevention takes place when parents and caregivers who, from the outset, learn how to care for, nourish, and meet the needs of their children with disabilities. In this way they promote their safety and success. Such simple acts as child-proofing a home lessen the potential for accidents and for potential accusations of abuse and neglect.

In summary, once identified with a disability, it is imperative that parents and caregivers embrace the unique and real needs of the children in their care. This may involve engaging in their own development as parents and caregivers while learning new ways to participate in the community. They acquire the information they need in order to understand their own as well as the unique needs of their children and families. Through such broad primary level educational programming, access to the resources and supports of local communities, as well as to those in the broader regional, state, national, and international levels is provided. Thus, at the primary level the prevention of ANCD is accomplished.

Law and Related Fields

The Child Abuse Prevention and Treatment Act (CAPTA) provides broad based legal support for primary level prevention of CAN. CAPTA was passed in 1974 and was reauthorized in 2003 as the *Keeping Children and Families Safe Act*. This law provides broad legal protection of children from abuse and neglect at the primary level. This law requires that caregivers and professionals fulfil their legal responsibilities toward children. Failure to execute these legal obligations, such as that of a mandated reporter, may have life changing consequences, not only for the child but also for offending adults. Furthermore, CAN is prevented when we engage in the continued development of our awareness of our legal responsibilities and when we advocate for the continued improvement of the legal protection of children with and without disabilities (Jones, 2006; Moxley, Squires, & Lindstrom, 2012).

CAPTA provides legal support for primary level assessment of children following a report that they might have been abused and neglected. This law, provides funding for further investigations when convincing evidence is present to suspect CAN. CAPTA also provides funds for the eventual prosecution of perpetrators when necessary. Finally, CAPTA supports the prevention of CAN at a primary level through its support of research, data collection activities, as well as program evaluation, and technical assistance.

Medicine and Related Fields

When children and their families have the medical care and attention they need, beginning prenatally, broad based primary level abuse and neglect prevention is in place. Through their involvement in proactive or preventative medical care they engage in either preventing or even reversing the effects of a host of potentially disabling conditions such as cerebral palsy, deafness, blindness, and autism. Conversely, neglectful medical care has potential to exacerbate children's medical needs and increase the complications of their disabilities.

Primary level prevention of abuse and neglect of children with disabilities involves parents, caregivers, and professionals in a variety of fields engaging in efforts to promote children's prosocial emotional, intellectual, and physical development. The prevention of ANCD is being accomplished at the primary level when caregivers and professionals educate themselves, clarify their knowledge and develop their skills relative to the disabilities of their children. Engagement in primary level prevention involves collaboration with others and engagement in a variety of interdisciplinary services.

Finally, we still have much to learn about what constitutes primary abuse and neglect prevention practices for children with disabilities (Moyer, 2013; Sanghera, 2007). We also have much to learn about the development of social and cultural awareness and about the implementation of effective primary practices that will ensure the prevention of CAN of all children and the unique ways it intersects with child disability. Continued research efforts as well as continued dynamic exchanges among professionals and child caregivers are essential to the development of primary level prevention in medicine and related fields.

Secondary Level Abuse and Neglect Prevention and Intervention Programming

Secondary level prevention involves focused and data based programming that is designed specifically to protect children with disabilities from abuse and neglect. In these programs groups of parents, caregivers, teachers, and other personnel learn how to address the needs of children with disabilities. Children with disabilities themselves learn self-awareness and self-advocacy skills, as well as a host of the unique social, emotional, and communication skills they need in order to facilitate their healthy social interactions. Secondary level prevention addresses the targeted needs of children with disabilities who are at-risk for abuse and neglect (Kenny et al., 2013; Ungar, 2013). At the secondary prevention level, educational programs, legal protection, and medical care enhance the care and protection of children with disabilities.

Education and Related Fields

Children with disabilities are taught in a variety of educational settings. They may be included in general education classrooms with their nondisabled peers, or engaged in educational programming in an assortment of environments that best meet their needs. A continuum of educational services is necessary in order to address the complex educational needs of children with disabilities. Secondary level prevention of abuse and neglect is accomplished when educational programs meet children's educational needs. When these programs do not meet the educational needs of children with disabilities they are at increased risk for abuse and neglect.

The educational outcomes of high school graduates with disabilities leave much to be desired. One third of young adults with disabilities live independently, many are unemployed, few participate in their communities, and many are engaged in the justice system eight years and less following high school graduation (Sanford et al., 2011). Young adults with EBD have most frequently been stopped by police officers for reasons other than speeding, arrested, spent a night in jail, and have been on probation for up to eight years following high school. These data indicate a continued need for relevant educational programming in the areas of academic skills, social skills, work skills, self-advocacy, and self-care skills. This programming enhances the lives of children who eventually become young adults with disabilities.

Law and Related Fields

Public Law 94-142 was first passed in 1975 and it was mandated for implementation in 1978. This law was reauthorized in 2004 and renamed the Individuals with Disabilities Education Act (IDEA). IDEA provides the legal foundation for the educational rights of children with disabilities. Based on its mandates, a free and appropriate public education in the least restrictive environment is the right of all children with disabilities.

For very young children with disabilities, secondary prevention is supported legally by Part C of the IDEA (PL 108-446). This involves the provision of early intervention for children from birth to 5 years old and their families. This is one of the finest legislative examples of secondary level prevention in relatively recent history. The legal mandate of early intervention programming provides family-centered service coordination that promotes child development and fosters the inclusion of children with disabilities from birth to 5 years.

Medicine and Related Fields

Early intervention programming is designed to begin upon the first recognition of disability potential prenatally. Caregivers prepare themselves to meet their child's needs and the needs of their families prenatally. They put in place the essential personnel, supports, and services needed in anticipation of the birth of their child.

It is not possible to anticipate the disabilities of most children prenatally. Caregivers, extended family members, medical teams, and other relevant professional and contextual personnel address children's needs on an hour-by-hour and day-by-day and basis. When child and family needs become evident and are addressed promptly, primary prevention and intervention programming may be sufficient. Targeted and specific secondary prevention programming becomes available when it is indicated.

Examples of secondary prevention and intervention programming for children with special needs include the services of home health care providers, home visits and the skills taught by such professional as feeding therapists, speech and language therapists and physical therapists. Other examples include caregiver support groups, care giving classes that focus on very specific child needs as well as the provision of respite care. Secondary prevention programming may also address issues related to poverty, ignorance, and isolation as these variables put children at-risk for abuse and neglect. Failure to develop secondary prevention and intervention programming puts children with disabilities at-risk for additional disabilities and instead of ameliorating the effects of a disability; the lack of such programming exacerbates disability effects (Bones, 2013). Consider the families in the following scenarios:

Exercise 10.4: Reflection Heather and John: Eager parents, Heather and Jon expect the birth of their first child, a baby girl in August. The pregnancy proceeded as planned until one day, following a doctor's visit; they are faced with the prospect of life as parents of a daughter with Down syndrome. Mom is an accountant and Dad is a primary care physican. Dad does not want to bring this baby to term and Mom does. Mom gives an ultimatum and says to her husband, "You are asking me to choose between our baby and you. I chose my baby." They decide to proceed with the pregnancy.

Maria and Isaac: Maria is a native of Mexico and speaks some English and her husband Isaac is a truck driver. Two months ago triplet boys were born to this couple and they are the younger brothers of their two older siblings. One baby has physical disabilities and medical complications such that Mom can no longer work. Doctor visits and hospitalizations are a common occurrence in this household. Money is tight now and Dad has to work longer hours in order to keep his family functioning. Mom spends many hours each day as the sole caregiver of these five children. Dad feels guilty being away from home so long each day and when he comes home he is tired and unable to participate in the family as fully as he wishes.

Which of these families is most vulnerable? What is the basis for your conclusion? What secondary prevention practices would you put in place in order to maximize the potential and capacity of these families?

In the case of the two scenarios above, both families are at risk for CAN for very specific reasons. Parent conflict and stress are risk factors and these stressors become even more pronounced when added stress is introduced to the home and family. Heather and John face many challenges in their marriage and they would be more prepared for the birth of their baby if, for example, they knew in advance that babies with Down syndrome are at risk for sleep apnea, and feeding disorders. Careful preparation to meet the child's needs will benefit all involved. Maria and Isaac are negotiating their way while living with new levels of stress and conflict and a lack of knowledge set the stage for even greater challenges which only escalate the challenges of an already strained family. Predictably ANCD will happen in contexts that are overwhelmed by human needs, isolation, ignorance and lack of appropriate resources. Secondary prevention capacity-enhancing programs for young children target their specific needs in the context of their families, such as, programs designed to encourage family participation in home and community activities that are designed specifically to address the needs of their children with disabilities (Khetani, Cohn, Orsmond, Law, & Coster, 2013).

Tertiary Level Prevention and Intervention Programming

Tertiary level prevention and intervention programming is focused and individualized and it is designed specifically to meet the needs of children with disabilities who have been abused and neglected. Tertiary level abuse and neglect prevention and intervention programming is intense and implemented at the individual level. It is by nature specialized, targeted, and expensive. It is designed to address unique and individual needs of children with disabilities relative to a specific incident or incidents that has or have actually occurred. Programming at this level will differ across age groups as well as across the specific incidents. It is designed to stall the effects of the harm that has occurred and prevent the reoccurrence of harm in the future. Tertiary level prevention and intervention programming is intense, individualized, long-term and labor intensive for all involved. Education, law and medicine, as well as an assortment of related fields in the social sciences all contribute to tertiary level prevention of ANCD.

Education and Related Fields

Who participates in educational programming, in education and related fields, which is designed to address the ANCD at the tertiary level? At this level the participants have either directly or indirectly experienced any form of abuse and neglect. They may have been victims or perpetrators of abuse and neglect or they may have been vicarious bystanders of abusive or neglectful behavior. Children with disabilities who have experienced abuse and neglect require focused and individualized educational programming in order to break the abuse cycle. If undone, abuse and neglect, as well as victim and perpetrator roles, cycle on randomly and unpredictably into generation after generation (Bones, 2013).

Educational programs at the tertiary level are designed to teach children with disabilities how to recognize abuse and neglect. They learn to recognize their own maltreatment or they may learn about when they themselves may be the perpetrators of maltreatment. They learn how to make a report and self-advocate in tertiary prevention programs. Children with disabilities learn to embrace their identities, as individuals with unique characteristics, in a healthy, accepting, and prosocial manner. They learn how their specific disabilities are manifested and how their unique emotional and behavioral characteristics may be negotiated on a daily basis. For example, children with autism may learn about their own unique needs for sensory breaks, for picture schedules, and for reliance on a trusted companion to navigate the ins and outs of daily life. Blindness, deafness, communication disorders, physical disabilities, intellectual, and emotional disabilities and more, that are mild, moderate, and severe bring with them inherently interesting unique human characteristics. Just as no two individuals are alike, neither are two individuals with any imaginable disability.

Educational programs that foster appreciation, acceptance, and embrace of inherent and unique characteristics build self-esteem, self-worth, and the celebration of each and every individual. Abuse and neglect prevention and intervention programming contribute richly to the education of children with disabilities and protects them from the potential of further harm.

Law and Related Fields

At the tertiary level, every child with a disability has legal rights. Young children have the right to an individualized family service plan (IFSP), and they have a right to an individualized education program (IEP) that is designed to address the child's unique educational needs beginning at three years old and until they are 21 years and 11 months. Students' educational goals and objectives outlined in these documents are designed to match the educational needs of each individual child. Just as no two children are the same, no two IEPs will be the same. Are the educational needs of one child with autism the same as those for other children with autism? Likewise, are the educational needs of a child with attention deficit disorder the same as those for other children with attention deficit disorder?

Exercise 10.5: Critical Thinking

Ms. Jones and Ms. Wang are friends. They both teach in the same district and are assigned to teach students with autism in the two high schools in the district. To make life easier, while completing their IEP development in the months of March and April every year, they organize work days during which they work side-by-side. They have strong beliefs about what students with autism need to learn before they graduate from high school. They manage to write students' goals and objectives with ease and haste. They have a set plan for what their students' will learn during each year of high school and they reflect these plans in the student' goals and objectives, during their freshman, sophomore, junior and senior years. *Is there a problem here? Defend your conclusions with at least three observations.*

The unique vulnerability of children with disabilities to abuse and neglect has been established for decades and now we work in a multidisciplinary, focused, and diligent manner to prevent it. Built into the IFSP and the IEP legal requirements are concerns about the individualized family service needs and the educational needs of children with disabilities. Johnson (2012) recommends that these documents also include statements that assure the safety and success of children with disabilities. Inclusion of safety and success assurances is being piloted in a program by Hands and Voices, "Observe, Understand and Respond: The OUR Children's Safety Project." When children with disabilities are safe and successful, they have a higher chance of being protected from abuse and neglect and in turn develop their unique potential as human beings.

Consider the following excerpt from a story by Christy Gutowski titled, "Kids get stuck in crowded shelter: DCFS houses babies, teens at same site; long stays not uncommon," published in the *Chicago Tribune* on January 8, 2013:

> The *Tribune* found no evidence of guns inside the facility, but two teens living there were arrested for having weapons elsewhere in the past two years.
>
> One, a 19-year-old boy, admitted he bought a .38-caliber revolver along with "some weed" and a box of bullets for $300 because the people who killed his cousin also were after him, according to court records. The teen said he had the gun for five years.
>
> In the other case, an 18-year-old who lived at the shelter was accused of threatening a police officer with a .25-caliber handgun in a nearby apartment, records show. The teen has bipolar disorder, intermittent explosive disorder and "mild mental retardation," court records said.
>
> Aunt Martha's separates children and older teens among three floors based on age and sex. It has staff and unarmed, off-duty Chicago police working security. There isn't a metal detector, but backpacks and other belongings are checked.

What options remain when children's safety and success appear to be a far-fetched dream? When children with disabilities are put in unsafe environments they are engaged in a cycle of abuse and neglect that may remain uninterrupted for far too long. The children and staff in the crowded shelter described above are at-risk for abuse and neglect either as victims, perpetrators, or both. Designated staff members who fail to carry out their professional responsibilities appropriately are putting themselves and others in harm's way, and they are at risk for potential serious legal consequences.

Legally, mandated reporters are required to act when they suspect CAN. This is necessary in order to bring perpetrators to justice and to protect children from further maltreatment. The protection of perpetrators is not an option. An observer, who has any reason to believe that a child, including a child with a disability, is maltreated, becomes a mandated reporter.

Prevailing evidence indicate that parents, teachers, and caregivers of children with disabilities must be particularly alert to the abuse and neglect potential of these children. They are mandated by law to call the National Child Abuse Hotline at 1-800-4-A-CHILD (1-800-422-4453) when they observe or even suspect CAN. In addition, the Child Welfare Information Gateway provides the available state-by-state contact information mandated reporters need in order to fulfil their responsibilities (U.S. DHHS, 2012).

Medicine and Related Fields

The first responsibility of professionals in the medical and related fields at the tertiary level is the careful assessment and documentation of the injuries children with disabilities sustained (Collin-Vézina, Coleman, Milne, Sell, & Daigneault, 2011; Kempe et al., 1985). In the mid-1980s Kempe and his colleagues described "the battered-child syndrome" as:

> The battered-child syndrome is a term used by us to characterize a clinical condition in young children who have received serious physical abuse, generally from a parent or foster parent. The condition has also been described as "unrecognized trauma" by radiologists, orthopedists, pediatricians, and social service workers. It is a significant cause of childhood disability and death. Unfortunately, it is frequently not recognized or, if diagnosed, is inadequately handled by the physician because of attention of the proper authorities.

Once the determination of abuse and/or neglect has been established, medical personnel engage in their roles as mandated reporters (Jenny, Crawford-Jakubiak, & Committee on Child Abuse, 2013; Paavilainen & Flinck, 2013).

In the assessment process, medical personnel first identify and then describe carefully in organized and detailed records, the children with and without disabilities who have been abused and neglected. They learn as much as possible about the context of their abuse and neglect and about the perpetrators who harmed them. Then these professionals proceed to provide medical attention for the actual injuries they observe. The careful physical examination of a child with a disability who has been abused and/or neglected may potentially reveal not only current injuries but past injuries which have healed.

Assessing the ANCD in a medical setting is complicated by disability characteristics. Children with communication disorders will have difficulty describing what happened to them; children with EBD may be withdrawn, anxious, and aggressive or otherwise compromise the rapport that may assist medical professionals during the assessment process. Children who are blind, deaf, or have physical disabilities may exhibit behaviors that are unfamiliar to many members of the medical profession. For example, Goldberg et al. (2009) examined the bruising frequency and patterns in children with physical disabilities. They found that functional mobility, challenges with self-care, cognition, or muscle tone did not contribute to bruising frequency. Among children with physical disabilities, bruising patterns were more frequently observed in the lower legs, knees, forearms and thighs.

Following abuse and neglect, the care of children with special health care needs often involves a long journey requiring additional medical care and rehabilitation as well as emotional and psychological interventions. No short-term fixes will address children's needs at this level of care. Children with disabilities who have been abused and neglected and are receiving medical intervention, at the tertiary level, may exhibit physical and emotional conditions that may last a life-time.

Giardino, Hudson, and Marsh (2003) examined the medical evaluations of children aged 3–16 years and who had special health care needs. They found that following the previsit screenings 54 % were males and 46 % were females and among the disabilities they exhibited were ADHD, autism, blindness, cerebral palsy, developmental delays, hearing impairment, intellectual disability, self-injurious behavior and speech and language delays. Forty two percent of these children were referred by personnel in the child protection services, 27 % were referred by physicians, 7 % by foster caregivers, 18 % by their own families, and 6 % were referred by an assortment of referral sources including child advocacy centers, informants, as well as school, residential treatment, and law enforcement personnel.

Among the children with special needs who referred for medical attention, 18 % had a history of abuse and neglect, 13 % had been determined to have been at high risk, 25 % had been determined to have been at low risk, and 44 % of these children were determined not to have been abused and neglected (Giardino et al., 2003). Upon follow-up, Giardino and his colleagues found that 76 % of the families involved remembered the recommendations made by the medical team. Of the 86 % who were referred for counseling, 48 % complied with this recommendation and 52 % did not follow through for different reasons, including inability to locate appropriate counseling services. All those contacted indicated that they were better able to identify the symptoms of abuse and neglect following the clinical evaluation.

The effects of abuse and neglect often disable healthy children and further disable children with disabilities. In Chap. 1, we discussed the complex relationship between abuse, neglect, and disability as a disposing variable as well as a consequence variable. Children not only need potential medical treatment and rehabilitation due to the characteristics of their disabilities, they may also need physical and/or emotional care and rehabilitation due to their exposure to any form of abuse and neglect.

The challenges to the medical profession involved in intervention and prevention of ANCD at the tertiary level include the contributing complications related to children's disability characteristics, the financial burdens imposed by the need for specialized staff members who know how to work with children with disabilities, and the challenges of locating appropriate medical personnel, and services once the children's needs have been identified. Bones (2013) reminds us that we have little choice but to continue the hard work of addressing these challenges in order to reverse these trends and protect the lives of children with and without disabilities for the losses incurred by their abuse and neglect.

The Story of Ellie

What does the prevention of ANCD look like in real life? For example, Ellie was adopted as a newborn baby girl. Upon arrival home, her parents found that she cried uncontrollably for hours and instead of reassuring her, touch increased her loud cries. In "Adoption interrupted: Parents' agonizing choice: Do they give up their adopted 7-year-old daughter?" Rubin (September, 2010) tells the story of a family who exhausted their savings as well as endured the life threatening gestures of their adopted daughter Ellie. Her parents received such pronouncements as, "The patient's mental illness has shown a deteriorating course" and that "At this point, residential treatment is strongly recommended as the best course of action."

Following years of medical attention a neuropsychologist from Chicago stated that Ellie "is at great risk of causing a tragic, irrevocable event (such as harming someone else or killing herself." Finally, following hurt and injury to her siblings and this child's alleged false reports that her mother was beating her and potential involvement of the Department of Children and Family Services, Ellie's family decided that she must go. Rubin reports that "Ellie is now living with another family in Washington state – 1,700 miles away from her comfortable Long Grove home, where she lived with her parents, two siblings and four dogs."

Exercise 10.6: Reflection

Read the newspaper article by Rubin (September, 2010). *Does this story surprise you? Do you know children like Ellie? In what way does this story illustrate the prevention of the abuse and neglect of children with disabilities? Who was at-risk here? Do we have heroes or heroines? What can we learn from this story? At what level of prevention would you place this story?*

Implications for Research and Practice – Let's Get to Work on Preventing Abuse and Neglect in the Lives of Children with Disabilities!

Children with and without disabilities are bearers of human rights and privileges. The dignity of each child prevails over their incidental attributes including race, culture, language, and disability. At a primary level of prevention of CAN, children with and without disabilities live in communities where child care is a priority. They live in communities where they are accepted and appreciated. Adults participate in the primary prevention of the abuse and neglect of children with and without disabilities when they integrate children into every facet of society and promote conditions that support their human growth and development, thus they:

Recommendation 10.1: Develop knowledgeable, caring, supportive communities where children with and without disabilities are valued and essential members.

∗∗∗

Secondary prevention of abuse and neglect in the lives of children with disabilities occurs in communities where members provide focused services to groups of children with specific and unique needs. Children who are blind learn braille, children who have cerebral palsy have access to the use of assistive technology – if it is recommended by a collaborative team that advocates for them and addresses their needs. Through collaborative decision-making the individualized needs of children are made known and they are addressed creatively. Community members, including parents and guardians as well as designated professionals either lead the way in advocating for the needs of children with disabilities or they participate in the provision of direct services to them. They make the emotional, intellectual and financial commitment to identify child needs, provide access to, and engage in the ongoing implementation of focused programming. This characterizes secondary prevention of abuse and neglect in the lives of groups of children with specific disabilities and requires that we:

Recommendation 10.2: Participate actively in building and supporting focused group efforts that address the unique needs of children with disabilities in the community.

∗∗∗

Prevention of abuse and neglect in the lives of children with disabilities occurs at the tertiary level of prevention when the individual needs of children with disabilities and their families are identified. Once these needs are known, individual access to appropriate programming is provided and sustained over time. Appropriate ongoing evaluation is essential to such tertiary programming. Does the child need continued services? Are the services a child is receiving sufficiently focused and individualized that they remain appropriate? Those involved in program development, planning, implementation, and evaluation employ innovative data-based methods and deliver age appropriate programs and services in tertiary prevention programs, thus:

Recommendation 10.3: Participate actively in building and supporting programs that are designed to meet the unique and individualized needs of children one-by-one.

∗∗∗

To what extent are the unique needs of children with disabilities understood and appreciated? Knowledge promotes understanding and acceptance. Data-based programs, such as New Kids on the Block demystify autism, cerebral palsy, learning disability, blindness, deafness, among other disabilities in childhood and thereby promote understanding and acceptance of childhood disability. Those who blame disability on some outside source, reject the real needs that arise based on child disability, deny its existence or ignore its effects actively or passively promote abuse and neglect. At best they delay prosocial responding and at worse they retrench, reverse, and weaken positive attempts to prevent abuse and neglect in the lives of children with disabilities. We recommend:

Recommendation 10.4: Actively participation in programs that raise awareness and promote acceptance of disability in childhood.

***

Two children with the same disability may exhibit its characteristics differently. For example, our best professional observations today conclude that autism occurs across a spectrum. Disability in childhood is dynamic and consensus about it among professionals often remains an illusion. The entry of abuse and neglect into the lives of children with disabilities further complicates professional consensus. To what extent did the disability contribute to abuse and neglect and vice versa?

Professionals foster the development of consensus when they engage in research, data based discussion, and debate. For example, despite what we know about fetal alcohol syndrome, professional debate remains about the use of alcohol during pregnancy. Continued debate about controversial issues keeps professional focus and attention where it is warranted and there we:

Recommendation 10.5: Work actively to build data based consensus on the prevention, when possible and intervention when necessary, of abuse and neglect in the lives of children with disabilities.

***

Children with disabilities are at particular risk of abuse and neglect. The effects of their disabilities often create unique social, emotional, educational, and medical needs, among other needs. These needs render children with disabilities uniquely vulnerable. For example, children with challenges to their communication skills may be unable to ask for help, even in an emergency. Children with physical disabilities may be rendered defenseless in the presence of perpetrators who have isolated them and rendered them entirely vulnerable. Thus:

Recommendation 10.6: Recognize the risks to which the lives of children with disabilities are exposed.

***

Focus on observable behaviors and provide specific evidence based on direct observations whenever possible. Behavioral observations may be documented using written, audio, or video recording. Establish access to and familiarity with a useful method of behavioral observation such as checklists or anecdotal records. Anecdotal records are commonly used when creating written documents about incidents that occur in children's lives at summer camps and school playgrounds. They involve the written documentation of factual information that may be observed by one or more staff members. They are clearly written statements, based on direct observations constitute anecdotal records. Conjecture, opinion, or bias have no place in an anecdotal record and serve only to undermine the potential contribution of the information contained in the record. Using an established behavioral observation tool to:

Recommendation 10.7: Pinpoint and document behavioral observations of children with disabilities who might have been exposed to abuse and neglect.

***

Who believes that corporal punishment is a legitimate method with which to discipline children? Who is aware that in the United States in 2014 this method is legally permitted to discipline children in schools in 19 out of 50 states? Who knows that in every state across the United States children with and without disabilities are legally unprotected from corporal punishment in their own homes? Who believes that, to this day, the corporal punishment of children with and without disabilities is permitted in many countries all over the world?

No data support the use of corporal punishment as an effective method to discipline children either with and without disabilities. Parents and child advocates in 31 states in the United States have managed to ban the use of corporal punishment in schools. During 2014, corporal punishment was banned in schools, child care settings, and in the homes of children in Argentina, Brazil, Bolivia, Estonia and Nicaragua. The most recent report of The Global Initiative to End All Corporal Punishment of Children (2014b) indicates that 91 % of the world's children remain legally unprotected from corporal punishment in their own homes.

Much work remains to be done in order to prohibit the corporal punishment of children in every institution and in every home in the world. When asked "Is there a legal defense for corporal punishment which must be repealed?" representatives of The Global Initiative to End All Corporal Punishment of Children (2014a, April) replied:

> Yes – State laws confirm the right of parents to inflict physical punishment on their children and legal provisions against violence and abuse are not interpreted as prohibiting all corporal punishment in childrearing. The near universal acceptance of corporal punishment in "disciplining" children necessitates a clear statement in law that all corporal punishment, however "light", is prohibited and the repeal of all legal defenses for its use. We recommend:

Recommendation 10.8: Active participation in legal reforms that support the prevention of abuse and neglect in the lives of children with and without disabilities.

***

Chapter 4 of this text focuses on the outcomes of abuse and neglect in the lives of children with disabilities. The findings in this chapter indicate that there are no positive outcomes of abuse and neglect for either victims or perpetrators and for anyone involved with children with and without disabilities who might be subjected to such abuse and neglect. To what extent are members of the general public aware of the extraordinary human toll of abuse and neglect in the lives of children with and without disabilities? Is the abuse and neglect of children with and without disabilities regarded differently among parents, caregivers, siblings, and extended family members? To what extent is there awareness that once children are victimized by abuse and neglect, they may become the future perpetrators? Many questions about the outcomes of abuse and neglect of children with disabilities need to be asked and answered, thus:

Recommendation 10.9: Engage actively in building knowledge and awareness of the outcomes of abuse and neglect.

***

Preventing the abuse and neglect of children with disabilities requires emotional, intellectual, and financial commitment. Emotionally this is a difficult subject. Few brave publishers and editors of professional journals take on this subject. Acceptance of this subject, as well as an intellectual understanding of the children, adults, and circumstances involved is essential in order to develop attitudes, behaviors, and programs that protect the lives of children with disabilities from abuse and neglect. It is also essential to make a financial commitment to support children with disabilities, their families, and their communities. Public and private funding sources are essential in the development and implementation of programs that prevent the abuse and neglect of children with disabilities when possible and intervene when necessary. We work to prevent the abuse and neglect of children with and without disabilities when we:

Recommendation 10.10: Actively engage in building support for the willingness to pay the price of prevention.

***

What organization do you know of is dedicated to preventing the abuse and neglect of children? Are you familiar with an organization that is dedicated to preventing abuse and neglect in the lives of children with disabilities? The

U.S. DHHS offers resources on the prevention of abuse and neglect in childhood through the Child Welfare Information Gateway. Prevent Child Abuse America offers its members a focused and dedicated organization that is headquartered in Chicago, Illinois. Prevent Child Abuse America is a national organization that was founded in Chicago in 1972. Prevent Child Abuse America:

> ... works to ensure the healthy development of children nationwide. The organization promotes that vision through a network of chapters in 50 states and nearly 600 Healthy Families America home visiting sites in 39 states, the District of Columbia, American Samoa, Guam, the Northern Commonwealth of the Marianas, Puerto Rico, US Virgin Islands, and Canada. A major organizational focus is to advocate for the existence of a national policy framework and strategy for children and families while promoting evidence-based practices that prevent abuse and neglect from ever occurring.

Prevent Child Abuse America promotes child "advocacy, public awareness, training/education, prevention programming, coalition building, and Child Abuse Prevention Month activities among others" (Prevent Child Abuse 2013). Through such endeavours we:

Recommendation 10.11: Participate in the work of dedicated organizations that focus on preventing the abuse and neglect of children with and without disabilities. Focus on increasing awareness of the unique needs of children with disabilities.

***

Exercise 10.7: Reflection Do you believe that there is a need for a dedicated organization that focuses on the prevention of abuse and neglect in the lives of children with disabilities? *Provide at least five observations to support your rationale.*

Earlier in this chapter we discussed the data on the frequency with which mandated reporters fail to report the abuse and neglect they observe. We might wonder why so many mandated reporters fail to come forward and risk the consequences of their own failure? What blocks, even mandated reporters from reporting CAN? We have much to learn in order to understand the issues which get in the way of mandated reporting? Advocates of universal mandated reporting laws would encourage us to:

Recommendation 10.12: Embrace the challenge to prevent abuse and neglect in the lives of children with and without disabilities. It is not someone else's business!

***

Chapter Summary

In this chapter, while using case examples, reflections, and analysis exercises, we discussed five major impediments that need to be addressed by the professional community in order to further the prevention of ANCD. Using these case examples, reflection, and analysis exercises we discussed abuse and neglect prevention programming at the primary, secondary and tertiary levels in the fields of education, law, and medicine. We concluded this chapter by discussing recommendations for researchers and practitioners.

References

Abel, E. L. (1984). *Fetal alcohol syndrome and fetal alcohol effects.* New York: Plenum.

Abel, E. L. (1998). *Fetal alcohol abuse syndrome.* New York: Plenum.

Black, L. (2013, September 10). *A glass of wine a day OK with baby on the way? Chicago Tribune.* Retrieved from http://articles.chicagotribune.com/2013-09-10/health/ct-met-pregnancy-alcohol-controversy-20130910_1_fetal-alcohol-spectrum-disorders-alcohol-consumption-book/2

Bones, P. D. C. (2013). Perceptions of vulnerability: A target characteristics approach to disability, gender, and victimization. *Deviant Behavior, 34*(9), 727–750. doi:10.1080/01639625.2013. 766511

Bonnie, M. R. (2010, October 6). The social homework. *Chicago Tribune.* Retrieved from http://search.proquest.com/docview/756550148?accountid=11578

Bowman, R. A., Scotti, J. R., & Morris, T. L. (2010). Sexual abuse prevention: A training program for developmental disabilities service providers. *Journal of Child Sexual Abuse, 19*(2), 119–127. doi:10.1080/10538711003614718

Carpenter, B., Blackburn, C., & Egerton, J. (Eds.). (2014). *Fetal alcohol spectrum disorders: Interdisciplinary perspectives.* New York: Routledge.

Chasnoff, I. J. (1998). Silent violence: Is prevention a moral obligation? *Pediatrics, 102*(1), 145–147. doi:10.1038/sj.jp.7211823

Chasnoff, I. J. (2010). *The mystery of risk: Drugs, alcohol, pregnancy, and the vulnerable child.* Chicago: NTI Upstream.

Chasnoff, I. J., McGourty, R. F., Bailey, G. W., Hutchins, E., Lightfoot, S. O., Pawson, L., ... Campbell, J. (2005). The 4P's plus screen for substance use in pregnancy: Clinical application and outcomes. *Journal of Perinatology, 25*(6), 368–374. doi: 10.1038/sj.jp.7211266

Chavis, A., Hudnut-Beumler, J., Webb, M., Neely, J., Bickman, L., Dietrich, M., et al. (2013). A brief intervention affects parents' attitudes toward using less physical punishment. *Child Abuse & Neglect, 37*(12), 1192–1201. doi:10.1016/j.chiabu.2013.06.003

Child Welfare Information Gateway. (2013). *Preventing child abuse and neglect.* Washington, DC: U.S. Department of Health and Human Services, Children's Bureau. https://www.childwelfare.gov/pubs/factsheets/preventingcan.pdf

Collin-Vézina, D., Coleman, K., Milne, L., Sell, J., & Daigneault, I. (2011). Trauma experiences, maltreatment-related impairments, and resilience among child welfare youth in residential care. *International Journal of Mental Health & Addiction, 9*(5), 577–589. doi:10.1007/s11469-011-9323-8

Collin-Vézina, D., Daigneault, I., & Hébert, M. (2013). Lessons learned from child sexual abuse research: Prevalence, outcomes, and preventive strategies. *Child & Adolescent Psychiatry & Mental Health, 7*(1), 1–9. doi:10.1186/1753-2000-7-22

Corso, P. S., Ingels, J. B., & Roldos, M. I. (2013). A comparison of willingness to pay to prevent child maltreatment deaths in Ecuador and the United States. *International Journal of Environmental and Research and Public Health, 10*(4), 1342–1355. doi:10.3390/ijerph10041342

De Bellis, M. D., Spratt, E. G., & Hooper, S. R. (2011). Neurodevelopmental biology associated with childhood sexual abuse. *Journal of Child Sexual Abuse, 20*(5), 548–587. doi:10.1080/10538712.2011.607753

Dunn, D. S., & Burcaw, S. (2013). Disability identity: Exploring narrative accounts of disability. *Rehabilitation Psychology, 58*(2), 148–157. doi:10.1037/a0031691

Fang, X., Brown, D. S., Florence, C. S., & Mercy, J. A. (2012). The economic burden of child maltreatment in the United States and implications for prevention. *Child Abuse & Neglect: The International Journal, 36*(2), 156–165. doi:10.1016/j.chiabu.2011.10.006

Gershoff, E. T. (2013). Spanking and child development: We know enough now to stop hitting our children. *Child Development Perspectives, 7*(3), 133–137. doi:10.1111/cdep.12038

Giardino, A. P., Hudson, K. M., & Marsh, J. (2003). Providing medical evaluations for possible child maltreatment to children with special health care needs. *Child Abuse & Neglect, 27*(10), 1179–1186. doi:10.1016/j.chiabu.2003.09.005

Goldberg, A. P., Tobin, J., Daigneau, J., Griffith, R. T., Reinert, S. E., & Jenny, C. (2009). Bruising frequency and patterns in children with physical disabilities. *Pediatrics, 124*(2), 604–609. doi:10.1542/peds.2008-2900

Gutowski, C. (2013, January 8). Kids get stuck in crowded shelter. *Chicago Tribune*. Retrieved from http://articles.chicagotribune.com/2013-01-08/news/ct-met-child-abuse-shelters-20130108_1_emergency-shelter-dcfs-aunt-martha

Herrenkohl, T. I. (2013). Person-environment interactions and the shaping of resilience. *Trauma Violence Abuse, 14*(3), 191–194. doi:10.1177/1524838013491035

Jenny, C., Crawford-Jakubiak, J. E., & Committee on Child Abuse. (2013). The evaluation of children in the primary care setting when sexual abuse is suspected. *Pediatrics, 132*(2), 558–567. doi:10.1542/peds.2013-1741

Johnson, H. (2012). Protecting the most vulnerable from abuse. *ASHA Leader, 17*, 16–19. Retrieved from http://www.asha.org/Publications/leader/2012/121120/Protecting-the-Most-Vulnerable-From-Abuse.htm?utm_source=asha&utm_medium=enewsletter&utm_campaign=leaderlive112112

Jones, W. G. (2006). *Working with the courts in child protection*. Office on Child Abuse and Neglect, Children's Bureau. Child Welfare Information Gateway. https://www.childwelfare.gov/pubs/usermanuals/courts/chaptersix.cfm

Kauffman, J. M. (1999). How we prevent the prevention of emotional and behavioral disorders. *Exceptional Children, 65*(4), 448–468. doi:10.1177/001440299906500402

Keeping Children and Families Safe Act. (2003). *Keeping Children and Families Safe Act*, PL 108-36. Retrieved from https://www.childwelfare.gov/systemwide/laws_policies/federal/index.cfm?event=federallegislation.viewlegis&id=45

Kempe, C. H., Silverman, F. N., Steele, B. F., Droegemueller, W., & Silver, H. K. (1985). The battered child syndrome. *Child Abuse & Neglect, 9*(2), 143–154.

Kenny, M. C., Bennett, K. D., Dougery, J., & Steele, F. (2013). Teaching general safety and body safety training skills to a Latino preschool male with autism. *Journal of Child Family Studies, 22*(8), 1092–1102. doi:10.1007/s10826-012-9671-4

Khetani, M. A., Cohn, E. S., Orsmond, G. I., Law, M. C., & Coster, W. J. (2013). Parent perspectives of participation in home and community activities when receiving Part C early intervention services. *Topics in Early Childhood Special Education, 32*(4), 234–245. doi:10.1177/0271121411418004

Leeb, R. T., Bitsko, R. H., Merrick, M. T., & Armour, B. S. (2012). Does childhood disability increase risk for child abuse and neglect? *Journal of Mental Health Research in Intellectual disabilities, 5*(1), 4–31. doi:10.1080/19315864.2011.608154

Mepham, S. (2010). Disabled children: The right to feel safe. *Child Care in Practice, 16*(1), 19–34. doi:10.1080/13575270903368667

Moxley, K. M., Squires, J., & Lindstrom, L. (2012). Early intervention and maltreated children: A current look at the Child Abuse Prevention and Treatment Act and Part C. *Infants & Young Children, 25*(1), 3–18. doi:10.1097/IYC.0b013e3182392ff0

Moyer, V. A. (2013). Primary care interventions to prevent child maltreatment: U.S. preventive services task force recommendation statement. *Annals of Internal Medicine, 159*(4), 289–295. doi:10.7326/0003-4819-159-4-201308200-00676

Oster, E. (2013). *Expecting better: Why the conventional pregnancy wisdom is wrong-and what you really need to know*. New York: Penguin.

Paavilainen, E., & Flinck, A. (2013). National clinical nursing guideline for identifying and intervening in child maltreatment within the family in Finland. *Child abuse review, 22*(3), 209–220. doi:10.1002/car.2207

Prevent Child Abuse America. (2013). *Prevent child abuse America: Home*. Retrieved from http://www.preventchildabuse.org/index.php

Rubin, B. M. (2010, September 21). Adoption interrupted. *Chicago Tribune*. Retrieved from http://articles.chicagotribune.com/2010-09-21/health/ct-met-disrupted-adoption-0921-20100921_1_ellie-family-constellation-new-jersey-woman

Sanford, C., Newman, L., Wagner, M., Cameto, R., Knokey, A.-M., & Shaver, D. (2011). *The post-high school outcomes of young adults with disabilities up to 6 years after high school: Key findings from the National Longitudinal Transition Study-2 (NLTS2)* (NCSER 2011-3004). Menlo Park, CA: SRI International.

Sanghera, P. (2007). Abuse of children with disabilities in hospital: Issues and implications. *Pediatric Nursing, 19*(6), 29–32.

Scheuermann, B. K., & Hall, J. A. (2012). *Positive behavioral supports for the classroom* (2nd ed.). Columbus, OH: Pearson.

Skarbek, D., Hahn, K., & Parrish, P. (2009). Stop sexual abuse in special education: An ecological model of prevention and intervention strategies for sexual abuse in special education. *Sexuality and Disability, 27*(3), 155–164. doi:10.1007/s11195-009-9127-y

Stalker, K., & McArthur, K. (2012). Child abuse, child protection and disabled children: A review of recent research. *Child Abuse Review, 21*(1), 24–40. doi:10.1002/car.1154

The Global Initiative to End all Corporal Punishment of Children. (2014a, April). *Corporal punishment of children in the USA*. Retrieved from http://www.endcorporalpunishment.org/pages/pdfs/states-reports/USA.pdf

The Global Initiative to End All Corporal Punishment of Children. (2014b, December). *Ending legalized violence against children*. Retrieved from http://www.endcorporalpunishment.org/pages/pdfs/reports/GlobalReport2014.pdf. doi: 10.1002/car.2207

U.S. Department of Health and Human Services. (2012). *State child abuse reporting numbers*. https://www.childwelfare.gov/pubs/reslist/rl_dsp.cfm?rs_id=5&rate_chno=W-00082

U.S. Department of Health and Human Services, Administration for Children and Families, Children's Bureau (U.S. DHHS). (2013). *Child maltreatment 2012*. Retrieved from http://www.acf.hhs.gov/programs/cb/research-data-technology/statistics-research/child-maltreatment

Ungar, M. (2013). Resilience after maltreatment: The importance of social services as facilitators of positive adaption. *Child Abuse & Neglect: The International Journal, 37*(2/3), 110–115. doi:10.1016/j.chiabu.2012.08.004

Walker, H. M., & Gresham, F. M. (Eds.). (2014). *Handbook of evidence-based practices for emotional and behavioral disorders: Applications in schools*. New York: Guilford.

World Corporal Punishment Research. (2014). *Corporal punishment in US schools*. Retrieved from http://www.corpun.com/counuss.htm

World Health Organization (WHO). (2011). *World report on disability*. Geneva, Switzerland: WHO Press. Retrieved from http://whqlibdoc.who.int/publications/2011/9789240685215_eng.pdf?ua=1

World Health Organization (WHO). (2014). *WHO global disability action plan 2014–2021*. Retrieved from http://www.who.int/disabilities/actionplan/en/

Helpful Resources for Further Study

Child Abuse Prevention Treatment Act (CAPTA). U.S. Code title 42, chapter 67. Retrieved from www4.law.cornell.edu/uscode/42/ch67.html

Gaffney, M. (2011). *Flourishing: How to achieve a deeper sense of well-being, meaning and purpose – Even when facing adversity.* London: Penguin.

International Society for the Prevention of Cruelty to Children http://www.ispcan.org/

Observe, Understand and Respond: The O.U.R. Children's Safety Project. Retrieved from http://www.handsandvoices.org/resources/OUR/

Organization for Autism Research. (2014). *Life journey through autism: A guide to safety.* Retrieved from http://researchautism.org/resources/reading/documents/LifeJourneyThroughAutism-AGuidetoSafety.pdf

Organization for Autism Research. (2014). Retrieved from http://www.researchautism.org/

The National Child Protection Training Center. Retrieved from http://www.ncptc.org/index.asp?Type=B_BASIC&SEC

Working with the courts in child protection. Retrieved from https://www.childwelfare.gov/pubs/usermanuals/courts/chaptersix.cfm